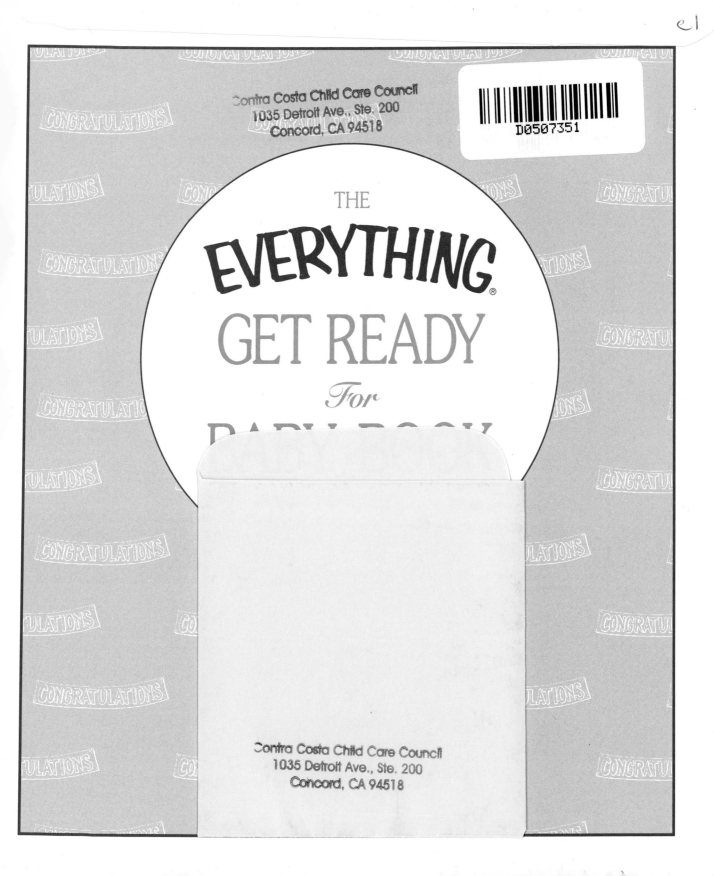

el

THE
EVERYTHING.
GET READY
For

The Everything Series:

The Everything® After College Book
The Everything® Baby Names Book
The Everything® Bartender's Book
The Everything® Beer Book
The Everything® Bicycle Book
The Everything® Casino Gambling Book
The Everything® Cat Book
The Everything® Christmas Book
The Everything® College Survival Book
The Everything® Dreams Book
The Everything® Etiquette Book
The Everything® Family Tree Book
The Everything® Games Book
The Everything® Golf Book
The Everything® Home Improvement Book
The Everything® Jewish Wedding Book
The Everything® Low-Fat High-Flavor Cookbook
The Everything® Pasta Cookbook
The Everything® Study Book
The Everything® Wedding Book
The Everything® Wedding Checklist
The Everything® Wedding Etiquette Book
The Everything® Wedding Organizer
The Everything® Wedding Vows Book
The Everything® Wine Book
The Everything® Get Ready for Baby Book

THE EVERYTHING®
GET READY
for
BABY BOOK

From Buying the Right Gear to Preparing a Room

Katina Z. Jones

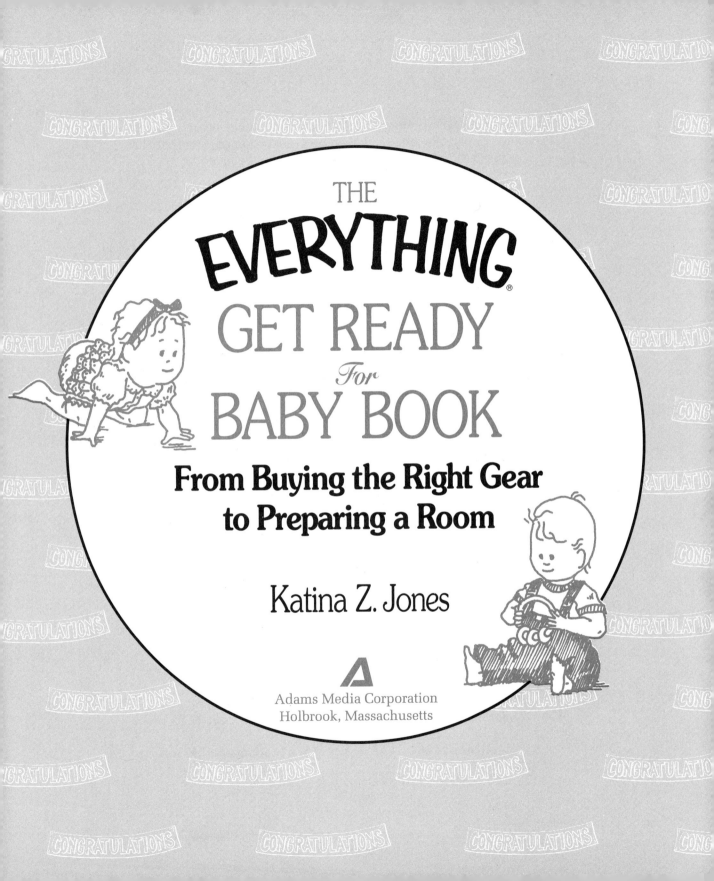

Adams Media Corporation
Holbrook, Massachusetts

An Everything® Series Book.
The Everything® Series is a registered trademark of Adams Media Corporation.

Published by Adams Media Corporation
260 Center Street, Holbrook, MA 02343

ISBN: 1-55850-844-9

Printed in the United States of America.

J I H G F E D C B A

Library of Congress Cataloging-in-Publication Data
Jones, Katina, Z.
The everything get ready for baby book / by Katina Z. Jones.
p.   cm.
ISBN 1-55850-844-9
1. Pregnancy.   2. Childbirth.   I. Title.
RG525.J677   1998
618.2'4—dc21   97-45898
CIP

Illustrations by Barry Littmann

This book is available at quantity discounts for bulk purchases.
For information, call 1-800-872-5627 (in Massachusetts, call 781-767-8100).

Visit our home page at http://www.adamsmedia.com

*For Madelyn Dela Yaceczko,
as you enter this world with nothing
but an eternity in your hands.*

—K. Z. J.

Contents

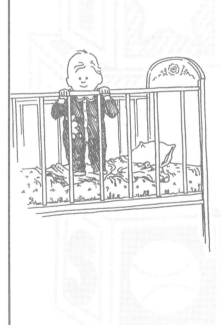

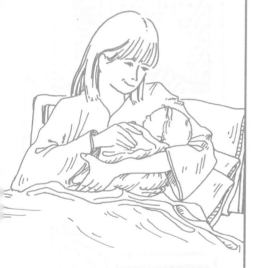

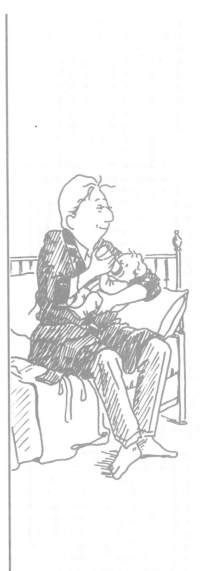

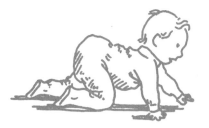

Acknowledgments

This book had an auspicious beginning, thanks to Madelyn Dela Yaceczko and John Yaceczko, Jr. Thanks to John for all of his sound advice and loving support. Of course, this book wouldn't have been possible without the editing supervision of Pam Liflander at Adams Media and the guidance of my agents, Frank Weimann and Catherine McCornack of The Literary Group International. Thanks also to Mary Lou Lund (part of my "village"), Kathy Baker of The Write Choice and Lilly Eleni Romestant, for being . . . well, herself.

Introduction

"Where did you come from, Baby Dear?
Out of the Everywhere, into the Here."
—GEORGE MACDONALD

When I had my first child, Lilly Eleni, in 1992, no one told me what a wonderful journey lay ahead. Sure, there were lots of birthing stories from other moms and unsolicited advice from complete strangers, many of whom also asked to touch my stomach for good luck. But with all of the advice and books out there on the topic of pregnancy, there wasn't anything that addressed what was really going on: the fact that I was part of a larger circle, a conduit through which past, present, and future would converge into one beautiful little life.

Now, as I near the end of my second pregnancy, I see the circle for what it is. I am a speck on the agenda sheet of a vast, unpredictable universe, a tiny part of an immense plan for the continuance of life on the planet. My purpose as a mother, as a life-giver, is to give back to the earth more than what I myself can leave behind: a new life, a new hope, a new beginning. My children are born holding the future in their tiny hands.

But while babies are a gift of the future, they are also a celebration of the past. They are the keepers of history, with everything from Great-grandma's curly auburn hair to Daddy's eyes. They are the pretty little ones we pass traditions, stories, and songs to across generations, building bridges that transcend time.

The Everything® Get Ready for Baby Book offers you hundreds of thought-provoking articles and tips to help you on your new life journey. It is filled with fun facts, useful information, and unusual ideas for celebrating the uniqueness of your parenting experience. There are plenty of places for you to record your own thoughts— places to capture the words that will spark the inevitable conversations beginning with "tell me again about the day I was born."

So, read on—and enjoy your part in the great circle of life!

KATINA Z. JONES

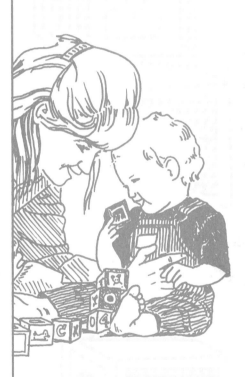

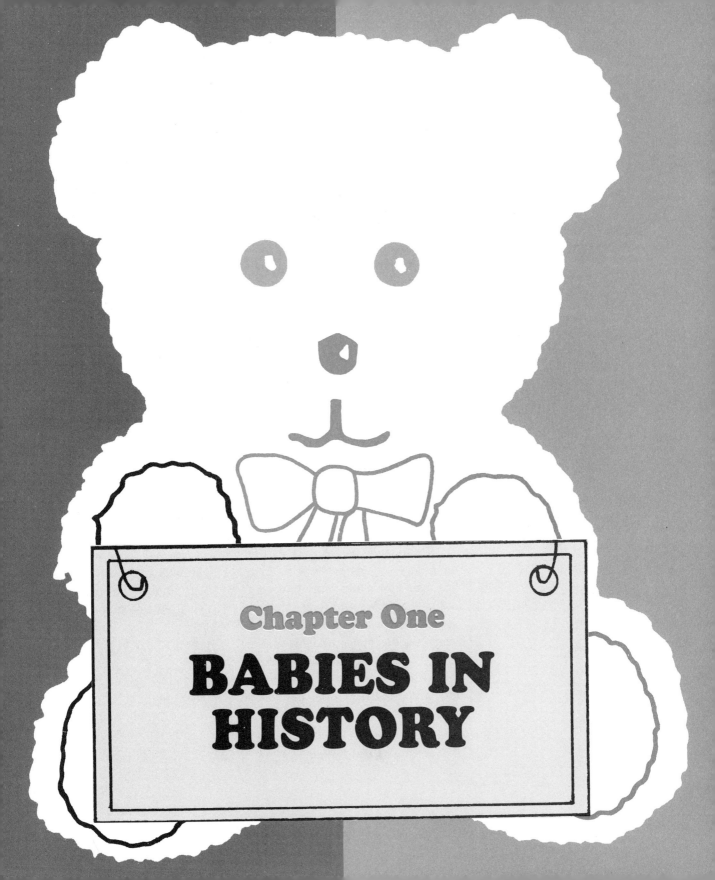

Chapter One

BABIES IN HISTORY

abies have been around since . . . well, prehistoric times. But did the cave dwellers adore their children the same way we do? Why did the ancient Egyptians shower their children with gifts? If the ancient peoples did love their children, how could they perform sacrifices that often involved their firstborn?

There is evidence that the cave dwellers held their children in high esteem. In fact, the hunters- and gatherers-to-be and their parents are the subject of many cave paintings. Some of these paintings show prehistoric man protecting his tribe; others show him mourning the loss of a child. Still others show a mother holding her child or a child acting out "the great hunt."

Egyptians, well known for worshipping cats, also worshipped their children as foreseers of the future and created statues of gods that were meant to protect their children from harm or death. They believed in reincarnation, and they felt that babies came directly from the "other world" and were thus more knowledgeable about future events. It is no coincidence, then, that among ancient Egyptian artifacts are elaborately carved baby gifts, which were given in celebration of the baby's "gift" of bringing the future to his or her parents.

In medieval times, plagues ripped through villages and wiped out many of the young. The surviving babies were believed to have been spared by God so they could perform a higher mission in life. Many parents gave their children to the monasteries as a way to thank God for sparing their precious little ones.

Renaissance babies were exalted through portraits. They were often depicted with white, cherubic faces with pink cheeks and red lips. Sometimes they wore tiny wigs, or caplets similar to the baby bonnets of today, and flowing velvet gowns covered with precious stones. Obviously, the parents of these babies believed their children were precious gems—and, like the cave dwellers, sought to preserve their youth through timeless works of art.

Victorian parents were not much different in that respect. They, too, wrapped their babies in cloaks of soft velvet and sat for elaborate portraits with their new families. They believed that once a child was born it should immediately be carried to the highest point in the house. Why? Victorians reasoned that the higher the baby was in its own house, the higher its supposed stature would be in life. Nurseries were thus designed to be in the attic rather than close to the parents.

In the early 1900s, particularly in the Southern United States, children were born into the farm economy. Parents had many children for a specific reason: to have enough hands to work the family business. It was not unusual for farm families to consist of fifteen or more members, all of whom contributed to the welfare and sustenance of the family. Many would inherit farms and continue the cycle.

Today's babies carry with them all of these interesting legacies, and yet they have an identity all their own. They remind us of babies past, with the same faces, angelic eyes, and sweet smiles; and yet they are tiny representatives of the future. Instead of relying on statues of gods to protect our children, we use baby monitors and video surveillance units. In place of the painted Victorian portraits are digitized, scannable images we can e-mail to all of our friends. For babies, it is certainly true that the more things change, the more they stay the same.

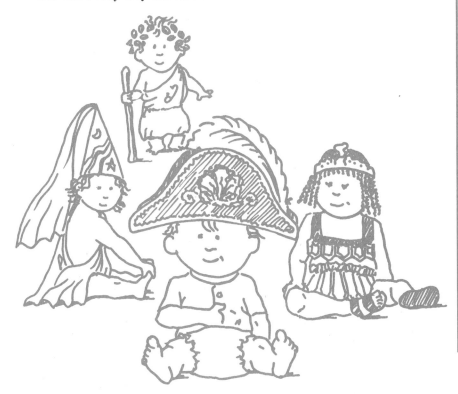

Highlights in Baby History

Native Americans believed that if a woman told her baby that a rattlesnake was on the way, the birthing process would speed up and she would have her baby much sooner.

In early American life, doulas (women helpers, not quite midwives) were far more common than doctors. Physicians were called on only when there were problems with the birth or in high-risk situations. Typically, births were attended by older, wiser women, since they had the knowledge and hands-on experience. More and more women are using doulas today for the same reason; it's a comfort to have another woman in the room who's been through the experience.

In colonial times, women often delivered their babies while in a sitting position—and even while sitting on their husband's lap. Such accommodation was considered the least the husband could do for his laboring wife. This runs contrary to the belief that men were not allowed in the room during birth in earlier times. Actually, they were included more often than not.

Africans believed that a pregnant woman was holy and to be exalted for bringing a new life into the world. This belief is still prevalent in South African culture today, as in many other cultures (whose people bring gifts to the new mother in honor of her life-giving ability).

Europeans made the first obstetric birthing chair in the mid-1500s. It had a back, and the bottom could be removed to accommodate the birth. This design is similar to the birthing chair of today, although more Europeans use these uniquely designed chairs than do Americans. Birthing chairs are most prevalent in Scandinavia; these countries place a high value on a birthing mother's comfort.

Catholics believe that a baby's spirit arrives at conception; some other religions believe that the spirit enters in the moments prior to birth.

Egyptians gave birth in a cross-legged position, as did many Native American women. American Indians believed that birth was a solitary event—and the women went off to a quiet, private spot to give birth to their babies. Since their culture was so closely tied to nature, it isn't surprising that the women would follow the example of animals in birthing their young.

In biblical times, women knelt or stood beside chairs for support during labor. Today, some women sit backward on a chair so that their partners can rub their backs and relieve some of the pain of labor. Chairs are often more comfortable for the mother than the lying-on-the-back-in-bed position.

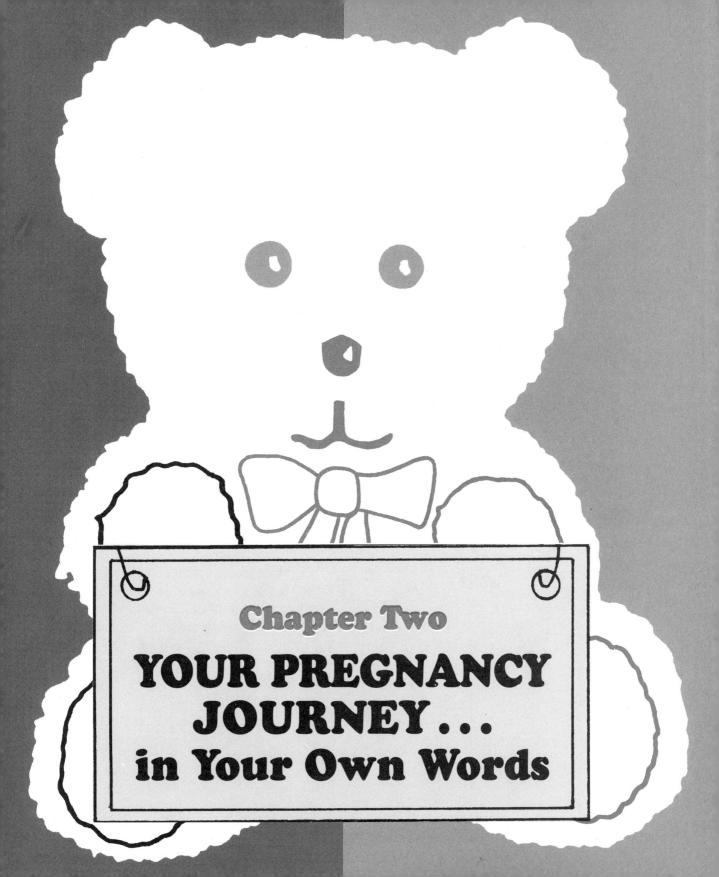

Chapter Two

YOUR PREGNANCY JOURNEY...
in Your Own Words

W hether it's your first, second, or fifth baby, you have within you a unique being with a distinct personality and its own set of hopes and dreams. But what are your own hopes and dreams during your pregnancy?

One of the blessings of pregnancy is that you have plenty of time to think, to dream, and to adjust to the idea of becoming a new mother. You've probably noticed a flood of emotions, worries, and thoughts about the impending birth; it may seem like you're spending too much time thinking about something that's still so far away.

Yet you can't stop thinking about this incredible little life inside you: What will he or she be like? Will the baby look more like you or your partner? Will it be healthy? Questions like these will fill your mind from time to time during this nine-month odyssey.

The best part about having plenty of time before baby comes is that you also have plenty of time to record your thoughts. A few years from now, when your new baby enters toddlerhood, you can pull out these notes for those inquiring eyes asking you to "tell me about the day I was born"—a moment that most assuredly will come. Whether you choose to create a pregnancy journal, time capsule, collage, book, or any other kind of memento to mark his/her important passage in your lives, this keepsake will become a treasure for many years to come. It's worth the time and effort to make it as complete a history of "time before baby" as possible!

Month 1

What's happening with you?

You are elated to discover you're pregnant! There is lots for you to tell others in your life; for example, how you found out you were pregnant, when the baby is due, and some of the names you have thought about. It's all a big ball of emotions for you this month. In fact, there's so much to think about, you hardly know where to start. Of course, physically, you're probably feeling a little tired and possibly even queasy, since morning sickness begins right away with some women.

What's happening with baby?

Baby is the tiniest little blip on an ultrasound machine at this point, something that looks more like a jelly bean than a baby. But so much is happening with baby, it's astounding. He or she has a head, a mouth, and eyes, and arms and legs are beginning to develop; a crude digestive system is already in place. Three-quarters of the way through this month, the baby's heart will begin beating, although it is still fairly tubelike rather than fully developed. Baby weighs less than an ounce now and isn't even an inch long.

What I was feeling this month:

_____

_____

_____

_____

_____

How I told my baby's father the news:

_____

_____

_____

_____

_____

When I told other people and who I told:

_____

_____

_____

_____

_____

_____

_____

What the first trip to the doctor was like:

_____

_____

_____

_____

_____

_____

_____

_____

The best part of knowing I was pregnant with my baby was:

_____

_____

_____

_____

_____

_____

_____

Month 2

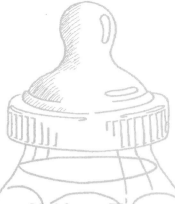

What's happening with you?

You may be more tired than you were during the first month, and the morning sickness could also be more pronounced. Then again, you could be having a great time and not have either of these problems. Every woman is different, and so is every pregnancy. Some women have to stop wearing their prepregnancy clothes at this point, although looser-fitting garments can often go the distance. You may develop cravings for unusual combinations of food and may avoid some foods that you previously enjoyed, since they make you nauseous. Emotionally, you might be worried about the baby's development—everything is so unknown at this point that it's hard for mothers-to-be to relax and enjoy this part of the process.

What's happening with baby?

Now baby's face is becoming a little more developed, as are buds for fingers and toes. Elbows and knees are beginning to show, too. All of the baby's major organs are present, though they are not fully developed. Baby is still less than an ounce in weight and is a little longer than an inch in length. But don't worry—greater growth spurts are only one month away!

What I was feeling this month:

_____

_____

_____

_____

Foods I could tolerate:

_____

_____

_____

_____

Making a Time Capsule for Baby

A time capsule is a keepsake for baby to enjoy as he or she grows older; it is a place for you to record the happenings, excitement, and triumphs of the days when baby was in the process of being born. You can include anything and everything you'd like; one friend of mine chose newspaper highlights, the *Billboard* 100 Top Hits list, and the *New York Times* best-seller list so that baby could know what was the popular fare of the day.

Here is what you'll need:

- Scissors and tape
- A decorated box (usually a shirt-size box or larger and covered in festive baby wrapping paper)
- Newspapers or magazines with the major stories of the day
- Pictures of yourself while pregnant
- Anything else you enjoyed or were a part of during your pregnancy (show programs, ticket stubs, sheet music, etc.)

Label each item with a brief description of its significance. Ask others in the family if they have anything they'd like to contribute.

Foods I absolutely could not be anywhere near:

_____

_____

_____

_____

What the doctor said at this month's checkup:

_____

_____

_____

_____

Month 3

What's happening with you?

Remember the emotional mood swings of premenstrual syndrome?—the ones you thought were gone, at least for nine months? Well, you may have a relapse this month, as hormones rush through your body at warp speed. It might make you a little irritable, a little restless . . . and, if you've had the other major discomforts of pregnancy, you might even be a little teary-eyed at times. However, the good news is that by the end of the third month, the morning sickness tends to subside. The trips to the bathroom haven't subsided, though, as increased pressure on your bladder will keeping you running.

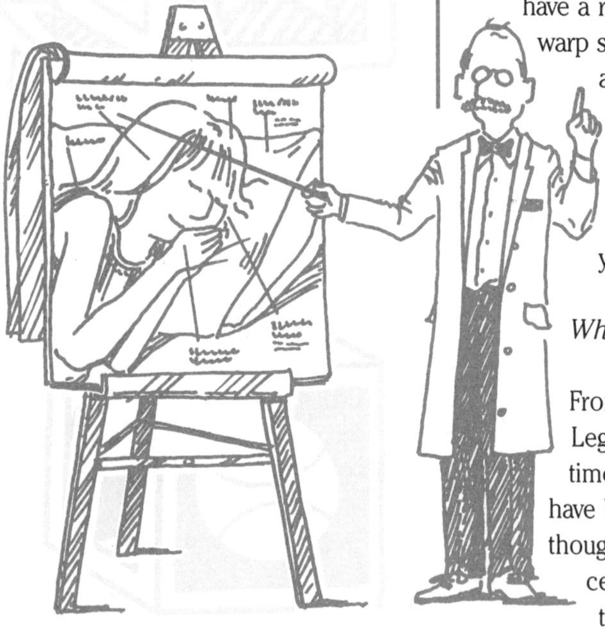

What's happening with baby?

Baby has graduated to a new classification: that of fetus. From this point on, more human-like features begin to appear. Legs begin to kick, arms to flutter . . . baby is having a great time, with plenty of room to begin moving. Teeth and genitals have begun to form. At this point, it's definitely a girl or a boy—though your doctor may not be able to tell yet without an amniocentesis. One thing is for sure: The baby is comfy in its own tiny bubble inside you, and it continues to thrive and grow.

What I remember thinking:

_____

_____

_____

_____

_____

Things I said to my baby:

_____

_____

_____

_____

_____

Special things I did for my baby this month:

_____

_____

_____

_____

_____

What the doctor said at this month's checkup:

_____

_____

_____

_____

_____

Letter to Baby

Write your baby a letter telling him or her what you looked forward to most after learning you were pregnant. Were you excited, nervous, or giddy? What kinds of thoughts ran through your mind? Whom did you think the baby would look most like? What other thoughts consumed you when you learned you had this precious little one growing inside you?

To give you an example of how you can write to your unborn child, here is the letter I wrote to my own baby just prior to her birth:

Dear Madelyn Dela,

My precious little one, you are not even born today, yet I feel such an incredible connection to you! When I first found out that I was carrying you, I was so happy—and so surprised. You came at a time in our lives when we had just embarked on a new beginning; we had been married only a short time and were hoping to have you soon afterward in spite of the fact that we already had four children from previous marriages. Little did we know that we would get this wish immediately!

It wasn't always easy, though. I was sick a lot in the beginning, and you were a feisty little thing, twisting and turning so that we were never really sure which way was up.

One of the best times your father and I had with you was the day we had our ultrasound. There you were, all curled up—my little lamb, my baby. And your daddy, who after three boys really deserved to have a girl of his own, was overjoyed when the doctor told us you were a girl. I thought he would cry he was so happy. I will never forget the proud look on his face.

You have been loved since the day you were created, Maddie, by two people who love each other a lot. Your brothers and sister love you, too, because you are the special link that builds a bridge between them. Thank you for coming into our lives.

Love, Mommy

Month 4

What's happening with you?

Congratulations! You're now in the second trimester of your pregnancy! You're nearly halfway there, and yet there is the growing frustration that this is taking too long. Impatience may rule the day, but there is still much work to be done. If the morning sickness is truly gone, you should eat better this month and your weight should begin to reflect this. Also, you look every bit as pregnant as you feel. If you're taking your prenatal vitamins, your energy level may seem to pick up this month.

What's happening with baby?

Movement! Now you know you're really pregnant, because you can feel the tiny kicks the baby is making. This is called quickening, and it will get stronger over the next few weeks, although no one else will be able to detect it except you. Baby weighs about 5 ounces and can be as long as 7 or 8 inches.

The first movements I felt with my baby:

_____

_____

_____

_____

_____

What I was feeling this month:

_____

_____

_____

_____

_____

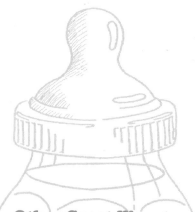

What the doctor said at this month's checkup:

_____

_____

_____

_____

_____

Other Great Ways to Capture Time for Your Baby

- **Videotape what life was like before baby.** Take him or her on a tour of your house, or interview others in your family about their feelings regarding the baby. Maybe Grandma would like to tell the baby her feelings about being a grandmother for the first time . . . or about her own grandmother. Maybe Daddy has a special message for baby. Some people even videotape their ultrasounds so that baby can get a glimpse of what he or she looked like before birth. Videos can be priceless in capturing family memories for future generations.
- **Tape-record your doctor's visits.** Well, not all of them . . . just the ones where baby's heartbeat was heard. I have a tape of my daughter Lilly's first heartbeats, and she loves to listen to it from

Month 5

What's happening with you?

With all of the increasing pressure you're likely to be feeling this month, it's no wonder that you'll have bowel troubles. Thankfully, there isn't much other discomfort—and the things that are slightly uncomfortable can be easily dealt with (i.e., drink more water if you're constipated). This month is, at least for some women, the highlight of pregnancy: You're showing, but you're not so big that you're uncomfortable; you're glowing but not tired looking. It's a beautiful in-between time, so enjoy!

What's happening with baby?

In the fifth month, the baby develops the "vernix" that will protect its tender skin; also, some hair follicles begin to fill. You will provide the necessary ingredients (vitamins and minerals) to nourish the baby from this point on, and baby will grow rapidly. In fact, he or she may reach the 1-pound mark and will grow to between 8 and 10 inches.

What I was feeling this month:

_____

_____

_____

_____

_____

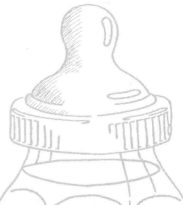

Some interesting things that happened to "us" this month:

_____

_____

_____

_____

_____

_____

_____

Things other people said to me:

_____

_____

_____

_____

_____

_____

_____

What the doctor said at this month's checkup:

_____

_____

_____

_____

_____

_____

_____

Other Great Ways to Capture Time for Your Baby
(continued)

time to time. For her, it's meaningful that I kept a record of her first moments; it makes her feel that much more special.

- **Make a collage.** Cut pictures from magazines depicting different aspects of your pregnancy, from Daddy's reaction to the news to your own hopes and dreams. You can also create really funny captions to go under each picture. Have fun with this project—it'll keep both you and baby laughing later on in life.
- **Keep a scrapbook of everything relating to baby.** From your positive pregnancy result to ultrasound photos to baby shower cards, your baby will appreciate knowing the "great anticipation" that everyone had for him or her. And you will appreciate knowing it's all in one place.

Month 6

What's happening with you?

About now, you're beginning to feel used to this pregnancy thing. You probably have your new, slightly larger wardrobe hanging in the closet and have gotten over the fact that you won't wear your favorite jeans again until sometime next year. You may experience some swelling in your legs, feet, or hands. Try to elevate your feet when you can; sleeping on your side with a pillow between your knees may become your new favorite sleeping position from now until delivery. Warning: Watch out for stretch marks—apply cocoa butter twice daily to avoid major wrinkles.

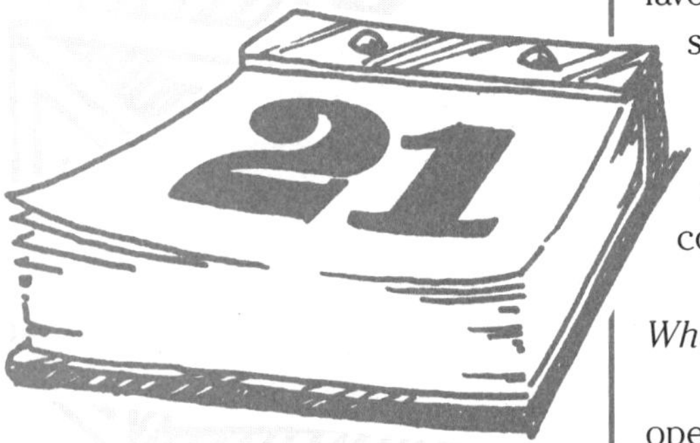

What's happening with baby?

Baby is becoming more of a person than ever, with eyes that open and close, ears that hear, and the ability to suck its thumb. This, of course, leads to hiccups, which you'll notice mostly by the rapid, repetitive movements you feel in your lower abdomen. At the end of this month, your precious cargo may be 1½ pounds and measure up to 13 inches in length.

What I was feeling this month:

_____

_____

_____

_____

_____

Funny dreams I had this month:

_____

_____

_____

_____

_____

New foods I ate:

_____

_____

_____

_____

_____

_____

_____

Things "we" did together:

_____

_____

_____

_____

_____

_____

_____

What the doctor said at this month's checkup:

_____

_____

_____

_____

_____

_____

_____

The "We" Thing: Connecting with Your Baby

One of the most unusual things about pregnancy is that you begin speaking in "we's" for the first time in your life. It's no longer "I don't want to have a hamburger tonight"; it's "We don't feel like hamburger tonight." It's no longer "I'm tired"; it's "We're tired."

Such connection, although at first awkward (not to mention a little funny), is understandable. After all, there really is another life inside you, someone to whom you grow closer with each passing day—someone with whom you are sharing all the precious resources your body has to offer.

As the pregnancy progresses and you begin feeling increased movement, you will also notice that the baby is starting to have a personality all its own: It sleeps, eats, reacts, and even sucks its thumb long before birth. It's only natural, then, for you to think of your baby as an extension of yourself. Your connection to your baby starts the instant you know you're pregnant and will likely continue throughout your child's life.

Moms in Dreamland

*"The baby's head was coming out,
and in this otherwise beautiful moment, I looked down in horror
to see that it was not a baby at all, but a monster."*

*"I went to the doctor, and he told me that I wasn't really pregnant . . .
that it was really just the flu."*

"The baby was born, and as I held it in my arms, it began speaking to me."

Are these experiences real? Of course not. Do they seem real to the pregnant woman who is dreaming them? You bet. Many an expectant mother has awakened in a cold sweat, shaking with fear and wondering just what made her dream such awful or strange things.

Strange, or even disturbing, dreams are not uncommon during pregnancy. In fact, nearly every mother will tell you she has had at least one dream that made her worry. Some tell their partners; others tell their doctors; but the response is likely to be the same: "Don't worry about it. It was only a dream." These words are easily said, but they are not so easily heeded by anxious mothers-to-be.

So what do these dreams mean? Should they be totally ignored, or do they really have meaning? Actually, they do have a meaning, and it's usually tied to your fears or anxieties about the baby's welfare or your own ability to be a good mother. Mind you, this does not mean that you are a sick, paranoid individual or that you really aren't cut out for the mothering thing. What it does mean is that you may have some underlying fears or doubts about motherhood; the dreams may be nature's way of encouraging you to give these worries a little more thought.

What can you do to overcome any fears you are having? Talk to other mothers and ask them to share their experiences with you. You might be surprised to find that they, too, worried about whether they might make good mothers. If you don't know any other moms to talk with (or that you feel comfortable enough to talk with), talk with your husband or obstetrician about your dreams. Getting to the heart of your fears as early as possible will help you conquer pregnancy nightmares and leave you feeling better about the new role you are about to take on.

Month 7

What's happening with you?

Can it really be that you are now in the last trimester of your pregnancy? Sometimes, an ultrasound will give you a clear picture of the baby's sex. Do you want to know, or do you want to be surprised? You and your partner should discuss things like this during the seventh month; it is hoped that you'll both agree on what you *do* and *don't* want to know at this stage of the pregnancy. This month, you may sign up for childbirth classes, start getting the baby's room ready, or maybe even do some shopping while you still have the energy. Some pregnant women enjoy their baby showers at some point from this month forward; generally, it's better to have your shower before the last month, since labor can really happen at any time. If you've got leg cramps, try drinking more milk from this point on; also exercise and stay off your feet as much as you can.

What's happening with baby?

Your baby is moving much more intensely than you know; his or her lungs are more developed, and much movement can be attributed to the baby's increased breathing capacity. Be careful what you say from this month on, since baby can hear sounds outside of its tiny bubble. The skin is red and appears wrinkled; it's just getting ready for deposits of baby fat to begin. Baby is now about 15 inches long and can weigh nearly 2 full pounds.

What I was feeling this month:

_____

_____

_____

_____

_____

Funny dreams I had this month:

_____

_____

_____

_____

_____

Songs I listened to this month:

_____

_____

_____

_____

_____

Things "we" did together:

_____

_____

_____

_____

_____

What the doctor said at this month's checkup:

_____

_____

_____

_____

_____

Month 8

What's happening with you?

Do you find yourself gasping for air sometimes? It could be that the baby is taking up some of your breathing space. Check with your doctor if you're worried. Even though the baby could be in ideal birth position, the blessed event is still at least one month away. Your back may be feeling the strain, too, as the baby grows and presses against your spinal column. Try to get as many back rubs as you can from your partner; they can really help minimize your discomfort. Wind down your work load if possible so that you can get the rest you'll need for next month's "Big Event." By the way, how have your dreams been? You might be experiencing an increase in dream activity, especially in relation to the baby and its welfare. Don't be worried if some of your dreams are frightening or disturbing; talking to your partner and other moms who've been there will help ease your fears. (For more on dreams, see "Moms in Dreamland.")

What's happening with baby?

The baby should be in a "presenting" position now, with head down. Not all babies do this, however, and some who decide to stay breech at this point have good reason for doing so (i.e., the cord is around its neck or a limb). Discuss with your doctor the pros and cons of turning a breech baby now; many doctors do not want to take the risk of hurting you or the baby and may recommend a Caesarean section to lessen the dangers. Baby can be 16 to 18 inches long and weigh about 3½ to 5 pounds.

What I was feeling this month:

_____

_____

_____

_____

_____

Dreams I had this month that worried me or made me laugh:

_____

_____

_____

_____

_____

Things "we" did together:

_____

_____

_____

_____

What "we" talked about this month:

_____

_____

_____

_____

What the doctor said at this month's checkup:

_____

_____

_____

_____

Eating for Two

Eating for one is sometimes challenging enough, with all of the tasty temptations currently offered. Here are some general guidelines that will help you make smart choices when it comes to your food intake.

Take the prenatal vitamins your doctor has prescribed. They contain all of the supplements you'll need during the pregnancy—and then some. Folic acid, now a mainstay in prenatal vitamins, has been shown to combat spina bifida, a disease affecting the baby's central nervous system. One word of caution: Don't rely solely on your prenatal vitamins to carry you through; you still need to eat well-balanced meals, since the vitamins are only a supplement to regular eating.

Eat foods from each of the food groups every day. Remember the food groups you learned about in grade school? Never have you needed them more than when your body is developing a healthy baby. You need at least four servings of protein foods (such as meat, cheese, eggs, milk, beans, and tofu); at least one vitamin C-filled food (including fruits and vegetables such as grapefruit, oranges, mangoes, papaya, cantaloupe, strawberries, cabbage, cauliflower, and spinach); two or three green leafy vegetables or yellow fruits or vegetables (such as peaches, raw carrots, broccoli, lettuce, spinach, and yams); four to five servings per day of breads, cereals, and grains (such as whole wheat bread, rice, grain cereal, wheat germ, and pasta). Snack on grapes, apples, nuts, and granola when you can; these foods are easy to pack and carry with you even if you're on the road or at work.

Consume more calories—but only the good kind. Simply eating more food than you usually do is not going to cut it; your body needs to have calories with high value—not the empty calories found in cakes, cookies, and pies. You don't have to gain a lot of weight to have a baby, and many doctors prefer that you eat better and weigh less rather than eat everything in sight and weigh more. Most women gain between 25 and 30 pounds during pregnancy. You need only an additional 300 to 500 calories per day for the baby's development. (But see your doctor for advice concerning your own individual requirements, as you may have underlying issues or health problems that require different plans of action.)

Drink plenty of fluids—especially water and milk. Water will flush out any impurities in your system, not to mention keep you hydrated. This is particularly important in early pregnancy, when your body is at work cleansing its system in preparation for building a new life. Especially in the last trimester, your milk intake should be three to four glasses per day; this helps your body build calcium levels sufficient for strengthening the baby's bones—with the added benefit of warding off those miserable leg cramps you might be getting. In fact, the leg cramps are nature's way of telling you to consume more calcium. (This also means you should limit the amount of caffeine you consume, since caffeine is notorious for depleting calcium levels in women.)

Watch your iron intake. If you're not getting enough iron, your doctor may put you on supplements. If this happens, be sure to take only what the doctor prescribes, since too much iron can damage a developing fetus.

Finally, your food selection is not as limited as you may think. For example, a Mexican meal consisting of refried beans (protein), avocados and salsa (fruit and vegetable), low-fat sour cream (protein), and flour tortillas (bread) offers a fairly nutritious meal.

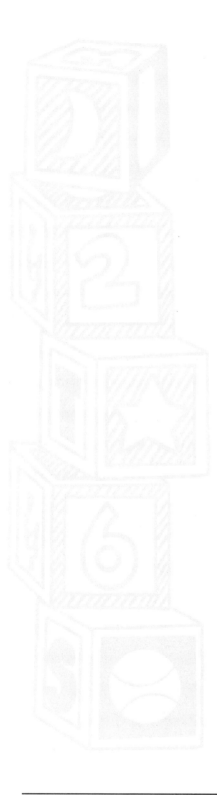

Month 9

What's happening with you?

You have finally made it this far. Can it be that in a few short weeks you'll be holding in your arms the little one you've been talking to and dreaming about all this time? The best part of the ninth month of pregnancy is knowing that the moment you've been waiting for is quickly approaching; the worst part is keeping your energy level high.

What's happening with baby?

This is the final stage of growth for the baby; most of its major organs are fully developed by now, except for the brain, which is now experiencing its largest growth spurt. The skin is smooth, and the skull will be soft and flexible enough to mold its way down the birth canal when labor approaches. As the baby begins its descent into the pelvis in preparation for birth, it continues to gain weight and muscle strength. Your baby may be 18 or more inches long and could weigh between 5½ and 8 pounds.

What I was feeling this month:

_____

_____

_____

_____

_____

Things people said about my baby in the last few days before the birth:

_____

_____

_____

_____

_____

What I thought about this month:

_____

_____

_____

_____

_____

What the doctor said at the last checkup:

_____

_____

_____

_____

_____

The "Big Day" and What Happened

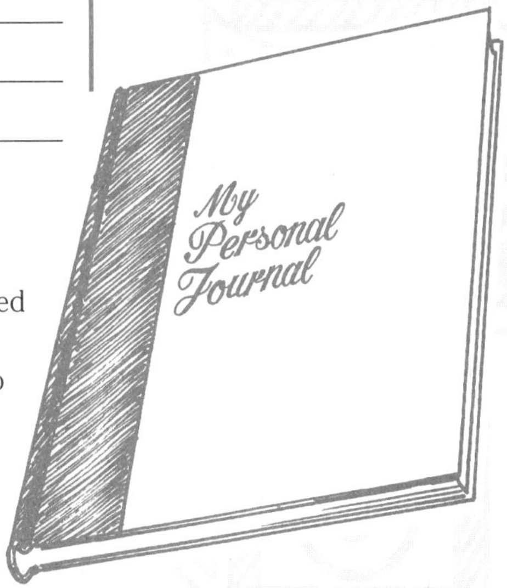

This is the part of your journal that is guaranteed to get dog-eared and worn out before any other. Children are fascinated by the birth process and, more specifically, the way that they came into the world. Try to jot down your responses to these items as soon as you can, so as not to forget the tiny details of this momentous occasion. If you don't feel like writing, ask your partner to do it for you as the two of you talk it through.

How I noticed labor was beginning:

_____

_____

_____

_____

_____

My Personal Journal

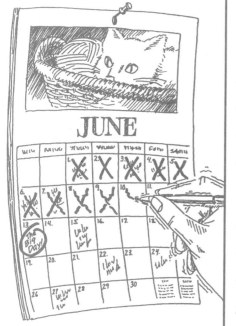

How my baby's father reacted:

_____

_____

_____

_____

What I was feeling and thinking:

_____

_____

_____

_____

Where my baby was born:

_____

_____

_____

Details my baby should know about the birth:

_____

_____

_____

_____

How we told the world the news of our baby's birth:

_____

_____

_____

_____

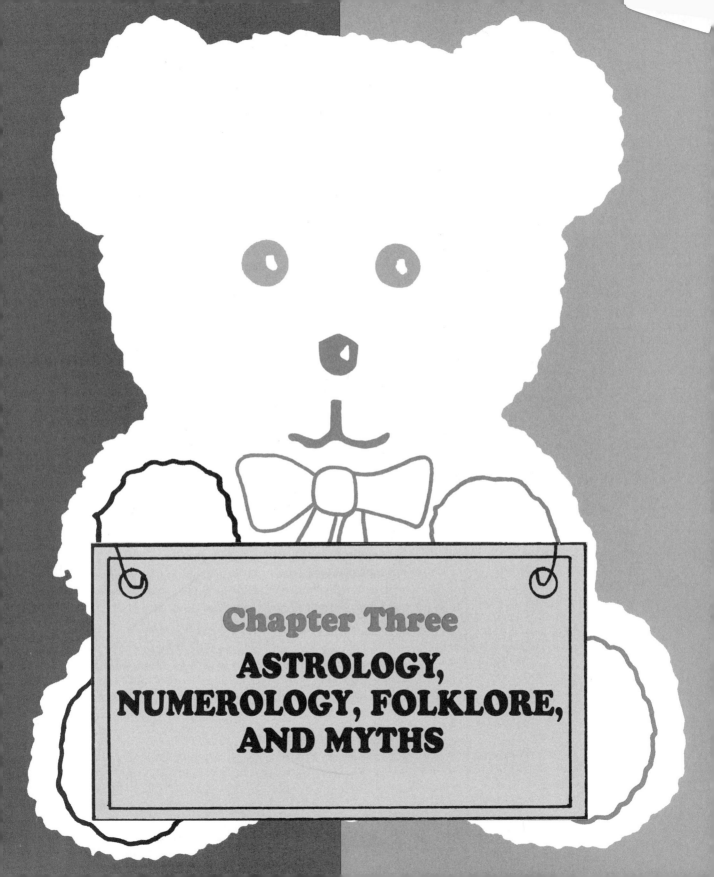

Chapter Three

ASTROLOGY, NUMEROLOGY, FOLKLORE, AND MYTHS

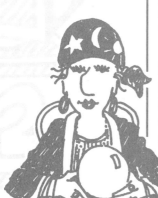

What parents can resist the temptation to delve into the future of their beloved new baby, especially in this New Age? Some even have their new baby's complete astrological chart produced by a psychic or astrologer. Whether you pay a professional or use one of the many books or software programs to cast an eye into baby's future, it is not at all uncommon to have an "inquiring mind" about your newborn's destiny.

The traditions of soothsaying and fortune-telling are ancient ones, built on the curiosity of parents wanting to know how their child might turn out. In classic Greek mythology, parents placed gifts at the temple of Delphi to seek information about their child's future. They weren't always pleased to hear the results; often they were told tales of war, rebellion, or scandal that would befall them. But occasionally there was that one child who would stand out in the crowd—the one who, due to the whim of a god, might become an Odysseus.

Whether or not it's accurate or whether or not it's fair to cast a baby's future into stone, parents have continued to peer into their child's future; and they likely will continue to do so well beyond this century. But if kept in the spirit of fun and entertainment, it can be fun for you to "guesstimate" your child's place in the world.

Astrology for Babies

For thousands of years, the superstitious have believed that the position of the stars and planets at the time of a child's birth determines the baby's personality and life path. It is a belief so entrenched in culture that it has survived many years, mostly due to our innate curiosity about the development of the self. (Oh, okay—maybe it's just for fun . . .) For your baby's astrological profile, read on.

Aries (March 22–April 22) babies are aggressive, restless, and strong willed. They are, after all, the born leaders of the zodiac. Aries babies are voted most likely to move on to potty training early; they are bored with the diapers they feel are holding them back from true greatness. Aries babies will be intelligent, physically strong, and assertive and are most compatible with Scorpio, Aquarius, and Gemini parents.

Taurus (April 22–May 22) babies are earthy, strong, and practical. There's no need to buy those fancy Baby Gap shoes when simple 100 percent cotton socks will do for this newborn. The sign of the bull leaves little room for adventure, as "bullish" baby doesn't fare well in the dining room china shop. Keep all breakables away from this active one. It's not that Taurus is hyperactive; he or she is just a tad clumsy. On the positive side, small Taureans are devoted to their families and love big reunion-type functions. Baby Taurus is most compatible with Gemini, Cancer, and Capricorn parents.

The **Gemini** child (May 22–June 22) seems okay to begin with, but then you notice that there are mixed messages coming from the child. One minute it's crying and the next minute it's laughing; it's almost as if your child has an evil twin. Maybe that's because Gemini is the sign of the twins, which means abrupt changes in temperament and unusual mood swings. Oh, well, at least such moodiness is short lived. Your Gemini baby will be off to giddyland again in a heartbeat; and this little one's good-natured disposition will be a godsend on those otherwise sleepless nights. Gemini babies are earthy, inquisitive, and adventuresome; they are most compatible with Aries, Capricorn, and Aquarius parents.

Cancer babies (June 22–July 22) are known for their mothering tendencies. This child will feel compelled at any early age to "mother" you! Cancerians are tenacious and extremely sensitive; and when they get "crabby," they are likely to experience all their turmoil in their tummies, making for some interesting diaper changes. Tiny moon-children are homebodies, yet they are artsy and creative; they relish connections to the past and will ask you repeatedly for stories about long-lost ancestors. They are most compatible with Taurus, Scorpio, and Pisces parents.

Leos (July 22–August 22) are voted most likely to roar when they're hungry, demand the undivided attention of Mommy or whoever else is within its "jungle," and strut their stuff across the living room without even bothering to crawl first. Leos are proud, loyal, and show-offish; they really do believe the world revolves around them (think of Leos Madonna and Mick Jagger and you get the picture). You can get some great home video footage of this baby, as baby Leo is a natural performer. They are most compatible with Aries, Taurus, and Libra parents.

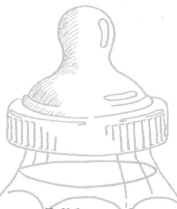

Folklore and Superstition . . . Timeless, in Any Language

Slovak tradition says if you put money in baby's hand soon after birth, the child will grow up to be wealthy and powerful.

Greek tradition says that a lock of baby's hair, snipped and preserved in wax paper, will protect the child from bad dreams, if placed under his or her pillow.

Native Americans made weblike dream-catchers to hang near their babies, in the hopes that their babies would be spared nightmares.

Gypsy folklore says that children born at three, six, nine, or twelve o'clock are extremely fortunate throughout life and have more intuition and instinct than others. Also, children born with teeth are said to be selfish in life; and children born with their hands wide open are said to be generous and giving.

Children who give way to crying during their christenings are said to be ridding themselves of evil spirits.

A baby's tooth worn in a ring, on a brooch, or hanging from a chain is said to bring good luck to the wearer.

Virgos (August 22–September 22) can't help themselves—they are the compulsive Felix Ungers of the zodiac and want everything to be perfect from the start. They simply can't stand an even slightly soiled diaper, and heaven forbid if they burp up anything on their little nightshirts. Buy lots of bibs, diapers, and clothes for these high-maintenance babies, and they'll be happy as clams. Virgo babies are, for all their fastidiousness, happy little spirits who are eager to learn. But do keep their rooms and toys clean. They are most compatible with Gemini, Cancer, and Taurus parents. (Warning: Watch out if you wind up with a Virgo baby and a Virgo parent—it could become a battle of the neatniks!)

Libra babies (September 22–October 22) like their lives to be well balanced; that is, they like sleeping and playing, eating and learning . . . you get the idea. They are charming, sweet, and giving; and, at the same time, they are manipulative and a little devious. You need to figure out which way the scale is tipping on a particular day before you decide a course of action. Librans are intelligent and require attention and encouragement to make the most of themselves. They are most compatible with Leo, Aquarius, and Sagittarius parents.

Some **Scorpios** (October 22–November 22) have been known to wait years to get back at you for all those humiliating bath-time photos and candid baby shots. Not known to be easily forgiving, these little ones are very sensitive and can get their feelings hurt with the greatest of ease. Tread carefully around the little Scorpion; they keep a mental diary that chronicles your every move. These babies are sensitive, dreamy, and creative and usually don't have motivational problems later in life. They are most compatible with Cancer, Pisces, and Virgo parents.

Sagittarius babies (November 22–December 22) can't get enough of toys such as gliders, Johnny Jump-Ups, or anything that even looks like an airplane. Perhaps it's because they are the quintessential air sign of the zodiac—free, fun loving, and unafraid of challenges. That could also be why they are the most accident prone of the zodiac. Buy a big box of Band-Aids and safety proof your house early—you're going to need it! Sagittarius babies are most compatible with patient Capricorn, Taurus, and Gemini parents.

Capricorns (December 22–January 22) are earthy, practical, and predictable. They can always be depended on to help with younger siblings and are the best at being Mommy's or Daddy's little helper. Baby Capricorns are most content when permitted to roam the grass in the backyard, and they love to go for hikes. If it's related to outdoors, they love it. They are most compatible with Aries, Gemini, and Virgo parents.

Aquarius babies (January 22–February 22) are inquisitive and highly intelligent. They may look at the black-and-white mobile for a week or so and then be ready to see what's behind door number two. You'll need to keep the toy supply current and make sure to change the pictures around in the nursery just to keep this baby interested and alert. Aquarians are the nontraditional, unpredictable sign of the zodiac—you will learn a lot from your Aquarius child (perhaps even stuff you never wanted to know). They will ask "Why?" a lot before the age of three. They are most compatible with Gemini, Libra, and Sagittarius parents.

The little **Pisces** (February 22–March 22) is emotional, pensive, and deep. Little Pisces sure can be moody; one minute, this baby is giggling hysterically, and the next minute it is awash in tears. Is the child manic? Not really—he or she is just more emotional than most. You need to ask this little one constantly if everything's okay; it may be a too-tight diaper, but it could just as easily be a bout of existential self-doubt. You may ride an emotional roller coaster with this one, but you'll have a devoted, loving child for eternity if you simply listen to him or her. They are most compatible with Cancer, Scorpio, and Virgo parents.

If baby is born on the cusp (on a twenty-second day of a month), he or she will carry some of the traits of both signs. Don't worry, though; astrology is something many of us only believe in when it is telling us the news we want to hear.

Chinese Astrology for Baby

The Chinese have their own method for divining a child's future, based not on the day of birth but on the year of birth. Chinese astrology focuses on animals and their relative traits in predicting

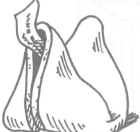

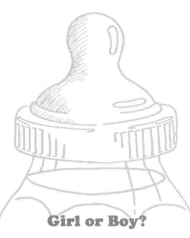

Girl or Boy?

Everyone wants to play the guessing game of determining the baby's sex before it is born. It's fun to let others have their say; and it's okay to let someone win the "baby pool" using whatever myth they believe in.

According to Greek folklore, if a pregnant woman walks away from you, then turns to her right to answer when you call her name, the baby is a girl. If she turns to the left, it is a boy.

According to Gypsy folklore, a baby born during a new moon will be a male; otherwise it will be a female.

Are you carrying extra "baggage" around your hips and rear? If so, it's probably a girl. If your weight is more up front, it's probably a boy.

Is your body hair growing faster (and heavier) than before pregnancy? Supposedly girls are behind this phenomenon.

Tie your wedding ring to the end of a string, dangle the string over your belly, and watch which direction it turns. If it goes around in a circular

a child's characteristics and fortune in life. For instance, we know that dogs tend to be loyal, dragons are believed to be fiery and temperamental, and rabbits tend to be meek and understated. Look below for the sign associated with your baby's birth year, and decide for yourself whether the ancient Chinese secret is on target.

Mouse/Rat (1996, 2007) babies are loyal and affectionate. They love to be held, sung to, rocked, and cradled in their parents' arms. Rats tend to be quiet, calm, and understated as little ones—perhaps they are conserving their energy for the leadership they will likely achieve as adults. They are also warm, intelligent creatures. Rats are most compatible with other Rats, Dragons, Monkeys, and Dogs.

Ox (1997, 2009) babies are quiet and very adaptable to unusual surroundings or situations. They are often very shy in their first few years, yet they are capable of building and drawing on their strong inner resources as they grow older. This makes them capable of achieving whatever they set their minds to; they often choose art, music, or sports-related professions and are extremely hard working once they get going. Oxen are most compatible with Rats, Monkeys, Roosters, and Pigs.

Tigers (1998, 2010) expect an undaunting spirit and a hungry sense of adventure. They are born explorers and have a strong sense of their place in the world. They are passionate and competitive from day one and later become fairly compelling individuals. Tigers are the luckiest sign in the Chinese zodiac. Tigers are most compatible with Dragons, Horses, Dogs, and Rabbits.

Rabbit (1999, 2011) babies are peaceful, docile creatures. These cuddly little bunnies are sensitive, soft, and even slightly fragile. They tend to cry often and easily but respond to the loving caresses of their parents. Don't worry about these "clingy" tendencies; your baby Rabbit will undoubtedly grow to become a strong individual later in life, if you provide a nourishing, stable environment. Many musicians and writers are born under this sign. Rabbits are very compatible with other Rabbits, Snakes, Sheep, and Pigs.

Dragons (2000, 2012) will make you forget that you are the boss, and you will often find yourself wondering how you were manipulated into giving this Machiavellian child his or her way yet another time.

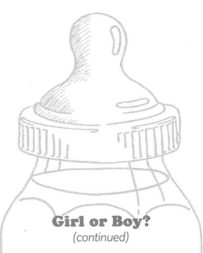

But you will always feel loved nonetheless. Dragons are flamboyant, strong willed, and dramatic, yet they have an uncanny way of making a lot of things seem like your idea. When they are being forceful about their own ideas, they take a firm stand and will not back down until they see the whites of your eyes; so get ready for some colorful discussions later on in this baby's life. Dragons eventually grow to become confident, successful business people. They are most compatible with Rats, Snakes, Monkeys, and Pigs—basically anyone who's willing to take a backseat to their ambitions.

Snake (2001, 2013) babies live in their own world. They need lots of time, room, and attention to flourish and will likely keep to a close inner circle of friends. These babies sulk or have a silent tantrum when they don't get their way and are as vengeful as the Western sign of Scorpio when they feel wronged. Still, if you give the Snake an opportunity to grow in his or her own time, you will have a young adult who is passionate and humorous (well, a dry sense of humor is better than none at all, right?). Snakes are highly compatible with Dragons, Monkeys, Dogs, and Rabbits.

Horses (2002, 2014) are full of the joy of living and blessed with intelligence and practicality. Yet, they are also notorious for making rash decisions; so keep your baby gate up just a little longer than you thought you should. Their quick little minds often take their bodies places where they shouldn't go; but on the positive side, they only need to learn a lesson once. Horses are individualistic and independent little creatures; you won't be called on until this baby is bored with a new concept or toy. They are most compatible with Tigers, Sheep, Pigs, and sometimes Dragons (although this combination could be a little too colorful and dangerous).

Sheep (2003, 2015) are family oriented from the start and will always insist that everyone go out together instead of separately. They are a tad too clingy for some of the other signs, but that is because they are very separation-anxiety ridden. Remember the nursery rhyme about Mary and her little lamb: ". . . everywhere that Mary went, the lamb was sure to go"? Well, this little lamb will follow you all over the house, if only to be constantly near you. Give Sheep as much encouragement as possible, and they may become more sociable.

Girl or Boy?
(continued)

pattern, it means you're carrying a girl. If it moves back and forth, it means you're carrying a boy.

Do you have cold feet? It could be a boy changing your body temperature.

Baby boys lie low in their mother's belly; baby girls are carried higher.

Extreme morning sickness means a girl child is on the way.

Is the baby's heart rate 140 or higher? Girls have racier hearts than boys, who supposedly rate lower than 140.

Are people complimenting you on your healthy glow? Rosier cheeks mean a girl is coming; mothers of boys favor the tired look.

Is the baby shaped like a watermelon? If so, it's a girl. Or is it shaped like a basketball? You guessed it—it's a boy.

Do you sleep on your left or your right side? "Right" means a girl; "left" means a boy is the object of your dreams.

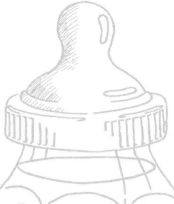

Pregnancy Myths

Low-carried babies mean early babies. It could be that your muscles are stretched from a previous pregnancy or that your body's weight distribution creates a low appearance. Many a low-lying baby has been late.

The more weight you gain, the bigger the baby will be. Most of your weight gain can be attributed to water, and some babies (even six-pounders) need more than others.

Morning sickness means a healthier baby. Folks have long said that this belief is true, and medical evidence finally supports the fact that bouts of nausea are meant to rid the mother's body of impurities that could negatively affect the baby.

Cravings should be ignored or made fun of. Actually, your body (or your baby) knows what it wants. If you're craving cream of broccoli soup, it could well be that your body needs it to combat nausea;

They are most compatible with Rabbits (the two can literally have a weep-fest together), Dragons, Horses, fellow Sheep, and Pigs.

Monkey (2004, 2016) babies are imaginative, resourceful, adaptable, and yet a little on the mischievous side. They are downright curious about everything, and you'll get the "Why?" questions streaming in at a pace that will make your head spin. Little Monkeys need to know everything, and they get restless when they have to wait for anything. But their memories can't be beat. Some Monkeys remember the tiniest of details from their youngest years; so watch what you say, as Monkeys make excellent parrots (if you know what I mean). A final word of caution: Your baby Monkey will be a quick learner with a wicked sense of humor. They are most compatible with Rats, Dragons, other Monkeys, and Pigs.

Rooster (2005, 2017) babies have a flair for the dramatic and can be a bit perfectionistic. They are alert, energetic creatures and, from an early age, can communicate well with others. Their charming nature makes them socially well adjusted and popular; balance that with their competitive nature, and you often wind up with little rivals. Don't worry, though—your little Rooster may get his or her feathers ruffled at times but will always find something else to crow about later. Roosters are most compatible with Oxen, Dragons, Dogs, and Pigs.

Dog (2006, 2018) babies are loyal, giving, and sincere; and they are capable of going to extreme lengths to keep everyone satisfied. They care about everyone else's feelings and often put their own on hold until the needs of others have been met. Dogs are blessed with common sense and the ability to amuse themselves as well as others. The one trait you'll appreciate most as parents of a Dog is his or her unbelievable honesty; if you ask who really broke the vase, you'll get the truth, and nothing but the truth. Dogs are very compatible with Tigers, Horses, other Dogs, and Pigs.

Pigs (2007, 2019) are happy, contented, and docile creatures—not to mention eternal optimists. They are born people-pleasers, always striving to serve the needs of everyone around them. They are generosity personified and often make excellent community servants (paramedics, teachers, etc.). If you haven't noticed by now, Pigs are compatible with darn near every other sign in the Chinese zodiac, which should come as no surprise given their altruistic, self-sacrificing nature. Just warn them not to be too giving; some naïve Pigs can lose themselves in the people they love and need to be encouraged to develop their own interests to keep it all in balance.

Whatever "animal(s)" you discover to have living under your roof, remember to know and love them for what they truly are; give your children the love, time, and space they need to step into themselves, and you will have beautiful and devoted friends for life.

Numerology for Baby

The science of numbers is not always 100 percent reliable in predicting a baby's future, but many a new parent has crunched the numbers anyway in the hopes of seeing into their child's future. Numerology assumes that the numbers relating to a baby's birth can tell something about the child's destiny and personality. The main number your child will have, then, is his or her "destiny" number.

Here's how to figure your baby's special number: Add all of the numbers of the baby's birthday together, and then reduce them to a single digit. For example, if baby was born on 7/10/97, its destiny number would be 7 + 1 + 0 + 1 + 9 + 9 + 7, or 34. To reduce 34 to a single digit, add 3 + 4 for a destiny number of 7. (If the number still has two digits at this point, add the digits together again for your baby's destiny number.)

Here's a quick guide to your baby's "numeric" personality.

Number One: Babies born with a destiny number of one are born leaders; they have courage, goals, and the tenacity to really accomplish whatever they set their minds to. They are reliable, strong, and considerate toward others; thus, they make excellent mentors (or big brothers and sisters!).

Number Two: Twos are incredibly calm, compassionate beings. They detest egotism and learn to share from an early age, since selfishness and injustice are completely foreign to them. They appreciate equality for all in the household—and in life. Twos are sensitive to the needs and desires of others and may actually be too sympathetic at times.

Number Three: The ancient Greeks believed that good things, especially useful ideas, happened in threes. Baby threes are the

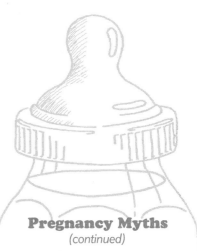

Pregnancy Myths
(continued)

broccoli contains vitamin B6, which is known to curb nausea to some degree. So, indulge yourself in (healthy) cravings—they may be your saving grace in the first few months of pregnancy.

Athletically inclined women have easier births. This belief is not necessarily true. Although athletes do have an endurance tolerance higher than that of nonathletes, some nonathletic women have shorter periods of labor and less difficulties than others run into. What does that say for "no pain, no gain"?

Raspberry tea, balsamic vinegar, or sex brings on labor. Nothing truly brings on labor as much as a willing (and ready) baby. You can try wild sex; bumpy roads; special teas, foods and spices; or even exercises, but the only one who really knows when it's time is the baby.

entrepreneurs and inventors on the numerology scale; they are the idea generators and are noted for their organizational abilities. They are exuberant, cheerful, and (some might say) overachievers. And they are always listened to, since they nearly always have ideas that can be immediately put to use.

Number Four: Fours are the backbone of numerology; they are strong, steady types who have their feet on terra firma from day one. They are hard working, determined, and honest—perhaps to a fault. And they are certainly practical and seldom given to criticizing others for sport. They would rather look on the bright side of everything.

Number Five: Here are the adventurers of the bunch—good luck trying to hold your little five down! They are brave, lively souls and love to overcome obstacles thrown their way. Typically, fives are healthy and athletic individuals, and they like variety in terms of tasks and companions. Many great explorers have a five destiny number.

Number Six: Sixes are idealistic and harmonious; they like everyone to get along and wish the world was as perfect as it is in the movies. They are loving and, from an early age, giving to others. They may make their mark in the world as great philanthropists; sixes can't stand to see anyone going without. They also make fine doctors, as they have a disdain for human suffering.

Number Seven: Babies with a seven destiny number are wise and unusually perceptive; they can make intelligent decisions and people will learn to rely on them for their problem-solving skills. Many great philosophers and thinkers have a seven destiny number. Sevens are notorious for being somewhat rigid and into the self-discipline thing; encourage your seven to get out and enjoy life a little.

Number Eight: As practical and down to earth as fours are, eights are double that. They are powerful individuals with a will to succeed in life, and they have little tolerance for others who don't work as hard as they do. These are not daydreamers in any sense of the word. Eights rise to the occasion so quickly that they can be a janitor one day and a company president the next.

Number Nine: Nines show tremendous intelligence and the ability to understand the complexities of life. They are artistic and make excellent and reliable friends. Nines like to help others succeed, too, and can be a source of great inspiration for their friends and family members. Many performers and artists have this destiny number.

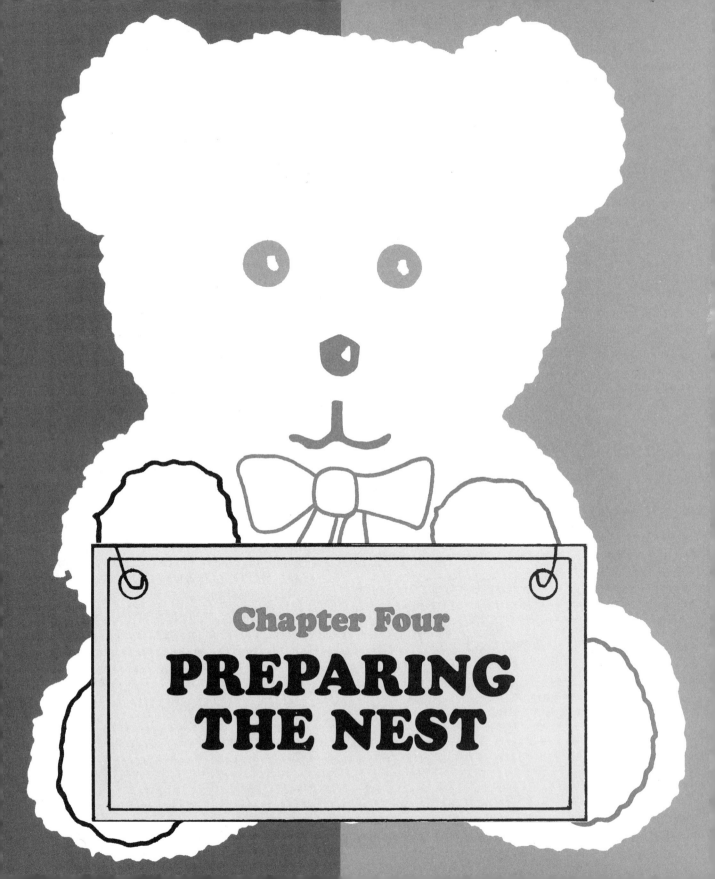

Chapter Four

PREPARING THE NEST

I n the animal world, the female prepares a special place for her young shortly before birth. In this "nest," she gives birth and at the same time provides a safe haven for her young to rest and grow in. In terms of your new baby's "nest," you and your partner will have the unique opportunity to create baby's first world outside of the womb—a place for it to dream, to experience, and to grow.

Since calm surroundings are so critical to a newborn's development, you should first give some serious thought to the location of the baby's room: Will it be on the same floor as your bedroom? If not, how will you monitor the room—with an audio or video monitor? Will the baby's room be near a busy, noisy street, or will it be facing a backyard where there is nothing but the sound of crickets?

Planning the best location for your baby's room is the starting point in designing the nursery. Once you have decided the space, then you can begin filling the room with plush toys and cool designs. Before you rush out to choose the décor, write down the room's dimensions; then, when you're at the baby furniture showroom, you'll have a clear idea of what pieces will fit. Such planning with regard to location and size of the baby's room will save you infinite amounts of time—and heartache, if the motif you like doesn't fit well within the parameters of the room.

Decorating the Nursery

Creating just the right aura or atmosphere for your baby's room can be one of the most exhilarating things for you to do in preparation for the "Big Event." It is, after all, one of the few things you actually have control over in this birthing odyssey.

Choosing a particular décor depends on a few variables, such as how much you want to spend, how much space you have for the baby's room, and whether you know for certain if it's a boy or a girl. The best option is to go with something that's generic enough for both sexes; you can always add more gender-specific items after the birth, in addition to personalized items with baby's name printed on them. Good gender-neutral colors are greens, purples, and reds.

As far as motifs go, it may be wise to visit a few baby stores to see how all of the components look together for each particular style. This will also give you hands-on experience with the equipment; if you don't feel comfortable with a particular crib style, for example, you can look around to see if there is another style that coordinates well with your selected motif.

Here are some traditional themes:

Animals. Kittens, puppies, teddy bears, and farm scenes are typical within this motif. The only thing as sweet as your own baby is a baby animal, right? You could purchase everything from the sheet and comforter set to coordinating wall hangings and wallpaper—nearly every baby store out there has at least one baby animal set in stock.

Three-ring circus. Clowns, lions, and tigers can fill baby's room with an exciting array of scenes; and you can create some of your own coordinating pieces—for example, fabric balloon wall hangings, crepe paper decorations for the window frame, and multicolor paint on pillars and trim.

Cartoon/TV characters. Bugs Bunny, Mickey Mouse, Winnie the Pooh, and the puppets on Sesame Street are just a few samples of what's out there in the baby department. You can choose a character you feel sentimental about yourself or simply one that's appealing to you and your partner. The big advantage to choosing this type of theme is that there are literally hundreds of licensed products that you can purchase from a wide variety of sources—and you're not limited to the baby shops for this one.

Sports teams. If you're certain about having a boy, you can decorate a room in the motif of your favorite team. You might have to order through a catalog to get some of the larger baby products (such as comforters and lamps) with the team logo on it. Smaller items can usually be purchased in the team's gift shop or at department stores.

Noah's Ark. This is a popular theme, and there are plenty of designs to choose from. You can coordinate with cute pictures of animals placed throughout the room, and it should be easy to find a nursery lamp to match.

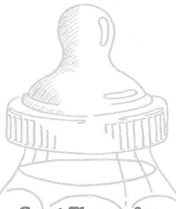

Great Themes for Baby Showers

Baby showers are still traditionally attended by women, but there is a growing trend toward coed showers. After all, it's Dad's baby, too—so why shouldn't he be there? For coed showers, you could opt for any of the following: a cookout, an ice cream social, a tea party, a Mexican fiesta, a picnic or potluck dinner, a pool party, or a even a baby film festival (rent any of the comedies out there about parenthood, or create your own film).

Showers typically begin with a meal and dessert and then move on to games (see Fun Shower Games on pages 44–45), opening gifts, and finally a thank you from the parents-to-be. Whatever you decide to do, plan to make it fun and to enjoy the excitement. And take lots of pictures!

Pastels. If you want to have a smooth, coordinated look that's a little on the conservative side, solid pastels might work best for you. This allows you tremendous flexibility in terms of coordinating items; you can mix and match pictures, lamps, wall hangings, and wallpaper borders in many different shades. Throw in a comforter or window treatment with an interesting pastel pattern to pull it all together.

Here are some nontraditional themes:

Suns, moons, and stars. Although popular among adults for decorating, the solar or planetary motif is still fairly new for baby's room. Set your baby's room apart from the rest by painting clouds on the ceiling and hanging fabric moons and stars from it as well. Just be sure to hang them in such a way that they don't interfere with baby's immediate area; hanging them too close to the crib would be dangerous, since they could fall or be pulled by baby into the crib. Keep it safe, yet interesting.

Geometric shapes. Geometric shapes work particularly well in black, red, and white, since many child-development specialists have recommended these contrasting colors for baby's early stimulation and brain development. Many mobiles are already sporting these colors, and there are plenty of baby toys in these shapes and colors, too. Paint the walls white, and then accentuate the windows and trim in black-and-white stripes with red highlights.

African safari. Cultural themes are growing increasingly popular in the new global village. You don't have to be African-American to appreciate African patterns or décor, such as a safari scene; likewise, you don't have to be British to enjoy a Victorian baby motif. Be creative—and think outside of your own heritage. We are all one in the world of babies!

Dolphins or underwater scene. These gentle mammals, usually in sea-blue coordinating materials, offer such a cool, refreshing feeling to a baby's room. You'll feel like diving right in—and baby will find the cool colors comforting, too. Use sea-related wall hangings, such as seahorses, sea shells, and waves, as a way of adding even more interest to the room.

Plain, bold colors. Don't fill the entire room with bright color; instead, use colorful accessories against off-white or light colored walls. You can mix and match accessory items such as balloons, animals, or basically anything in the list of motifs, as long as it's colorful and fun.

Denim. Not usually associated with babies, denim can give you an interesting dimension from a design standpoint. For instance, think of mixing a denim crib sheet set with white lace trim and lace accessories. Basically anything you could match with your jeans would work in this baby's room, leaving you lots of options.

Crayons. It all started with those giant crayon-shaped banks . . . and now you can add those banks as accessories to a room painted white and highlighted by primary color accents on the walls (perhaps in the shape of handprints—or use a stencil of your choice), on the window frames, or even on the entire closet door. The choices are up to you; the good news is that Crayola has come out with paints in their famous colors made specifically for baby's room. Check your local paint store for availability.

Carousel. Although the carousel is not exactly nontraditional, it can be enhanced by painting wall posts in pastel colors and by adding fabric with a spiral pattern to the wall to create a merry-go-round effect. You might even be able to find larger carousel music boxes to place around the room to create an even more realistic effect.

Baby Equipment: What You Need to Buy or Borrow

Now that you've got the baby's room decorated, you'll need to fill it with some major pieces of equipment. But with all of the equipment out there, it's hard to know what you absolutely need and what's optional. For instance, do you really need a room monitor, or is this something you can do without?

Here are some general guidelines that will help you determine which items you really need to have in your baby's life:

Bassinet or cradle: *Optional.* Some parents feel better when the baby is sleeping closer to their bed; that's why bassinets or cradles work so well in the first few weeks after birth. On the downside, you may spend a lot of money for something the baby can stay in only a short period of time (up until the third or fourth month). The bassinet or cradle doesn't replace the crib by any means. A bassinet will also require a separate mattress, sheets, and bumper set that can not be used in the crib. ($30–$225)

Crib with mattress: *Required.* Whatever your taste in crib furniture, try out the floor model to see how easily the side rail comes down. This is an important feature: Look for ease of use and safety for the baby. Most makes and models conform to U.S. standards; check labels to be certain. In the crib itself, look for the following features: adjustable mattress heights, wheels, and the ability to convert to a toddler bed, if you are not planning on having other children. ($200–$600)

Mattresses for cribs come in foam or innerspring options. They need to fit the crib properly (check dimensions) and should be covered with a waterproof cover. Foam mattresses are lighter and easier to change than innerspring mattresses; also, they tend to be more economical. ($50–$200)

Cribs also require fitted sheets, a bumper, and a cotton or wool blanket. Bedding accessories such as a dust ruffle or matching comforter are optional. ($50–$200)

Stroller: *Required.* Carriage strollers are beautiful in appearance but can be heavy in reality. A carriage stroller is defined by the feature of allowing the baby to rest in a flat, horizontal position. The seat is supported by a frame that moves on four wheels. Large, set wheels allow for a smoother ride, and are recommended for mothers planning on lots of walking activities. Carriages set on smaller, swiveling wheels are better suited for quick turns and shopping. Carriage or full-size strollers are recommended for at least the first six months, as the baby will need to fully recline. Carriage strollers also usually come with some sort of basket—either mesh or a wire rack—that is handy when hauling lots of extra items, or for shopping excursions. The size of the basket is often a selling feature. These strollers can weigh as much as 25 pounds, so consider how much you can lift in and out of your trunk before purchasing.

Umbrella strollers are designed for portability. They are completely compact, and fold into themselves for easy storage. These strollers do not typically recline to a flat position. However, they can weigh as little as seven pounds, and are great for traveling. They usually do not come with a basket attachment.

The combination stroller/car seat is useful and especially good for first-time moms, since it covers all the stages of growth to toddlerhood and is multipurpose. ($25 umbrella to $425 top-of-line carriage)

Car seat: *Required by law.* You have the option of buying a car seat that is strictly for infants (rear-facing only, and handles an infant up to 20 pounds) or one that is for both infants and toddlers (can convert to front-facing and holds an infant or a toddler to 45 pounds). The benefit of buying

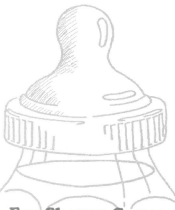

Fun Shower Games

What fun is a baby shower without games? The sillier the game, the more fun you'll have. Here are ideas for games you can either use or suggest for your next shower:

Baby naming: With a timer in hand, ask the guests to write down as many girl and boy names as they can in one minute. Whoever comes up with the most names wins. Make this game more challenging by limiting names to those beginning with a specific letter.

Total recall: Place a dozen baby-related items on a tray, and then let the guests see the items for thirty to forty-five seconds. Cover the tray; whoever remembers and writes down the most items wins a prize.

So big: How big is the mom-to-be's belly? If you were to wrap toilet paper around her, how many squares do you think it would take?

Mystery food: Put twelve baby-food jars—labels hidden—on a tray, and place the tray in the center of a table for fifteen minutes (use more

one at a time is that you can make the toddler seat purchase to accommodate needs you know your child has; for instance, if he or she likes to look at books while in the car, a booster-type car seat for toddlers is what you'll need. If it's sheer economy you're going for, however, a combination infant/toddler car seat will probably do the trick. Keep in mind that some of the combination seats lack portability—an important consideration for some. You must have a car seat to take baby home from the hospital, and most states require that babies ride in approved car seats for travel by car or airplane. In sedans, or cars with airbags in the front passenger seat, any carseat must be placed in the back seat of the car. ($35–$80)

Changing table or dresser/changing table combo: *Optional—but extremely useful.* Some new mothers prefer changing their babies on a table. You may, on the other hand, feel more comfortable changing baby on a floor mat. Either way, you're going to need a place to store baby's clothes and diaper paraphernalia; so decide which method will work best for you as soon as you can. In the worst-case scenario, if you choose later on not to use a changing table, you'll have a lovely piece of furniture that you can re-sell later. ($35–$400)

Baby carrier: *Optional—but useful.* These kangaroo-like carriers strap around your waist and shoulders and hold baby close to your chest. They are very useful when baby is still too small for a stroller, and they are amazingly easy to tote baby around in. And dads can get that "bonding" feeling from carrying baby around. ($15–$70)

Playpen or porta-crib: *Required.* Baby needs a safe place to play during the daytime, especially when you're busy. You can choose from either a stationary fold-up playpen or a porta-crib. The obvious advantage with the porta-crib is its ability to be transported to Grandma's or to any other visiting

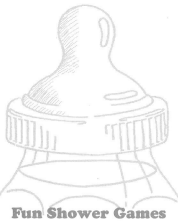

spot on baby's busy schedule. Whichever style you choose, stock the playpen with soft, safe toys. ($45–$175)

Rocker: *Optional—but oh so nice.* There's nothing in the world like soothing a crying baby by rocking it back to sleep. You can choose either the old-fashioned wooden high-back rocker or the more modern (and some say more comfortable) glider with ottoman variety. ($200–$500)

Baby monitor: *Optional.* For years, mothers and fathers have been able to raise children without these types of products. And let's face it, you should always be close enough to monitor the baby yourself. However, they may occasionally come in handy. There have been some product recalls and problems associated with monitors, so it's worth looking into before making a purchase. Check out *Consumer Reports* before buying audio or video monitors. Definitely stay away from used or older models unless you're absolutely certain they're safe. And if you have portable phones already, make sure the monitor is compatible. ($45–$200 for video monitors)

Sling carrier: *Optional.* Sling carriers keep baby in a good position for breastfeeding and are useful for carrying baby around the house with you as you go about your household duties. You can buy one of these used (and in good condition) at a consignment store, or you can purchase one new and resell it later at a consignment store. If you have a history of back trouble, this item is a skip. ($15 used–$40 new)

Backpack: *Optional.* Some parents are more outdoorsy than others; if you like hiking in the park with baby, this is a terrific product for you. If, on the other hand, your major explorations take place in the mall, it's better to have a carrier that keeps baby in front of you. Backpacks are convenient; yet they can be a little dangerous since baby can't tell you if a branch is about to hit his or her face. Backpacks cannot be used with newborns. ($40–$75)

Fun Shower Games
(continued)

trays for larger groups). Whoever can identify all or most of the "mystery foods" wins a prize.

Pin the diaper on the baby: No, I don't mean the *real* baby—just a large picture of a baby. Mount the picture on a piece of cardboard, and then give each guest a picture of a diaper with tape on the back. See how close to the target area they can "pin" the diaper—while blindfolded, of course.

Guess how many: Put as many pieces of candy into a large baby bottle as you can; whoever guesses the right amount wins the candy as a prize.

Name that tune: Using a spoon or similar object, play lullabies and other well-known baby songs by tapping the spoon on an oatmeal container. Whoever can guess the most songs wins.

Special day: Whoever's birthday is closest to the baby's due date wins a prize for sharing their special day.

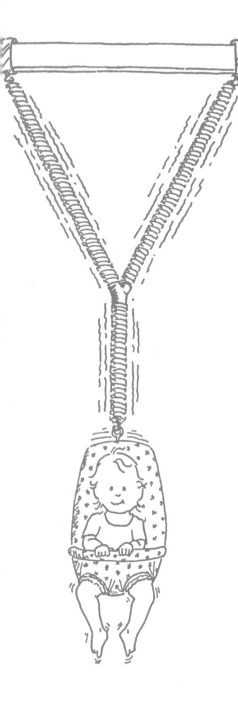

High chair: *Required.* Although you won't need it at first, since baby can't even hold its head up until about three months, you will eventually get lots of use out of your high chair. Baby does need to be confined during feeding time, and high chairs accomplish this most safely. Plus, there's a tray to protect you from wearing all of the food baby doesn't take a liking to. The tray will also serve as a "finger food" testing ground for baby. ($45–$200)

Swing: *Optional.* This is a battery- or crank-powered ride that keeps baby in continuous motion. Some babies like them and some don't. You can't really know until you try; so it might be wise to take baby for a test-drive. This is a good piece of equipment to borrow! ($45–$125)

Walker/bouncer: *Optional.* The walkers with wheels have long been considered culprits in terms of baby safety, since many a baby (including my own) has gone headfirst over a stair. It's better to stick with the bouncer/saucer variety, which offer baby a view and mobility in all directions, yet spin and tilt in place. ($35–$90)

Jumper: *Optional.* A jumper hangs from a doorway and allows baby to swing, or push off the floor. My daughter loved her jump-up; to this day, I attribute her strong legs to the hours of exercise she got swinging from the doorway. Some children like them; others aren't the least bit interested. The safest variety are those with "bumper guards" that keep baby's body from making contact with the wall. This is another good item to borrow. ($20–$45)

Booster seat: *Optional—but nice to have.* After about six months, baby will be able to sit up. And a booster seat (with a safety belt, of course) would be especially nice for travel. They're perfect for restaurants—or when visiting relatives—that don't have their own high chairs. ($20–$50)

Safety gates: *Required.* Gates need to go at both ends of any staircase, as well as in rooms you don't want baby to have easy access to. You should equip your nest with gates, electric-socket covers, and other precautions to keep baby from doing himself or herself harm. Safety precautions need to be taken care of as soon as baby is in any way mobile. Total baby-proofing costs could run anywhere from $40–$250.

Bouncing seat: *Optional—but extremely useful.* As soon as the baby comes home from the hospital, you will need a quick, safe place to put it down. Our bouncing seat was a godsend. Otherwise, you will end up lugging your car seat in and out of the house. Bouncing seats are more comfortable for the baby, too, as they are usually made of cotton instead of the rigid plastic of a carseat. ($20–$40)

Diaper pail: *Required.* No matter whether you use cloth or disposable diapers, you'll need something to put the dirty ones in. Deciding which to choose will depend on your choice of cloth or disposable. ($10–$35)

When buying any piece of equipment, you need to consider safety and convenience first. Price should really be your last concern; after all, what good will that used $15 stroller do you if it folds up while baby's still in it? Before buying any piece, read the chapter on baby safety to find out what to watch out for and how to protect your baby from potential harm.

Best (and Worst) Shower Gifts

It's not that you're ungrateful, but some gifts are generally better than others. Here's a list of the best gifts:

Clothes in the 12- to 24-month size range. Many moms and well-meaning friends purchase 3- to 6-month clothes, which don't last long on a growing baby.

Theme gifts. Fill a diaper bag with all diaper-related items, put feeding-related items in a large basket, fill a baby bath tub with tub toys and cleaning supplies, or buy a large plastic baby bottle filled with miscellaneous baby items (such as pacifiers, bibs, toys and nail scissors).

Anything for moms and their life after birth. Gift certificates for clothing, day spas, or even a trip to the movies for Mom and Dad make fine gifts. Offer to baby-sit as an added bonus.

Toiletries for baby, including baby shampoo, lotion, a hair brush, and baby nail scissors. With shampoo and cleaning products, stick with brand-name, hypoallergenic items—you never know what sensitivities the baby will have.

Special gifts for smaller siblings (so they don't feel left out of the experience). These small tokens can be tucked in with your gift to the baby—and will be much appreciated by the new mom.

Gift certificates for baby. As carefully as new parents shop for their babies, there's always that one thing that needs to be bought when baby comes home. It's a godsend, then, to have a few gift certificates on hand. If you want to do something a little different, purchase a gift certificate for a baby-related service, such as a diaper service or play group.

Here's a list of the worst gifts:

Any toys that are inappropriate for the baby's near-future age range. Sure, toys that are for children five or older are neat, but the baby won't get any immediate benefit from them. In fact, it will be a long time before baby can even touch such toys.

Toys or items with small parts. These parts could become dislodged and find their way easily into baby's mouth.

Toys that don't stimulate baby's brain or senses. Believe it or not, there are plenty of toys out there that try to do everything for children except teach or stimulate them. If it has lots of bells, buttons, and whistles, it's probably too much. There's nothing else for baby to do except stare.

Toys that overstimulate. Don't overdo it with lots of noisy or brightly colored toys or decorations. Babies need contrast; but too much color, music, and noise can become unnerving to a little one.

Baby's Basic Layette

You've got the nursery decorated and the furniture and equipment all set up. What else do you need? Here is a list of items you can fill baby's drawers with:

Clothes: You'll need five or six undershirts (both full-snap and half-shirt varieties), nightgowns with pull strings at the bottom, and non-flammable sleepers/rompers with covered feet. You will also need at least four pair of socks or booties (depending on the climate), one sweater or light jacket, two to four waterproof diaper covers, and one snowsuit (again, depending on the climate or the time of year).

Bath time items: You'll need a plastic bath tub or tub liner, baby soap, baby shampoo, baby lotion, two to four bath towels (preferably with a hood) or receiving blankets, three to four washcloths, sterile cotton balls, and alcohol (to keep the umbilical cord area clean until it heals).

Sleepy time items: You'll need a crib set (including a bumper pad, three to four fitted sheets, and two comforters), a bassinet sheet (if you're using a bassinet), waterproof crib liners, a light blanket or sheet for cover, a baby roll for propping baby to sleep on a particular side, and a music box or mobile.

Eating time items: You'll need four to six bottles (in both 4- and 8-ounce sizes for water, breast milk, formula, or juice), a bottle brush, a bottle rack (for easy—and sterile— dishwasher cleaning), six to eight bibs and burping cloths, and, if nursing, at least two nursing bras, breast pads and a breast pump (either manual or electric).

Changing time items: You'll need to stock your changing table with four or five undershirts or stretchies, petroleum jelly, baby wipes (alcohol free and hypoallergenic), a thermometer, a nasal aspirator, a pair of baby nail scissors, cotton balls and swabs, washcloths, diaper rash ointment, and, of course, hundreds of diapers!

Preparing You: What to Bring to the Hospital

Here is a list of items your bag should include:

- *A robe and nightgown.* If you're going to breastfeed, you'll need one that opens easily in the front.
- *Nonskid slippers.* You'll want to make sure that they are non-skid, since hospital floors can be slippery—and you'll be walking to the nursery at least once during your stay.
- *A nursing bra.* Throw in some nursing pads, too, in case your milk comes in sooner than you expect. If you're not going to breastfeed, bring a bra that's slightly smaller than you would normally wear; this will help your breasts return to their prepregnant state sooner.
- *Toiletries.* Include your toothbrush, toothpaste, hair brush, makeup, and deodorant. Also pack a box of large maxi pads with wings, as you'll need them after the birth.
- *Comfortable clothing.* You'll need one outfit to come home in after the delivery; make sure it's loose enough to accommodate your body comfortably, as you will not loose incredible amounts of weight immediately upon delivery. Include a few pairs of maternity panties and several pairs of socks—you'll need them for the delivery and afterward.
- *A picture or calming image to focus on.* When you're in labor, it helps to have something special to focus on, other than a hospital wall. Bring a favorite nature photo or maybe one of your pet.
- *Books, tapes, or magazines.* After the birth, you might have a little time to yourself for relaxation. Bring anything you'd like to help you accomplish that.
- *A tennis ball or back massager.* Especially in labor, you may need your partner to give you a strong back rub. These items will help him provide extra pressure—a godsend if you have back labor.
- *A bottle of champagne.* Or bring whatever you'd like to drink to celebrate baby's arrival.

❀ *Your call list.* Having all of the names and phone numbers of your friends and family handy will speed the announcements along. You'd be surprised how many new parents become so overwhelmed by the birth experience that they forget the numbers of their families and friends; so don't rely on your memory.

❀ *Nonperishable snacks for your birthing coach.* Your baby's father is bound to get hungry, especially during a long labor, and you don't want him having to spend time waiting on line at the hospital cafeteria when he could be rubbing your back instead. Hospital staff will probably not let *you* eat during your labor, but there is no reason your partner should starve as well.

❀ *A portable CD or tape player and your favorite soothing music.* Music during labor can be a big help for relaxation. Your hospital may allow you to play one of these at a low volume, or you could bring along some headphones.

❀ *A nursing pillow.* If you are planning to nurse, these can be a huge help, and your hospital is unlikely to have them on hand.

❀ *Lansinoh or another lanolin-based nipple protectant.* If you are planning to nurse, this soothing ointment can be a lifesaver, and your hospital may not provide it.

Here is a list of items for baby's hospital bag:

❀ *Two nightshirts.* Pack the gowns that are open at the bottom or that have a pull string.

❀ *Diapers.* If you are planning to shy away from disposables, bring four or five, and be sure to include a waterproof diaper cover to catch any diaper leakage. The hospital will provide all the disposable diapers you will need.

❀ *A going-home outfit.* By now, you should have lots to choose from. Decide what you want to dress the baby in for its first pictures, since Dad will probably take several shots of you leaving the hospital.

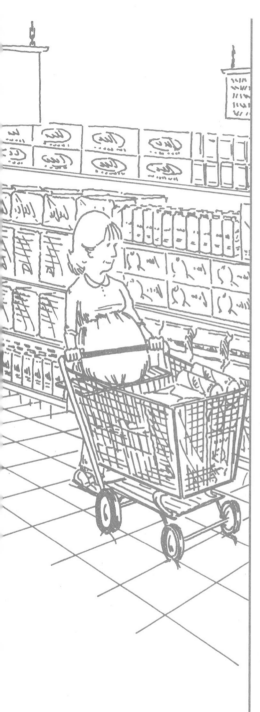

- *A blanket.* Bring a light or heavy one, depending on the climate or the time of year.
- A *snowsuit.* Bring this item only if it's wintertime, of course.
- A *pacifier.* The hospital may give you one; but in case they don't, bring one that's sterilized. Don't use one for baby if you're planning to breastfeed, however. It could cause nipple confusion.
- *Nail scissors.* Most hospitals won't cut baby's nails, which grow quite long in utero. Special baby scissors with clean, sharp edges are the best buy.
- A *baby hat.* The hospital may give you one, but your newborn's head needs to be covered when you walk out the door, no matter what season it is.

Shopping for Baby

One of the best parts of having a new baby is having a new excuse to shop. After all, there are so many things baby truly needs—and so many interesting and cute things that baby might want. The baby industry is booming, largely because manufacturers have finally figured out what motivates parents to buy for their babies: ego. We all want our babies to have the best and to look their best. But what do we really need to buy, and how much should we expect to spend at each stage of baby's development?

Buying Baby's Clothes—the Smart Way

Buying clothes for a growing baby is a bit of a challenge at first; for many new parents, none of the sizes printed on the label correspond to the baby's actual age. Particularly if the baby was large at birth (8 to 9 pounds or more), you might have to skip the 0- to 3-month-old clothing right from the start in favor of a roomier 3- to 6-month wardrobe.

So, what should you buy, and when should you buy it? Well, you already have your layette in place by now; so you should be okay for the first few weeks. What to buy after that time depends on the baby's growth spurts and your financial limitations. Not everyone can afford to buy brand-new clothes every few weeks, and not everyone can afford state-of-the-art baby toys.

If the baby is progressing as most do, you should expect to buy larger sizes of clothing (including diapers) every few months. Purchasing brand-new clothes will cost you an average of $60 to $200 per spree; so you can see the advantage of using hand-me-downs or scavenging garage sales for real bargains. New or used, be sure you wash all clothing with a gentle laundry detergent before putting it on baby.

You would also do well to shop at consignment stores; most major cities have these, and they are well worth it, since they screen out the worn clothes in favor of the "gently used." There's also the added advantage of being able to return good-quality items for resale to get even more of your money's worth. You could spend $20 to $30 per month on clothes and slightly used toys, but you stand a chance of getting 20 percent back on a resale of the same item.

Which Toys for Which Stage?

With so many different toys available (your first trip through Toys-R-Us will take hours!), you can't help but be confused about which toys go with which stage of your baby's development. Thankfully, most toys are clearly marked for different age groups right on their boxes. But to avoid having to read every box, here are some general guidelines about what's appropriate for each stage of baby's development:

- **One month.** Your newborn is still getting used to light, sound, voices, and general comfort. The best thing you can do at this stage is provide all the comfort you can and don't expect much in the way of fun and excitement. Remember, the first month is about getting to know each other. This doesn't mean, however, that you shouldn't sing to baby; it simply means that you shouldn't expect much interaction from baby at this point. The crib mobiles, music, and perhaps a rattle or two will be all you'll need. Buy toys or mobiles in sharply contrasting colors that are easier on baby's eyes—black, white, and red work best.

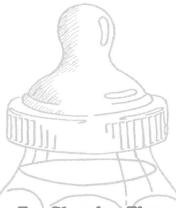

Toy Cleaning Tips

Clean baby's toys with antibacterial soap at least once a month; germs can grow easily on toys and babies have a tendency to put toys in their mouths. Particularly if your baby shares toys with other children, you'll need to keep a watchful eye out for places where germs can grow (the inside of dark toy boxes seems to be a favorite spot). If you feel you've got too many toys to keep clean, pack away some of them in a sealed plastic container; then rotate the toys every few weeks. Your baby will think he or she has a constant supply of new toys.

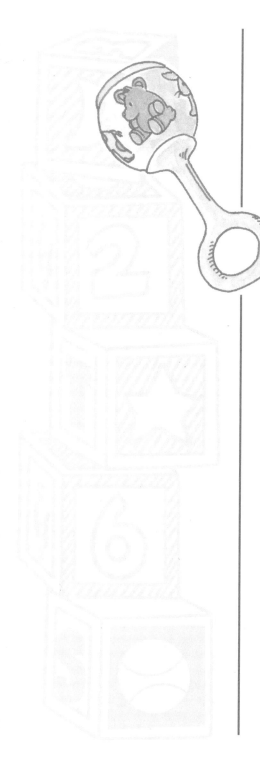

❧ **Two months.** Baby begins to wake up to the colors and sights around him or her—much to your delight! At this stage, you might still be using rattles, music, and maybe a stuffed animal in bright or contrasting colors. Babies at this stage become more responsive to sounds, too. So you could try toys that make simple noises—remember that babies might be frightened by loud noises.

❧ **Three months.** This is a fun stage because it's the time when your baby begins to notice more of the world around him or her. Babies start to notice other babies at three months and can likely hold their heads up by now. Bouncing chairs, crib gyms, baby swings, and teething rattles can provide hours of fun, but so can a mirror strategically placed by the crib. Faces are most interesting to baby now—his or her own, and, in particular, yours. Try some toys with faces, too.

❧ **Four months.** As soon as babies unclench their fists, they are ready for touching and feeling; they want to reach out and experience what things feel like. You could, at this stage, invest in some rattles and teething toys.

❧ **Five months.** Baby is better able to grasp with his or her hands this month and will appreciate toys like cups, balls, blocks, and spheres that spin on the end of a stroller or swing. There will be a lot of pounding going on, as baby's hands are truly his or her new favorite toy.

❧ **Six months.** The baby is now getting more and more mobile; this would be a good time to put baby in a saucer-bottom exerciser or a doorway jumper to see whether he or she likes such activities. Continue with cups, balls, stuffed animals, rattles, and nursery rhymes as well.

❧ **Seven months.** This is the stage where baby is getting interested in playing with you; get ready for "This Little Piggy" and "Peek-a-boo!" You can also bring out the wooden spoon and pots or pans, since baby will be ready to make some music!

❧ **Eight months.** Uh-oh—is baby starting to crawl around the house already? If so, he or she will likely want to play with the things you are using (don't worry, the wooden spoon is still a favorite!). This might be a good time to let baby have a big plastic bowl, a wooden spoon, and items to put inside larger ones; stacking bins are ideal for this stage. A favorite of Lilly's was the wooden spoon/empty oatmeal box combination.

- **Nine months.** Babies gets stronger and more mobile at nine months; they also don't seem to mind the louder toys. Toys that have electronic buttons that make sounds would be most appreciated from this stage on. Also, blankets with Velcro-attached toys would be popular items among nine-monthers.

- **Ten months.** Your baby can make some interesting sounds now and is most curious about items you use on a regular basis. Buy toys like large wooden puzzles, dolls that play music, and push/pull toys (the toy telephone with the pull string was my own personal favorite back in 1965, and it's still popular today).

- **Eleven months.** Baby is either walking or close to it at this stage; buy toys that will help him or her along in mobility, such as a rocking horse with cushioned seat, a small trampoline, and push/pull toys. Board books are also good at this stage, since baby can't rip up or eat the pages.

- **One year.** Baby is starting to explore the idea of independence, walking throughout the house with help or by himself or herself. Besides buying all of the safety latches you'll need, you should start a collection of toys that baby can grow into over the next year. Toys that teach sounds and toys that baby can ride on will be most appealing.

Books, Books, Books

Don't forget that you should begin reading to baby anytime from conception on. Invest in a small library of books; often you can find great books at bargain prices at your local library book sales. At first choose books with simple pictures and as few words as possible. Gradually work up to books with simple story lines—and rhymes or poetic language. Babies respond well to sounds that are alike, and for that reason rhyming stories tend to be most popular with the younger set.

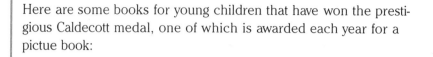

Here are some books for young children that have won the prestigious Caldecott medal, one of which is awarded each year for a pictue book:

1997: *Golem* by David Wisniewski (Clarion)

1996: *Officer Buckle and Gloria* by Peggy Rathmann (Putnam)

1995: *Smoky Night*, illustrated by David Diaz; text: Eve Bunting (Harcourt)

1994: *Grandfather's Journey* by Allen Say; text: edited by Walter Lorraine (Houghton)

1993: *Mirette on the High Wire* by Emily Arnold McCully (Putnam)

1992: *Tuesday* by David Wiesner (Clarion Books)

1991: *Black and White* by David Macaulay (Houghton)

1990: *Lon Po Po: A Red-Riding Hood Story from China* by Ed Young (Philomel)

1989: *Song and Dance Man*, illustrated by Stephen Gammell; text: Karen Ackerman (Knopf)

1988: *Owl Moon*, illustrated by John Schoenherr; text: Jane Yolen (Philomel)

1987: *Hey, Al*, illustrated by Richard Egielski; text: Arthur Yorinks (Farrar)

1986: *The Polar Express* by Chris Van Allsburg (Houghton)

1985: *Saint George and the Dragon*, illustrated by Trina Schart Hyman; text: retold by Margaret Hodges (Little, Brown)

1984: *The Glorious Flight: Across the Channel with Louis Bleriot* by Alice and Martin Provensen (Viking)

1983: *Shadow*, translated and illustrated by Marcia Brown; original text in French: Blaise Cendrars (Scribner)

1982: *Jumanji* by Chris Van Allsburg (Houghton)

1981: *Fables* by Arnold Lobel (Harper)

1980: *Ox-Cart Man*, illustrated by Barbara Cooney; text: Donald Hall (Viking)

1979: *The Girl Who Loved Wild Horses* by Paul Goble (Bradbury)

1978: *Noah's Ark* by Peter Spier (Doubleday)

1977: *Ashanti to Zulu: African Traditions*, illustrated by Leo and Diane Dillon; text: Margaret Musgrove (Dial)

1976: *Why Mosquitoes Buzz in People's Ears*, illustrated by Leo and Diane Dillon; text: retold by Verna Aardema (Dial)

1975: *Arrow to the Sun* by Gerald McDermott (Viking)

1974: *Duffy and the Devil* illustrated by Margot Zemach; retold by Harve Zemach (Farrar)

1973: *The Funny Little Woman*, illustrated by Blair Lent; text: retold by Arlene Mosel (Dutton)

1972: *One Fine Day*, retold and illustrated by Nonny Hogrogian (Macmillan)

1971: *A Story A Story*, retold and illustrated by Gail E. Haley (Atheneum)

1970: *Sylvester and the Magic Pebble* by William Steig (Windmill Books)

1969: *The Fool of the World and the Flying Ship*, illustrated by Uri Shulevitz; text: retold by Arthur Ransome (Farrar)

1968: *Drummer Hoff*, illustrated by Ed Emberley; text: adapted by Barbara Emberley (Prentice-Hall)

1967: *Sam, Bangs & Moonshine* by Evaline Ness (Holt)

1966: *Always Room for One More*, illustrated by Nonny Hogrogian; text: Sorche Nic Leodhas, pseud. (Leclair Alger) (Holt)

1965: *May I Bring a Friend?* illustrated by Beni Montresor; text: Beatrice Schenk de Regniers (Atheneum)

1964: *Where the Wild Things Are* by Maurice Sendak (Harper)

1963: *The Snowy Day* by Ezra Jack Keats (Viking)

1962: *Once a Mouse*, retold and illustrated by Marcia Brown (Scribner)

1961: *Baboushka and the Three Kings*, illustrated by Nicolas Sidjakov; text: Ruth Robbins (Parnassus)

1960: *Nine Days to Christmas*, illustrated by Marie Hall Ets; text: Marie Hall Ets and Aurora Labastida (Viking)

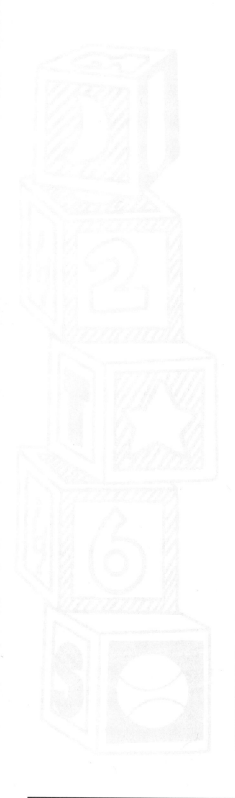

1959: *Chanticleer and the Fox*, illustrated by Barbara Cooney; text: adapted from Chaucer's *Canterbury Tales* by Barbara Cooney (Crowell)

1958: *Time of Wonder* by Robert McCloskey (Viking)

1957: *A Tree Is Nice*, illustrated by Marc Simont; text: Janice Udry (Harper)

1956: *Frog Went A-Courtin'*, illustrated by Feodor Rojankovsky; text: retold by John Langstaff (Harcourt)

1955: *Cinderella, or the Little Glass Slipper*, illustrated by Marcia Brown; text: translated from Charles Perrault by Marcia Brown (Scribner)

1954: *Madeline's Rescue* by Ludwig Bemelmans (Viking)

1953: *The Biggest Bear* by Lynd Ward (Houghton)

1952: *Finders Keepers*, illustrated by Nicolas, pseud. (Nicholas Mordvinoff); text: Will, pseud. (William Lipkind) (Harcourt)

1951: *The Egg Tree* by Katherine Milhous (Scribner)

1950: *Song of the Swallows*, by Leo Politi (Scribner)

1949: *The Big Snow* by Berta and Elmer Hader (Macmillan)

1948: *White Snow, Bright Snow*, illustrated by Roger Duvoisin; text: Alvin Tresselt (Lothrop)

1947: *The Little Island*, illustrated by Leonard Weisgard; text: Golden MacDonald, pseud. (Margaret Wise Brown) (Doubleday)

1946: *The Rooster Crows* by Maude and Miska Petersham (Macmillan)

1945: *Prayer for a Child*, illustrated by Elizabeth Orton Jones; text: Rachel Field (Macmillan)

1944: *Many Moons*, illustrated by Louis Slobodkin; text: James Thurber (Harcourt)

1943: *The Little House* by Virginia Lee Burton (Houghton)

1942: *Make Way for Ducklings* by Robert McCloskey (Viking)

1941: *They Were Strong and Good* by Robert Lawson (Viking)

1940: *Abraham Lincoln* by Ingri and Edgar Parin d'Aulaire (Doubleday)

1939: *Mei Li* by Thomas Handforth (Doubleday)

1938: *Animals of the Bible, A Picture Book*, illustrated by Dorothy P. Lathrop; text: selected by Helen Dean Fish (Lippincott)

List compiled by the American Library Association

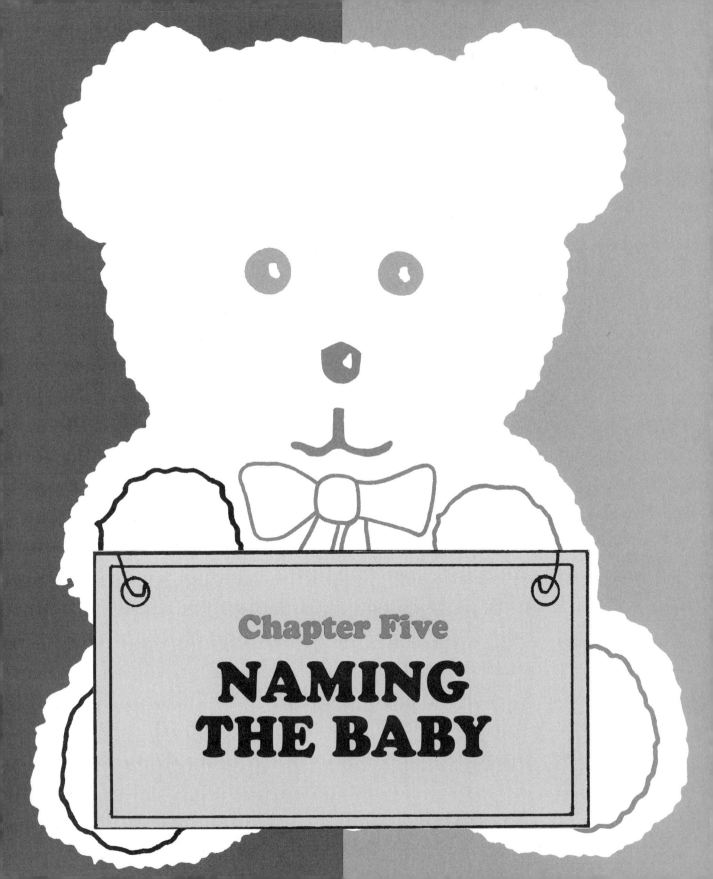

Chapter Five

NAMING
THE BABY

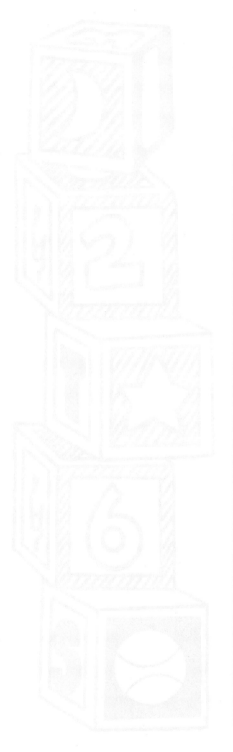

During the process of pregnancy and getting everything ready for the baby, deciding what you're going to name the baby can sometimes seem like just another chore to fit into your overpacked schedule. How can you make choosing a name for your baby less like work and more like the joy it should be? Here are some ideas you can try:

- Leaf through all the entries in baby name books (such as *The Everything® Baby Name Book*). Try to figure out the names your friends and family would pick if they were allowed to name the baby.

- Hold a lottery. Tell all your friends and relatives that you're looking for suggestions and that you'd like their input. Of course, you don't have to commit to any of the names provided to you, and indeed, some of the entries will be good for a laugh or two. Put all of the entries into a box, and pick the winning entry out of the hat a week before your due date or at your baby shower. Make the prize relevant to the birth of the baby. The winner gets to serve as baby's first sitter when you and your spouse find the time and energy to go out for your first dinner alone after baby arrives.

- Pick five names that just sound good when you say them. Write them down on a card; and every day for a month, pull the card out and read the names aloud to hear how they sound. At the end of the month, one will probably become your favorite.

- Go through the phone book or the newspaper (the wedding announcements page can be a help) to see if any first names jump out at you.

- Practice yelling different names out the back door, loudly and several times in a row, just before dinnertime. Then ask your neighbors which ones they like best.

As an uncle once told me, in the end it doesn't matter what you name your child, because you'll always wind up calling the child by a nickname, a middle name, or even some shortened variation of his or her full name. What matters most is how lovingly you say the name.

When you finally do settle on a first name, you may be dismayed to discover that you're still not done. You need to choose a middle name—and to see how these two names fit with your last name.

The middle name is where you can be really creative. True, some people believe that the middle name should flow naturally from the first, as in the name Mary Ann; but there is a select group of people who believe that when it comes to the child's middle name, anything goes.

Of course, in these days of hyphenated last names, the first half of the combined last name could rightly be considered to be the middle name. But many of these kids get a middle name as well. This practice, as well as the Catholic tradition of providing a child with a number of names depending on his or her age in the church, has opened the floodgates to the trend of children having not one but several middle names.

I heard about a kid in St. Paul, Minnesota, who has a total of ten middle names. Why? Because *Eric Michael David Stephen Joshua Kevin Carl Quentin Jesse Alexander William Peters* had six siblings when he came into the world, and each one wanted to give him a name. Plus, the parents say they like round numbers. Needless to say, Eric got more names than anyone had bargained for.

Time will tell exactly how many of these names the parents will have the patience to use on a daily basis. Most parents only call a child by his or her full name when the child has done something wrong. By the time the angry parent has finished reciting the child's full name, he or she will have forgotten what to be angry about.

This naming business may not be as easy as it seems, since people frequently have different ideas about what works and what doesn't. When both the first and last names have multiple syllables and the pronunciation emphasis is on the first syllable of both, the combination seems to work well. However, when the number of syllables in each name differs, primarily when one of the names has only one syllable, it's a good idea that the other name have more than one.

Pay attention to how the names sound together: Watch for rhymes, alliterations, and onomatopoeia. Billy Joel once said he decided to go by "Billy" instead of Bill Joel because he thought Bill Joel sounded like the sound of a doorbell.

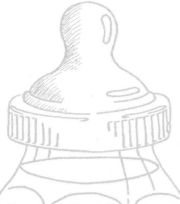

Getting Dad Involved

Many times, amid the monthly obstetrician visits, the baby showers, and all the attention that's paid to the mother-to-be, the prospective father feels a bit left out. Here are some suggestions for ways Dad can become involved in naming the new baby:

- If you know your baby is going to be a boy, consider naming him after his father. It's a misconception that this practice is most common among country-club families; many families from a variety of ethnic backgrounds feel that the best way to feel proud of a son is to give him his father's name.
- Split the responsibilities, and let Dad pick the baby's first name or middle name entirely on his own.
- Sit down together with a baby name book, and leaf through it to look for names you like. Discuss why you like certain names the other person has selected. Then try to come up with a name that combines both of your preferences.

Narrowing Down Your Choices

Okay, so you've started to spend some serious time flipping through pages of baby name books and have marked some of the names that sound particularly attractive to you. Some parents will glance at a name and know instantly that it's the perfect name for their baby. However, if you're like most parents-to-be, you're not in that category. Some names sound great; others are definite possibilities. Some parents feel that there are so many choices it's close to impossible to decide.

So what do you do? From the hundreds of names available, how do you begin to choose the right one for your baby? The first thing you should do is write down the names that sound good to you with your last name. Your partner should do the same thing, but separately. It's a good idea to see what the other person thinks; if, by chance, you share some of the same names on your lists, you could choose a name from your mutual selections.

After you've drawn up a list, you should say the full names out loud to hear how they sound. After all, your child will hear that name directed at him or her tens of thousands of times over the next several decades or more. You have to make sure that the first and last names at least sound like they're part of the same name.

You may have a middle name in mind, too. Though it's less important than the first name you select, it's still a good idea to hear how everything fits together. So after you have some solid candidates for your first name picked out, go ahead and see how some possible middle names fit into the mix.

To further narrow down your choices, you may want to ask some friends or relatives what they think; but to tell the truth, picking a name is such a personal matter that I think the more people you involve in your search, the more confused you're going to be. So take time on your own to get to your short list. If, at that point, you still don't have a favorite, you might just need a dart board to finalize things.

Family Ties: Junior, Senior, III, Etc.

Some people believe that the biggest honor that can be given to another person is to name their newborn baby after him—or her. Though I am aware of several cases in which a daughter was given the same name as her mother, this is a relative rarity. Most often, a son is named after a father, with the appropriate suffix after the name to indicate the position in the family.

Although this can be a great source of pride for the family, it can also be a living nightmare for the U.S. Postal Service and other government agencies, who rarely indicate such distinctions on important documents. It can also create problems for children if they are made to believe that (1) they have to live up to their fathers' accomplishments, or (2) they come to equate their identity with their dads' and never really have a chance to develop their own unique personas.

This was the case with artist Vincent Van Gogh, whose parents gave birth to a stillborn child almost exactly one year prior to his birth; they named the first child Vincent, and when the artist was born one year later, they chose to name him after the first Vincent. This was said to create a lifelong inner turmoil for the artist, who struggled with identity issues in addition to his battle with epilepsy and mental illness.

If you are absolutely set on successions, it is customary to use *Jr.* when the son is second in line and Roman numerals for each successive child with the same name. However, the current generation may tire of the repetition—putting a *V* after a kid's name just starts to seem silly. I've never seen this practice carried beyond the fourth generation . . . except, of course, for Catholic popes, whose numbers have gone into the double digits. Then again, they don't have sons to pass their names on to. Aside from popes, royalty are the only others who tack big numbers onto their children's names.

Of course, you can always do what former boxer George Forman did. He named all of his sons George and then numbered them successively. That doesn't seem egotistical, does it?!

The Trend Toward Ethnic Names

If you want to give your baby a name that sounds a bit exotic but is really just a variation of a true-blue American name, you might want to think about giving him or her a particular nationality's version of that name. For instance, the Spanish variation of William is Guillermo; Paul becomes Pavel and John becomes Janich in Polish; and Jane is Juana in Spanish and Jana in Hungarian.

Of course, you could also pick a name from your own ethnic background that doesn't necessarily correspond with any American equivalent. Or you could select a name from an ethnic group other than your own just because you like the name. Welsh and Irish names are currently popular, as well as names from African countries. I chose "Dela" as a middle name for my daughter; it is from a Zulu word meaning "sublime contentedness."

The good news about giving your baby an ethnic name is that there are no rules; if you like the name, then choose it. As more Americans travel to all corners of the globe and as more people from foreign places are living and working in the United States, we will continue to be exposed to an increasingly wide community of people. This will continue to be reflected in the names we choose for our kids.

In addition, once these previously exotic names are used more in the United States and start to become more a part of the American mainstream, they won't stand out as much in the coming years. Thus, parents thirty years from now who want something new and different for their kids will continue to push toward increasingly exotic baby names.

Superstitions about Names

On the face of things, a name is simply an amalgam of letters arranged in a certain way so that the person who has the name can assume some kind of identity through the name; it's a symbol of sorts. That's the scientific side of things. The truth is that generations of parents in every country and in every faith have superstitions about what they should and shouldn't name their babies. A traditional Ashkenazi superstition dictates that if you name a baby after a living person, that person would instantly fall ill and die, since the baby needed more of the energy and so would suck the life force out of the adult. (However, Sephardic Jews believed the opposite!) Many cultures also chose names from nature, names of flowers, for example, so that the baby would be sure to blossom and grow.

Today many of us scoff at these beliefs, but the truth is that individuals hold their own peculiar superstitions about names. For instance, you may choose not to name a baby after an elderly relative because you didn't like the way the older person smelled or behaved while you were growing up; and you may be worried that your child will grow up to be like that person. Or you may hate a name your spouse loves because a friend's mother with the same name died when you were only thirteen and you don't want a similar fate for your child. Or maybe the name is one of an ex-girlfriend or ex-boyfriend, making it unacceptable to both parents because of jealousy.

Don't name your child after a relative who's currently in prison, many people say, no matter how much you love your relative, because your child may end up with the same lifestyle. Some superstitions relate to particular names; you may have been brought up to believe that people named Benjamin cannot be trusted or that many criminals and notorious folks have the middle name of Wayne (John Wayne Gacy, John Wayne Bobbitt).

The superstitions that swirl around the names we do and don't choose for our kids most often involve unreasonable associations. No matter how unreasonable these associations might be, no one can tell you to get rid of your superstitions about names or anything else. And you should know that you're in good company around the world if you choose to abide by them.

The Most Popular Names from the 1990s, So Far

Many parents are turning back to names from an earlier era. The jury is still out as to why this is so. Perhaps parents are looking back to simpler times and choosing names from the years they perceive as having been easier to live in. Boys' names for the '90s also are heavy in Biblical influence—Daniel, Matthew, John—and girls' names have a wealthy sound to them—Ashley, Amanda, Brittany.

No matter what the reason, the only thing that you can be sure of is that parents will continue to select names for their kids that reflect the times they're living in—or the years they're nostalgic about

Boys Names

Michael	Corey	Kyle
Kevin	John	Derek
Christopher	Aaron	Sean
Adam	Steven	Jared
Matthew	Mark	William
Tyler	Robert	Patrick
Joshua	Alexander	Brandon
Jacob	James	Scott
Andrew	Richard	Eric
Jeffrey	Nicholas	Charles
Daniel	Cody	Zachary
Jason	Joseph	Dustin
Justin	Jeremy	Thomas
Timothy	Brian	Jordan
David	Nathan	Anthony
Benjamin	Jonathan	Jesse
Ryan	Travis	

Girls Names

Ashley	Kimberly	Lily
Rebecca	Katherine	Kelsey
Jessica	Allison	Emily
Michelle	Caitlin	Andrea
Amanda	Erica	Carly
Kelly	Lauren	Alexandra
Sarah	Alicia	Melissa
Chelsea	Rachel	Christine
Brittany	Jamie	Tiffany
Courtney	Samantha	Angela
Megan	Katie	Lindsey
Crystal	Heather	Jacqueline
Jennifer	Erin	Kristen
Amy	Elizabeth	Casey
Nicole	Mary	Kayla
Laura	Danielle	Shannon
Stephanie	Alyssa	

A Short List of Possible Baby Names

Boys Names

AARON (Hebrew) Lofty or exalted. The older brother of Moses, appointed by God to be his brother's keeper. Aaron has actually been one of the more popular names since the early days of the United States in the 1600s. Perhaps the early colonists felt that they needed to name their newborns after strong Biblical figures in order to make it through the hardships of settling a new land. Famous people from the past and present with the name include a vice-president, Aaron Burr, the American composer Aaron Copland, and the singer Aaron Neville. Variations: *Aarao, Aharon, Arek, Aron, Aronek, Aronne, Aronos, Arran, Arren, Arrin, Arron.*

ABDUL (Arabic) Servant.

ABDULLAH (Arabic) Servant of God. Variation: *Abdulla.*

ABEL (Hebrew) Breathing spirit or breath. In the Bible, Abel was the second son of Adam.

ABID (Arabic) One who worships Allah. Variation: *Abbud.*

ABNER (Hebrew) Father of light. Biblical. Variations: *Aviner, Avner.*

ABRAHAM (Hebrew) Father of many. If the name Abraham conjures up an image of a wise old man to you, you may scoff at the idea of making an infant put up with the name until it fits, say, oh, in sixty years or so. But as more and more parents decide to give their children names that conjure up American history, Abraham will continue to have a growing place in baby names. Variations: *Abe, Abrahamo, Abrahan, Abram, Abramo, Abran, Abrao, Avraham, Avram, Avrum.*

ACE (English) Unity. Nickname given to one who excels. It's also the name of a member of the rock group Kiss.

ACTON (English) Town in Great Britain.

ADAM (Hebrew) Man of the red earth. Adam was the first man who made it into the world, and his name has always been popular in many countries and in many religions. In this country, the popularity of Adam increased during the '60s with a slew of positive, almost macho associations in the entertainment world. Adam West, who played Batman in the television series, undoubtedly served as the inspiration for many men named Adam today, while the cop show *Adam-12* also did its part. Parents also have chosen this name to honor the late congressman Adam Clayton Powell. Many parents pick the name for their first son. Variations: *Adamec, Adamek, Adamh, Adamik, Adamka, Adamko, Adams, Adamson, Adamsson, Adan, Adao, Addam, Addams, Addamson, Addie, Addis, Addy, Adhamh, Adnet, Adnot.*

ADDISON (English) Son of Adam.

ADISA (African: Nigerian) One who is clear.

ADOLPH (German) Noble wolf. Variations: *Adolf, Adolfo, Adolphe.*

ADRIAN (Latin) Black; dark. Variations: *Adrean, Adren.*

AHMAD (Arabic) More deserving. Variation: *Ahmed.*

AHMED (Arabic) Praise. Variation: *Ahmad.*

AIDAN (Irish, Gaelic) Warm. Aidan has become popular in recent years due to the success of the ice-blue-eyed actor Aidan Quinn. It is also the name of an Irish saint from the year 600 A.D.

AJANI (African: Nigerian) He fights for possession.

AKAMU (Hawaiian) Red earth. Variation: *Adamu.*

AKIM (Russian) God.

ALAN (English, Celtic) Fair; handsome. Some may think of Alan as somewhat of a name of the '50s and '60s, since so many of the kids back then were named Alan, as well as popular TV stars, like Alan Carr, Alan Sues, and Allen Ludden. For this reason, some parents might shy away from the name, and never even consider it, but if you want a steadfast name that will stand out, Alan is a good choice. Today, famous Alans include Alan Jay Lerner, Alan Alda, and Allen Ginsberg. Variations: *Ailean, Ailin, Al, Alain, Aland, Alano, Alanson, Alao, Alen, Alin, Allan, Allayne, Allen, Alleyn, Alleyne, Allin, Allon, Allyn, Alon, Alun.*

ALBERT (Old English) Bright; brilliant. Variations: *Alberto, Albie, Albin, Albrecht.*

ALDRICH (English) An old and wise leader.

ALEXANDER (Greek) Protector; helper and defender of mankind. Alexander is one of those great, strong names that stands well on its own as well as in one of its many versions. So if you like the name as is, fine. If your boy later decides that he'd rather be called Alex, Alek, or chooses the wonderfully sensual Spanish name Alessandro, it's all possible. Famous Alexanders include Alexander the Great, Alexander Hamilton, actor Alec Baldwin, Alexander Haig, and Aleksandr Solzhenitsyn. Variations: *Alasdair, Alastair, Alaster, Alec, Alejandro, Alejo, Alek, Alekos, Aleksander, Aleksandr, Alesandro, Alessandre, Alessandri, Alessandro, Alex, Alexandre, Alexandro, Alexandros, Alexei, Alexi, Alexio, Alik, Alisander, Alissander, Alissandre, Alistair, Alister, Alistir, Allistair, Allister, Allistir, Alsandair, Alsandare, Sacha, Sande, Sander, Sanders, Sanderson, Sandey, Sandie, Sandor, Sandy, Sascha, Sasha, Sashenka, Sashka (Russian), Saunders, Saunderson.*

ALI (Arabic) Elevated.

ALPHONSE (German) One who is ready to fight. Most adults today who have the name are commonly known as Al, but when it comes to naming their own kids, it's Alphonse, probably after a grandfather. Variations: *Alfonse, Alfonso, Alfonze, Alfonzo, Alonzo, Alphonso.*

ALTAIR (Greek) Bird.

ANDRE (French) Manly. French version of Andrew. Variations: *Ahndray, Andrae, Andray, Aundray.*

ANDREW (English) Manly; brave. Andrew has always been a popular name for boys in this century, not only in English but in many languages. A recent study at Harvard found that Andrew is the name that mothers who have at least a bachelor's degree choose for their sons most often. The name Andrew conjures up both dignity and informality, traits that served United States Presidents Andrew Johnson and Andrew Jackson. Other famous Andrews include Andy Warhol, Andrew Wyeth, Andy Griffith, Prince Andrew, Andy Rooney, and Andy Hardy. Variations: *Aindrea, Aindreas, Anders, Andi, Andonis, Andor, Andre, Andreas, Andrei, Andres, Andrey, Andy.*

ANGELO (Italian, Portuguese, Spanish) Messenger; angel. Though the name Angel used to be the most popular form of this name, Angelo has come into favor because Angel has been used more often as a girls' name. Variation: *Angel.*

ANTHONY (Latin) Praiseworthy; valuable. Saint Anthony was a hermit who lived in the third century in what is today Italy; he is the patron saint for poor people. Today, even though the name Anthony may often conjure up images of Little Italy and doo-wop singers in the 1950s, it is one of the more popular names of the last twenty-five years. A list of famous people who have Anthony as their first names is a veritable *Who's Who* of class: Anthony Quinn, Anthony Hopkins, Anton Chekhov, and Anthony Perkins. Variations: *Andonios, Andonis, Anntoin, Antin, Antoine, Anton, Antone, Antonello, Antoney, Antoni, Antonin, Antonino, Antonio, Antonius, Antons, Antony, Antos.*

ARLO (Spanish) Bayberry tree. Even though the only Arlo you may have heard of is Arlo Guthrie, the name is actually a common Italian version of Charles.

ASHER (Hebrew) Happy. Asher was one of Jacob's sons in the Bible. One of the most common nicknames for Asher—along with the other names listed here that start with "A-s-h"— is Ash, which has an interesting superstition connected with it. The ash tree supposedly brings good luck; one belief is that if you give a bit of sap from an ash tree to an infant, he will be lucky the rest of his days. Variations: *Anschel, Anshel, Anshil, Ashu.*

AUSTIN (English) Majestic. Austin, along with its variants, is currently one of the more popular names. Especially with the recent newfound popularity of writer Jane Austen, this name seems to be at the forefront of an explosion in "veddy British" names on these shores. Austin has recently held the honor of being the most popular name for newborn boys in a few of the western United States. Famous Austins are still few and far between, until those in the current crop hit their stride. Variations: *Austen, Austyn.*

AVERY (English) Counselor. Perhaps the most famous Avery today is Murphy Brown's baby in the hit TV series. This name fits tidily into the trend of naming a baby after a town or place, and also as an androgynous name that suits both boys and girls equally well.

BAILEY (English) This name has become popular for girls in the last decade; it originally meant a steward or bailiff. Variations: *Bailee, Bailie, Baillie, Baily, Baylee, Bayley, Bayly.*

BALDWIN (German) Brave friend. Variations: *Bald, Baldovino, Balduin, Baldwinn, Baldwyn, Baldwynn, Balldwin, Baudoin.*

BARRY (Gaelic) Pointed object. Barry is also increasingly being used as a girls' name with the spelling of Barrie. The name, however, is not as popular as it was a couple of decades ago. Variation: *Barrymore.*

BARTHOLOMEW (English) Farmer's son. The basic version of this English surname may be given as a first name, usually after a family member. There are countless derivatives that come from Bartholomew, which was the name of one of the twelve apostles. Today, the most famous celebrity who goes by a shortened version of Bartholomew is none other than Bart Simpson. Variations: *Bart, Bartel, Barth, Barthel , Barthelemy , Barthelmy, Barthlomeo, Bartholome, Bartholomieu, Bartlett, Bartoli, Bartolo, Bartolomeo, Bartram.*

BARTON (English) Field of barley.

BEAU (French) Beautiful. Variation: *Bo.*

BENJAMIN (English) In the Bible Benjamin was the youngest son of Jacob. The name translates to son of my right hand. The name Benjamin has become extremely popular in recent years, but it has been a great American staple since the days of Benjamin Franklin. Other famous Benjamins include Benjamin Disraeli and Dr. Benjamin Spock. Benjamin is a great name not only for a toddler running around in tiny overalls but also for a sensitive teenage poet. Variations: *Benejamen, Beniamino, Benjaman, Benjamen, Benjamino, Benjamon, Benji, Benjie, Benjiman, Benjimen, Benjy, Bennie, Benny, Minyamin, Minyomei, Minyomi.*

BENSON (English) Son of Ben. Last name. Variations: *Bensen, Benssen, Bensson.*

BERNARD (German) Brave. Bernard has a long and illustrious history, even though it is not frequently on the top fifty lists. Two saints from medieval days went by the name of Bernard, as does the heroic type of dog that is considered to be the patron saint for hikers. Variations: *Barnard, Barnardo, Barney, Barnhard, Barnhardo, Barnie, Barny, Bernardas, Bernardel,* *Bernardin, Bernardino, Bernardo, Bernardyn, Bernhard, Bernhardo, Bernie, Berny, Burnard.*

BEVAN (Welsh) A son of a man named Evan. Its usage today is becoming popular among parents who like the name Evan, but are looking for something a little different. Variations: *Beavan, Beaven, Beven, Bevin, Bevon.*

BILL (English) Bill is rarely a given first name. It is a variation of the more formal name William, which most parents of "Bills" choose to name their boys. Variations: *Billy, Byll.*

BLAKE (English) This name could be given to both boys and girls, and strangely enough, could mean either light or dark. Blake is a name that became synonymous with the most famous TV character of the '80s, *Dynasty*'s Blake Carrington, who was played by John Forsythe. The husband of actress Julie Andrews, Blake Edwards, has long been known for his offbeat movies. Variations: *Blaike, Blayke.*

BOB (English) Bright; famous. Like its common counterpart Bill, Bob is rarely given as the name that will appear on the birth certificate; Robert is typically the given name of choice. Variations: *Bobbey, Bobbie, Bobby.*

BOYD (Gaelic) Blonde. Variation: *Boid.*

BRADLEY (English) A wide meadow. Bradley is one of those names that seems to always skirt the edge between extreme popularity and obsolescence. In the '70s, it seemed like a slightly nerdy name but was saved by the virile sound of its nickname: *Brad.* Undoubtedly, its growing popularity today is due to the fame of movie star Brad Pitt. Variations: *Brad, Bradlea, Bradlee, Bradleigh, Bradlie, Bradly.*

BRADY (English) Wide island.

BRANDON (English) Sword; hill afire. Brandon is one of those names that appears to be suddenly cool. Famous Brandons include Brandon Cruz, who played Bill Bixby's son in the TV show *The Courtship of Eddie's Father*, and network heads Brandon Tartikoff and Brandon Stoddard. Variations: *Bran, Brandan, Branden, Brandin, Brandyn.*

BRANT (English) Proud. Variation: *Brannt.*

BRAXTON (English) Literally, Brock's town.

BRENDAN (Irish) Foul-smelling hair. It's likely that most parents who give their sons this name haven't a clue what it really means. Famous Brendans include

Brendan Gill, Brendan Frasier, and Brendan Behan. Brendan was also an Irish saint nicknamed the Voyager who, rumor has it, was the first Irishman to sail to America. Variations: *Brenden, Brendin, Brendon.*

BRENT (English) Mountaintop. Though Brent is very popular today, it has been used as a first name only for the last fifty years or so. Famous Brents include Brent Musburger, Brent Scowcroft, and the fictional character Brent Tarleton. Variations: *Breneon, Brentan, Brentin, Brenton, Brentyn.*

BRETT (English) British man. Brett is a name that is more popular in Australia than it is on these shores. Brett is also frequently used as a girls' name today, which unlike many popular androgynous names, hasn't diminished its popularity among boys. Bret Harte is a famous Brett, as are Bret Easton Ellis and James Garner's cowboy character. Variations: *Bret, Brette, Bretton, Brit, Britt.*

BRIAN (Celtic) Brave; virtuous. If English names are currently popular among American parents-to-be, Irish names are a close second, and Brian leads the pack. Brian seems to be popular because it's a solid name with lots of possibilities for variety, yet it has a bit of a lilt to it, and it doesn't seem overexposed—*yet.* There are many famous Brians, including Brian Adams, Brian Wilson, Brian Boitano, Bryan Ferry, Brian De Palma, and Brian Dennehy. Variations: *Briano, Brien, Brion, Bryan, Bryon.*

BRIGHTON (English) Town in Britain.

BRODERICK (Scottish) Brother. Variations: *Brod, Broddy, Broderic, Brodric, Brodrick.*

BRONSON (English) Dark man's son. With the popularity of other boys' names that start with "B-r-" and have two syllables, Bronson certainly seems like a candidate for an increase in usage. Actor Bronson Pinchot may help further the cause. Variations: *Bron, Bronnson, Bronsen, Bronsin, Bronsonn, Bronsson.*

BROOK (English) Brook; stream. Variations: *Brooke, Brookes, Brooks.*

BRUCE (English) Thick brush. Variations: *Brucey, Brucie.*

BRYSON (English) Nobleman's son.

BYRON (English) Cow barn. Variation: *Biron.*

CALDWELL (English) Stream; cold well. Variation: *Cal.*

CALEB (Hebrew) Brave; dog. Caleb was a popular name among Puritans in the United States, since the Biblical Caleb was one of the people who spent time wandering with Moses on his excursion in the wilderness. Starting in the nineteenth century, common usage of the name began to fall off. However, in the current trend to look for baby names that are traditional yet different, the prevalence of Caleb among American boys has grown. Variations: *Cale, Kalb, Kaleb.*

CALEY (Irish) Slender.

CALVIN (English) Bald. There have been a wide variety of Calvins who have been on the pinnacle of fame since the twentieth century began. The great thing about them is that they're all radically different from one other: Calvin Coolidge, Calvin Klein, Cal Ripken, and last but not least, Calvin of the late, great comic strip "Calvin and Hobbes." Variations: *Cal, Calvino, Kalvin.*

CAMERON (Gaelic) Crooked nose or river. Though the name is very popular today, it was rare until the 1950s, when it began to show up as the name of characters on TV shows. Variation: *Camron.*

CAREY (Welsh) Near a castle. Variation: *Cary.*

CARL (English) Man. Nickname for Charles. Carl is one of those names that rolls off the tongue and sounds like it has more than one syllable. Famous Carls include Carl Sagan, Carl Sandburg, and Carl Bernstein. Variation: *Karl.*

CARLOS (Spanish) Man. Spanish version of Charles. Variations: *Carlino, Carlo, Carolo.*

CARSON (English) Son who lives in a swamp. Variation: *Karsen.*

CASEY (Irish) Observant. Popular among both girls and boys, Casey is being chosen by many parents today because it sounds like a name that suits both a kid and an adult. Some names are great for children but falter when you try them out on an adult, and vice versa. Casey works well for all ages, and both sexes, which will only continue to contribute to its popularity. Famous Caseys include Casey Stengel, Casey Kasem, and infamous engineer Casey Jones. Variations: *Cacey, Cayce, Caycey, Kasey.*

CASSIDY (Irish) Smart. It literally translates from O'Caiside, which means one who dwells in an area of Ireland called Caiside. Caiside itself means bent love, which somehow turned into smart. Cassidy is another wildly popular name for both boys and girls that may have begun to bloom at the peak of the TV show *The Partridge Family*, back in the 1970s. Variation: *Cassady.*

CHAD (English) Protector. Strong, one-syllable names became popular for a while in the late '60s and early '70s, mostly owing to TV actors with such names. Among the most popular was Chad Everett of the show *Medical Center*. Variations: *Chadd, Chadwick*.

CHANCE (English) Good fortune.

CHANDLER (English) Candle maker. This name has become popular in the last few years, due perhaps to its appearance as first and last names among both male and female TV characters.

CHAPMAN (English) Peddler. Variations: *Chap, Chappy*.

CHARLES (English) Man. Charles has spawned a number of variations in all cultures throughout the centuries. The name has a rich and varied history, as the name of the patron saint of Catholic bishops, cartoon characters, and a slew of actors, from Charles Bronson to Charlie Chan. Prince Charles and the unfortunate events at Windsor Castle may diminish the popularity of the name in Great Britain, but it doesn't seem to be affected on these shores. Other famous Charleses include Chick Corea, Charles Darwin, Charley Weaver, Charles Dickens, and Charlie Chaplin. Variations: *Charley, Charlie, Chas, Chaz, Chick, Chip, Chuck*.

CHARLTON (English) House where Charles lives. Variations: *Carleton, Carlton*.

CHASE (English) Hunter. Variations: *Chace, Chaise*.

CHASIN (Hebrew) Strong. Variations: *Chason, Hasin, Hassin*.

CHEN (Chinese) Great.

CHESTER (English) Campsite. Chester seems to be a fussy name that conjures up Victorian tea in the afternoons and bow ties. What's more popular, however, is one of Chester's nicknames: Chet. Chet Huntley and Chet Atkins are two celebrities with the name. Variations: *Cheston, Chet*.

CHIP (English) Nickname for Charles that is sometimes given as the full name.

CHRISTOPHER (English) One who holds Christ in his heart. Famous Christophers include St. Christopher, the patron saint of people who travel, the actor Christopher Plummer, Winnie-the-Pooh's friend Christopher Robin, and explorer Christopher Columbus. Christopher just started to become popular among new parents in the '80s; now classrooms are filled with Christophers and its variations. Variations: *Chris, Christof, Christofer,*

Christoff, Christoffer, Christoforus, Christoph, Christophe, Christophoros, Christos, Christos, Cris, Cristobal, Cristoforo, Kit, Kitt, Kristofer, Kristofor.

CLARENCE (English) Clear. Variations: *Clair, Clarance, Clare, Clarey*.

CLARK (English) Scholar. Variations: *Clarke, Clerc, Clerk*.

CLAY (English) Maker of clay. Clay can stand on its own, but it's also short for some of the following names that have Clay as their first syllable.

CLIFFORD (English) Place to cross a river near a cliff. Cliff has been a good name for celebrities: think of Cliff Richard, Clifford Irving, Cliff Robertson, and Cliff Claven from *Cheers*. Variations: *Cliff, Clyff, Clyfford*.

CODY (English) Cushion. Cody used to be known as a town in Wyoming and the name of various Western outlaws from the second part of the nineteenth century. Today, however, it is undoubtedly most famous for being the name of Kathie Lee Gifford's baby, which is all it took for the name to skyrocket in popularity in the mid-'90s. Cody is not only popular for boys but also for girls. Years ago, Cody—actually, Coty, one of its variations—got most of its recognition as a brand of nail polish, which just goes to show you how much things change in a short period of time. Variations: *Codey, Codie, Coty, Kodey, Kodie, Kody*.

COLBY (English) Dark farm. Variation: *Collby*.

COLIN (English) Triumphant people; also, young boy. Colin and its various spellings have become popular for boys, and to a lesser extent, girls, in the last ten years or so. The name sounds British and worthy of respect. Another reason for its popularity is that General Colin Powell has become an American hero since his victory in the Gulf War. Variations: *Colan, Cole, Collin, Colyn*.

COLWYN (Welsh) River in Wales. Variations: *Colwin, Colwynn*.

CONNOR (Irish) Much desire. Another popular name that could serve as last name or first, male or female; it is starting to appear in both sexes more frequently. Variations: *Conner, Conor*.

COREY (Irish) The hollow. This name is red hot and it's not difficult to see why. It fits several of the criteria for why certain names are popular today: it's unisex—both girls and boys are comfortable with the name. It originates from across the big sea, and in the '90s in

America, anything British or Irish is much sought after. In addition, a number of popular young actors and singers have the name: Corey Feldman, Corey Haim, and Corey Hart. However, it does show signs of being overtaken by other popular names. Variations: *Corin, Correy, Cory, Korey.*

COSMO (Greek) Order. Cosmo is the Patron Saint of Milan and of doctors. Variations: *Cos, Cosimo, Cosme.*

CRAIG (Welsh) Rock. Craig was once very popular, with actors Craig Stevens and Craig Lucas claiming it for themselves. Variation: *Kraig.*

DAKOTA (Dakota) Friend. Dakota is also used as a name for girls, as are many of the other currently popular names that describe locations.

DALE (English) One who lives in a dale or valley. Variations: *Dal, Daley, Daly, Dayle.*

DALLAS (Scottish) Town in Scotland. Dallas can also be used as a name for girls. Dallas Green and Dallas Townsend are two big reasons for the popularity of the name.

DALTON (English) A town in a valley. Variations: *Dallton, Dalten.*

DAMIAN (Greek) Tame. Damian was a popular name in the 1970s, until its appearance in several horror movies. The name isn't used much for boys for fear that the child might actually live up to the potential of his name. Damian is also the name of the patron saint of hairdressers. Variations: *Dameon, Damiano, Damien, Damion, Damyan, Damyen, Damyon.*

DANIEL (Hebrew) God is my judge. Daniel has always been one of my favorite names. Every time you use the full, formal version, it sounds somewhat distinguished and knowing, yet a bit mischievous. The name is Biblical in origin—as in the tale of Daniel being thrown to the lions—but it is an approachable name, not stuffy at all. There are a slew of famous Daniels to help cement your choice: Danny DeVito, Danny Kaye, Danny Thomas, Daniel Webster, Daniel Boone, Daniel Barenboim, and Daniel Day-Lewis. Variations: *Dan, Danakas, Danek, Dani, Daniele, Daniels, Danil, Danila, Danilkar, Danilo, Danko, Dannie, Danniel, Danny, Dano, Danya, Danylets, Danylo, Dasco, Donois, Dusan.*

DANTE (Latin) Everlasting. Some parents might shy away from this name for their newborn boys because

of its association with hell from Dante's *Inferno*, but this name is actually a sound choice for those who like the name Damien but are looking for something a bit less threatening. Variations: *Dontae, Donte.*

DARIN (Greek) Gift. Variations: *Dare, Daron, Darren, Darrin, Darron.*

DARNELL (English) Hidden area. Variations: *Darnal, Darnall, Darnel.*

DARREN (Gaelic) Great. Variations: *Daran, Daren, Darin, Darran, Darrin, Darron, Darryn, Daryn.*

DARRYL (English) An English last name. Darryl was a popular name in the '80s. Famous Darryls include Darryl Strawberry, Darryl Hall, and Darryl and Darryl on the *Newhart* show. Variations: *Darrel, Darrell, Darrill, Darrol, Darryll, Daryl, Daryll.*

DAVID (Hebrew) Cherished. Even though the name David has been in this country since the 1700s, it has never really gone out of style. The fact that David is a Biblical name—David opposed mighty Goliath—and that so many famous people have lived with the name may combine to account for its continued popularity: David Bowie, David Mamet, David Cassidy, David Letterman, Davy Jones, and Dave Winfield. The name has significance in both the Christian and Jewish religions: David is one of the patron saints of Wales, while the Star of David is the cornerstone symbol of Judaism. Variations: *Dave, Daveed, Davi, Davidek, Davie, Davy, Dewey, Dodya.*

DAVIS (English) Son of David. Variations: *Davison, Dawson.*

DEAN (English) Valley. Dean was wildly popular back in the '50s and '60s, probably because of actor Dean Martin, but today no such actor carries the torch for the name. However, the name is coming back in style anyway. Variations: *Deane, Dene.*

DELANEY (Irish) Child of a competitor. Variations: *Delaine, Delainey, Delainy, Delane, Delany.*

DELBERT (English) Sunny day. Though Delbert seems a bit old-fashioned, singer Delbert McClinton and baseball player Del Unser keep this name in the public consciousness.

DELMAR (Spanish) Oceanside. Variations: *Delmer, Delmor, Delmore.*

DEMARCO (African-American) Demarco is a newly created name that literally means of Mark.

Variations: *D'Marcus, Damarcus, Demarcus, Demario, Demarkis, Demarkus.*

DEMETRIUS (Greek) Lover of the earth. Variations: *Demeter, Demetre, Demetri, Demetrio, Demetris, Demetrois, Dimetre, Dimitri, Dimitry, Dmitri, Dmitrios, Dmitry.*

DENNIS (Greek) One who follows Dionysius, the Greek god of wine. Denis is also the patron saint of France. Dennis the Menace is undoubtedly the most famous Dennis around, but a number of other Dennises have made their mark on the world: Dennis Weaver, Denis Diderot, Denis Papin, and Dennis O'Keefe, among others. Variations: *Denies, Denis, Denka, Dennes, Denney, Denny, Dennys, Denys.*

DENZELL (African-American) Unknown definition. Variations: *Denzel, Denziel, Denzil, Denzill, Denzyl.*

DEREK (English) Leader. Eric Clapton and his group Derek and the Dominoes probably gave Americans their first exposure to this name. It is also distinguished by the many British actors who share it: Derek Bond, Derek Jacobi, Derek Farr, and Derek de Lint are just a few on this prestigious list. Variations: *Dereck, Derick, Derik, Derreck, Derrek, Derrick, Derrik, Deryck, Deryk.*

DERMOT (Irish) Free of jealousy. Variations: *Dermod, Dermott.*

DESHAWN (African-American) Newly created. Variations: *D'chaun, DaShaun, Dashawn, DeSean, DeShaun, Deshaun.*

DESMOND (Irish) From South Munster, an old civilization in Ireland. South African Archbishop Desmond Tutu and author Desmond Morris have helped to make this name more visible in the last decade. Variations: *Desmund, Dezmond.*

DEWAYNE (African-American) Newly created. Dewayne is one of many popular African-American names that are created by adding the prefix "De-" to another name, most often with one syllable. No one knows exactly how this custom started, but it certainly helps to set these names apart, and the practice creates hundreds of new names to play with. Variations: *D'Wayne, DeWayne.*

DEXTER (Latin) Right-handed. Variation: *Dex.*

DILLON (Irish) Loyal. Variations: *Dillan, Dilon, Dilyn.*

DION (African-American) God. Variations: *Deion, DeOn, Deon.*

DOMINICK (English) Lord. Variations: *Dom, Dome, Domek, Domenic, Domenico, Domicio, Domingo, Domingos, Dominic, Dominik, Dominique, Domo, Domokos, Nic, Nick, Nik.*

DONOVAN (Irish) Dark. Variations: *Don, Donavan, Donavon, Donoven, Donovon.*

DOUGLAS (English) Dark water. River in Ireland. Common Scottish last name. It was used as frequently for girls as for boys when it first began to catch on back in the seventeenth century. Famous Douglases include General Douglas MacArthur, Douglas Fairbanks, Douglas Edwards, and Douglas Moore. Variations: *Doug, Douglass.*

DREW (English) Wise. Diminutive of Andrew. Drew also became a popular girls' name in the '80s. Variations: *Drewe, Dru.*

DYLAN (Welsh) Son of the ocean. Variations: *Dillan, Dillon.*

EARL (English) Leader; nobleman. Famous Earls include Erle Stanley Gardner, Earl Warren, and Earl Scruggs. Rarely used as a first name these days; Earl is often chosen as a good middle name. Variations: *Earle, Earlie, Early, Erl, Erle, Errol, Erryl.*

EATON (English) Town on a river. Variations: *Eatton, Eton, Eyton.*

EDEN (Hebrew) Delight. Variations: *Eaden, Eadin, Edan, Edin.*

EDGAR (English) Wealthy man who holds a spear. Edgar Winter, Edgar Allan Poe, and Candice Bergen's father, Edgar, are all notable men with this name. Variations: *Edgard, Edgardo.*

EDISON (English) Edward's son. Variations: *Ed, Eddison, Edson.*

EDWARD (English) Guardian of property. Edward has a touch of nobility to it, along with a number of famous, distinguished men who go by the name: Edward Albee, Edward Hopper, and Edouard Manet. Of course, some of the more exotic spellings can only help to enhance the image of Edward. Variations: *Ed, Eddie, Edouard, Eduardo, Edvard.*

EDWIN (English) Rich friend. Variation: *Edwyn.*

ELAN (Hebrew) Tree. Variation: *Ilan.*

ELDRIDGE (German) Wise leader.

ELI (Hebrew) God is great. Variations: *Elie, Ely.*

ELIJAH (Hebrew) The Lord is my God. Variations: *Elek, Elias, Eliasz, Elie, Eliya, Eliyahu, Ellis, Elya.*

ELLERY (English) Island with elder trees. Last name. Variation: *Ellary.*

ELLIOT (English) God on high. Variations: *Eliot, Eliott, Elliott.*

ELMORE (English) Valley with elm trees.

EMANUEL (Hebrew) God is among us. The name given to the Messiah. Biblical names are hot, and Emanuel, which appears in Isaiah 7:14, signifies prophecy and promise and is given by parents to a son who they believe is capable of accomplishing great things. Though the shortened versions of Manny and Manuel are directly derived from Emanuel, today's parents are tending toward the full, more formal version. Variations: *Emmanuel, Emmanuil; Immanuel, Manny, Manuel.*

EMERY (German) Leader of the house. Variations: *Emmery, Emory.*

ENNIS (Gaelic) Only choice.

ENZO (Italian) To win.

ERIC (Scandinavian) Ruler of the people. Eric is a very popular name that appears to have reached its peak in the mid-'70s, helped along, no doubt, by the fame of Eric Clapton, Eric Severeid, and speedskater Eric Heiden. Like its feminine counterpart, Erica, Eric first became popular in the United States in the mid-nineteenth century as the result of a popular children's book called *Eric, or Little by Little*, by an author named H. Rider Haggard. Variations: *Erek, Erich, Erick, Erico, Erik.*

ERROL (Scottish) Area in Scotland. Variations: *Erroll, Erryl.*

ERWIN (English) A boar and a friend. A number of men with the name Erwin have been involved behind the scenes in movies, including producer Erwin Allen. Author Irwin Shaw wrote the book *Rich Man, Poor Man.* Variations: *Erwinek, Erwyn, Erwynn, Irwin.*

ESTEBAN (Spanish) Crown. Variation of Stephen.

ETHAN (Hebrew) Steady. The novel *Ethan Frome* and the Revolutionary War hero Ethan Allen are the best-known examples of this name. It should be among the top contenders for parents who are looking for a dignified name that fits a child as well as it does an adult. Variations: *Eitan, Etan.*

ETIENNE (French) Crown. Variation of Stephen.

EVAN (Welsh) God is good. Evan is a version of John that is picking up speed as a common name for American boys today. However much they like the name, we wouldn't suggest that parents with the last name of Evans go so far as the parents of Evan Evans, a Welsh poet from the eighteenth century. Variations: *Ev, Evann, Evans, Evin, Ewan.*

EVANDER (Scottish) Good man.

EVERETT (English) Literally, boar plus hard. Everett is most commonly known as a last name. Variations: *Everard, Everet, Everhard, Everitt.*

EZEKIEL (Hebrew) The strength of God. Variation: *Zeke.*

EZIO (Italian) Unknown definition.

FABIAN (Latin) One who grows beans. The singer Fabian from the '50s—whose full name was Fabian Forte—may make this name a good choice for parents who fondly remember that decade. Variations: *Faba, Fabek, Faber, Fabert, Fabiano, Fabien, Fabio, Fabius, Fabiyan, Fabyan, Fabyen.*

FABRON (French) Blacksmith. Variations: *Fabre, Fabroni.*

FAGAN (Irish) Eager child. Variation: *Fagin.*

FAHIM (Hindu) Intelligent.

FAIRLEIGH (English) Meadow with bulls. Variations: *Fairlay, Fairlee, Fairlie, Farleigh, Farley.*

FALKNER (English) Falcon trainer. Falkner is a first name/last name that is ripe for an increase in use among parents who are looking for something distinctive and distinguished. Variations: *Falconer, Falconner, Faulkner, Fowler.*

FARAJ (Arabic) Cure. Variation: *Farag.*

FARIS (Arabic) Knight.

FARON (English) Unknown definition. Last name. Variations: *Faran, Farin, Farran, Farrin, Farron, Farrun, Farun.*

FARRELL (Irish) Courageous man. Variations: *Farall, Farrel, Farrill, Farryll, Ferrel, Ferrell, Ferrill, Ferryl.*

FARROW (Irish) Unknown definition. Last name.

FENTON (English) Town by a swamp.

FERDINAND (German) Brave traveler. Ferdinand is a very old name. It was used by Shakespeare in *Love's Labour's Lost* as well as *The Tempest.* More recently, Fernando Lamas and Jelly Roll Morton—whose real name was Fernando—are the most stellar examples of the name. Parents who wish to have a calm son may name their baby after the main character in the children's book *Ferdinand the Bull*, where the bull would rather smell flowers and loll in the forest than fight. The name is currently enjoying a renaissance in some of its variations. Variations: *Ferdinando, Ferdynand, Fernand, Fernando.*

FIELDING (English) In the field. Variation: *Field.*

FINIAN (Irish) Fair. The musical *Finian's Rainbow* is how most people were first exposed to this name. Its wonderful lilt and Irish connotations may cause Finian to become more popular than it's been. Variations: *Finnian, Fionan, Fionn.*

FINNEGAN (Irish) Fair. Like Finian, Finnegan seems to be poised for an increase in popularity among boys' names because it meets the popularity criteria of last name, unisex usage, and the association with Ireland. Variation: *Finegan.*

FITCH (English) Name of a mammal similar to a ferret.

FITZPATRICK (Irish) Son of a statesman.

FLANNERY (Irish) Red hair. Though Flannery is more popularly known as a girls' name, the choice seems appropriate for a red-haired boy. Variations: *Flaine, Flann, Flannan.*

FLETCHER (English) One who makes arrows. Actor Chevy Chase has helped to make the nickname of Fletcher more visible through his *Fletch* movies, but the full name is also an attractive choice for a boy today. Variation: *Fletch.*

FLOYD (Welsh) Gray hair. Boxer Floyd Patterson was the antithesis of this almost-feminine name, but his reputation hasn't increased the popularity of the name very much.

FLYNN (Irish) Red-haired man's son. Variations: *Flin, Flinn, Flyn.*

FOREST (French) Woods. Forrest Gump isn't the only popular figure with this name: Forrest Sawyer, Forrest Whittaker, and Forrest Tucker were around long before Tom Hank's character was. Variations: *Forester, Forrest, Forrester, Forster, Foster.*

FRANCIS (Latin) Frenchman. Francis and its derivatives were very popular earlier in this century; top names include Frank Sinatra, Franco Zeffirelli, Franco Harris, Frank Lloyd Wright, Frankie Valli, Frank Capra, and Frank Loesser, among many others. Though Francis was frequently in the top ten list of names from the late nineteenth century through the 1940s, it doesn't even crack the top fifty names today. All that may be about to change, however, as more parents

opt for traditional names from their own family trees. Variations: *Fran, Franc, Franchot, Francisco, Franco, Francois, Frank, Frankie, Franky.*

FRANKLIN (English) A free property owner. Variations: *Frank, Franki, Frankie, Franklyn, Franklynn, Franky.*

FRANZ (German) Frenchman. Franz Kafka and composers Franz Liszt and Schubert are the men who come to mind with this name. Variations: *Frans, Franzen, Franzl.*

FRASER (English) Town in France. Undoubtedly, Fraser will become a popular name in the next decade, due to the success of the TV character played by Kelsey Grammer. Variations: *Frasier, Fraze, Frazer, Frazier.*

FREDERICK (German) Merciful leader. Fred Astaire, Fred Mertz, Fred MacMurray, and even Mister Fred Rogers serve as the most popular men with this name. Variations: *Fred, Freddie, Freddy, Fredek, Frederich, Frederico, Frederik, Fredric, Fredrick, Friedrich, Fritz.*

FRITZ (German) Peaceful ruler. Fritz started out as a nickname for Frederick, but started to appear as an independent name among babies born in the late nineteenth century. Variations: *Fritzchen, Fritzroy.*

FULLER (English) One who shrinks cloth.

GABRIEL (Hebrew) Man of God. Gabriel is a wonderfully diverse name with plenty of choices for the parent—and later, the son—who wants a variant of the name, yet wishes to remain true to the root. Famous Gabriels include Gabe Kaplan, Garbriel Garcia Marquez, and Gabriel Byrne. Variations: *Gab, Gabby, Gabe, Gabi, Gabko, Gabo, Gabor, Gabriele, Gabrielli, Gabriello, Gabris, Gabys, Gavi, Gavriel.*

GALEN (Greek) Healer. Variation: *Galeno.*

GALLAGHER (Irish) Foreign partner.

GALVIN (Irish) Sparrow. Variations: *Gallven, Gallvin, Galvan, Galven.*

GARETH (Welsh) Gentle. Variations: *Garith, Garreth, Garyth.*

GARRICK (English) He who rules with a spear. Variations: *Garreck, Garryck, Garyk.*

GARTH (English) Gardener. Garth is most popular today because of the country singer Garth Brooks, but it was even more popular in the nineteenth century, when a number of writers, from George Eliot to

Charlotte Yonge, chose the name for main characters in their novels.

GARY (English) Spear. Gary Cooper is singlehandedly credited with creating this name as a possibility for modern use in the '40s and '50s. Before he began using it as his first name—his real name was Frank—its only use was as a last name and as a town in Indiana immortalized in the musical *The Music Man*. Today, while Gary isn't as popular as it was in the middle part of this century, celebrities currently in the spotlight include Garry Trudeau and Garry Shandling. Variations: *Garey, Garrey, Garry*.

GAVIN (Welsh) White falcon. Variations: *Gavan, Gaven, Gavyn, Gawain, Gawaine, Gawayn, Gawayne, Gawen*.

GAYNOR (Irish) Son of a pale man.

GEARY (English) Changeable. Variation: *Gearey*.

GENE (English) Well born. Derived from Eugene. Gene is a friendly, approachable name, probably made so by actors Gene Kelly, Gene Wilder, and Gene Hackman. Variations: *Genek, Genio, Genka, Genya*.

GEOFFREY (German) Peace. Alternative spelling for Jeffrey.

GEORGE (Greek) Farmer. While George as a given name has not been the most popular choice in the last couple of decades, it seems to be making a mini-comeback, particularly among parents who wish to honor an older relative with the name. Famous Georges include George Washington, George Patton, Giorgio Armani, and George Bush. Although a woman novelist in the nineteenth century became famous under the pseudonym George Sand, the name George is overwhelmingly more popular for boys than for girls. Variations: *Georg, Georges, Georgi, Georgios, Georgy, Giorgio, Giorgos*.

GERALD (German) Ruler with a spear. The fact that a recent president had this name may have increased its popularity among parents who like the nicknames that are created from Gerald, but prefer something a bit more formal as the given name. Once a particularly popular choice among African-American families, today it is chosen equally frequently by parents of many backgrounds. Variations: *Geralde, Geraldo, Geraud, Gerrald, Gerrold, Gerry, Jerald, Jeralde, Jeraud, Jerold, Jerrald, Jerrold, Jerry*.

GERARD (German) Brave with a spear. Variations: *Garrard, Gerhard, Gerrard, Gerrit, Gerry*.

GERONIMO (Native American: Apache) A famous Apache Indian chief.

GERSHOM (Hebrew) Exile. Variations: *Gersham, Gershon, Gerson*.

GIANCARLO (Italian) Combination of John and Charles.

GILBERT (German) Bright pledge. In the past, Gilbert hasn't been a name to choose if you're looking for your son to grow into a suave, debonair adult, but Johnny Depp's role in the recent movie *What's Eating Gilbert Grape?* may do a lot to change all that. Variations: *Gib, Gil, Gilberto*.

GILES (English) Young goat. Variations: *Gil, Gilles, Gyles*.

GILMORE (Irish) Servant of the Virgin Mary. Variations: *Gillmore, Gillmour, Gilmour, Giolle Maire*.

GLEN (Irish) Narrow valley. In the past, parents have chosen Glen for their children—boys and, to a lesser extent, girls—because the name is a smooth one, non-threatening, and already claimed by such equally unflappable celebrities as Glenn Miller and Glen Ford. Today, it may seem to be a bit plain for some parents, but others are choosing it just for that reason alone. Variation: *Glenn*.

GORDON (English) Round hill. A relative of Gordon—Jordan—is currently popular and making the rounds among new parents. Those who want to be a bit different might choose Gordon, the original. Famous Gordons include Gordon Lightfoot and Gordie Howe. Variations: *Gordan, Gorden, Gordie, Gordy*.

GRAHAM (English) Gray house. Singer Graham Nash and novelist Graham Greene, as well as the graham cracker, make this name a possibility for parents who are looking to give their sons a name that couldn't be mistaken for anything but British. Variations: *Graeham, Graeme, Grahame, Gram*.

GRANT (Scottish) Great.

GRAYSON (English) Son of a man with gray hair. Variation: *Greyson*.

GREGORY (Greek) Observant. Gregory and its off-shoots have been popular in this country since Gregory Peck appeared in *To Kill a Mockingbird*. Before that watershed event, it was more frequently chosen by popes—sixteen of them, to be precise. Today, the most famous Gregorys include Greg Louganis, the Olympic diver, and Greg Brady. Variations: *Greg, Gregg, Gregoire, Gregor, Gregorio, Gregorios, Gregos, Greig, Gries, Grigor*.

GRIFFIN (Latin) One with a hooked nose. Variations: *Griff, Griffon, Gryphon.*

GUNNAR (Scandinavian) Battle. Variations: *Gun, Gunder.*

GUS (English) Majestic. Gus was originally a shortened form of Augustus, but came into its own as an independent name over the course of the last century.

HABIB (Arabic) Dear.

HAKEEM (Arabic) Wise. Hakeem is common in Muslim countries, as it is one of the ninety-nine qualities of Allah that are detailed in the Koran, but it is becoming more popular here, particularly among African-American and Muslim families. Variations: *Hakem, Hakim.*

HALSEY (English) The island that belongs to Hal. Variations: *Hallsey, Hallsy, Halsy.*

HAMID (Arabic) Greatly praised. Derivative of Mohammed. Variations: *Hammad, Hammed.*

HAMILTON (English) Fortified castle. Variation: *Hamelton.*

HAMISH (Scottish) He who removes. Hamish, which is appearing more frequently among parents who want their son's name to convey an Arabic feel—even though it originates in Scotland—also has its roots in Yiddish, where it means comfortable.

HANK (English) Ruler of the estate. Diminutive of Henry. Hank is a down-home, unpretentious name that, because of the famous men who have lived with the name—Hank Aaron and Hank Williams—is a good choice for parents who are also down-home and unpretentious. However, most people use Hank as the nickname and instead give Henry as the full name.

HARLAN (English) Army land. Variations: *Harland, Harlen, Harlenn, Harlin, Harlyn, Harlynn.*

HAROLD (English) Army ruler. The name Harold conjures up a feel of the good life as it was experienced about a hundred years ago, in smoking jackets and booklined parlors. Harold was also the name of the boy on TV and in the movies who was always getting picked on by the bullies in his neighborhood, which may be the reason that it isn't selected more often today. Variations: *Hal, Harailt, Harald, Haraldo, Haralds, Haroldas, Haroldo.*

HARPER (English) Harp player. Harper is a great name for parents who are looking for an androgynous last name as first name that hasn't gotten around much yet and possesses no negative connotations. Harper is also used as a girls' name.

HARRISON (English) Harry's son. Variation: *Harrisen.*

HARRY (English) Ruler at home. Variation of Henry. Today Harry seems to be one of those previously nerdy names that is on its way back in style. Britain's young Prince Harry may have something to do with the revival. Variations: *Harrey, Harri, Harrie.*

HARTWELL (English) Well where stags drink. Variations: *Harwell, Harwill.*

HARVEY (French) Eager for battle. Although the name has had a nerdy image in the past, Harvey is back with a vengeance, and growing in popularity. Playwright Harvey Fierstein may have helped the reputation of the name, with his activism and outspokenness. Variations: *Herve, Hervey.*

HASIM (Arabic) To determine.

HAYDEN (English) Hill of heather; (Welsh) Valley with hedges. Though Hayden and its variants are quite popular across the ocean in Great Britain and Wales, the name is just beginning to catch on in this country. Parents-to-be whose childhoods were filled with piano lessons are familiar with another spelling of the name, Haydn, as in Franz Joseph, but kids today are more likely to know it through actor Aidan Quinn. Variations: *Aidan, Haddan, Haddon, Haden, Hadon, Hadyn, Haydn, Haydon.*

HAYWARD (English) Protector of hedged area.

HEINRICH (German) Ruler of the estate. Variation of Henry. Variations: *Heinrick, Heinrik, Henrik, Henrique, Henryk.*

HELMUT (French) Helmet. Helmut Kohl and Helmut Newton have made this name visible, but it tends not to be too popular in this country.

HENRY (German) Ruler of the house. Like Harry, another previously unpopular name in recent decades, Henry is one of the more popular choices around. Famous Henrys include Henry L. Mencken, Henry James, and Henry Longfellow. But perhaps an unconscious influence for the name's increasing popularity is Henry David Thoreau, who seems to be in the environmental news on a regular basis all over the country, which is pretty good considering that he's been dead for more than a hundred years. Variations: *Henery, Henri, Henrik, Henrique, Henryk.*

HERBERT (German) Shining army. Variations: *Heibert, Herb, Herbie.*

HERMAN (German) Army man. Herman Munster and Herman Melville, the author of *Moby Dick*, are among the most famous recipients of the name. Variations: *Hermann, Hermon.*

HILLEL (Hebrew) Highly praised. Jewish families are choosing this name more frequently for their sons. Hillel was the name of one of the first great Talmudic scholars.

HIRSH (Hebrew) Deer. Variations: *Hersch, Herschel, Hersh, Hershel, Hersz, Hertz, Hertzel, Herz, Herzl, Heschel, Hesh, Hirsch, Hirschel.*

HOLBROOK (English) Brook near the hollow. Variation: *Holbrooke.*

HOLDEN (English) Hollow valley.

HORACE (Latin) Old Roman clan name. Neither Horace nor its variant, Horatio, has ever been a wildly popular name. But Horatio actually has a bit of potential these days, as its illustrious past shows: Navy hero (Nelson), composers (Palmer), and aircraft pioneer (Phillips). Variations: *Horacio, Horatio.*

HOSEA (Hebrew) Deliverance. Variations: *Hoseia, Hosheia.*

HOWARD (English) Observer. Last name. Howard isn't widely used in the United States today, but earlier in the century it was chosen with great frequency in Britain because people felt that it had a decidedly aristocratic feel. Howard is a saint as well as, and perhaps most famously remembered, an eccentric billionaire by the name of Hughes. It's not clear why this name went out of fashion after being one of the top twenty names for boys from the late nineteenth century through to the 1950s. Variation: *Howie.*

HOWELL (Welsh) Exceptional.

HOYT (Irish) Spirit.

IAN (Scottish) God is good. Ian is perhaps the most quintessentially British name you could give a boy. Ian Fleming is the writer who penned all of the James Bond stories, which could be the reason why Ian and England are so intertwined in our American minds. Ian hit its peak in both Britain and the United States in the mid-'60s. Variations: *Ean, Iain, Iancu, Ianos.*

IBRAHIM (Arabic) Father of many. Variation of Abraham.

ICARUS (Greek) Greek mythological figure who flew too close to the sun; his wings, attached to his body with wax, fell off and he plummeted to earth.

IMRAN (Arabic) Host.

INCENCIO (Spanish) White one.

INGHAM (English) Area in Britain.

INNES (Scottish) Island. Variations: *Inness, Innis, Inniss.*

IRA (Hebrew) Observant. Famous Iras include Ira Gershwin, brother of George, and Ira Allen, brother of Ethan.

IRVIN (Scottish) Beautiful. Variation: *Irvine.*

IRVING (English) Sea friend. Though Irving is not as popular as the other previously nerdy names that seem to be making a comeback these days, there is no doubt that it is being selected more in the '90s than it was ten or twenty years ago. Famous Irvings include Irving Berlin, Irving Stone, Irving Thalberg, and Irving Wallace. Variation: *Irv.*

ISAAC (Hebrew) Laughter. One way it's obvious that people have become more aware and proud of their ethnic heritage is by choosing names that have clear connections to their backgrounds. Isaac is a great example of this trend, as it is beginning to appear with greater frequency at synagogues and playgrounds alike. Isaacs who have made a name for themselves include Isaac Stern, Isaac Asimov, Isaac Hayes, and Isaac Bashevis Singer. Variations: *Isaak, Isak, Itzak, Ixaka, Izaak.*

ISAIAH (Hebrew) God helps me. Variations: *Isa, Isaia, Isia, Isiah, Issiah.*

ISHA (Hindu) Lord.

ISHMAEL (Hebrew) God will hear. Variations: *Ismael, Ismail, Yishmael.*

ISRAEL (Hebrew) Struggle with God. The country. Israel has been given to both Jewish boys and African-Americans in the last few decades. Variation: *Yisrael.*

IVAN (Czech) God is good. Variations: *Ivanchik, Ivanek, Ivano, Ivas.*

IVES (English) Yew wood; archer. Variations: *Ivo, Ivon, Yves.*

IVORY (African-American) Ivory.

JABBAR (Hindu) One who comforts.

JACKSON (English) Son of Jack. Variation: *Jakson.*

JACOB (Hebrew) Supplanter or heel. Jacob first appears in the book of Genesis in the Bible; Jacob was the youngest son of Isaac and Rebecca. It is very popular among parents these days, possibly because it displays a sense of forthrightness and openness. No upper-crust pretentions here. Perhaps the most famous literary Jacob was created by Charles Dickens in *A Christmas Carol.* Variations: *Jaco, Jacobus, Jacoby, Jacquet, Jakab, Jake, Jakie, Jakiv, Jakob, Jakov, Jakub, Jakubek, Kiva, Kivi.*

JAGGER (English) To haul something.

JAKEEM (Arabic) Noble.

JAMAL (Arabic) Handsome. Variations: *Gamal, Gamil, Jamaal, Jamahl, Jamall, Jameel, Jamel, Jamell, Jamil, Jamill, Jammal.*

JAMES (English) He who replaces. Variation of Jacob. James—by itself and in its many incarnations—has never really gone out of style. It can be formal or casual, and a boy with the name of James will either love it or prefer one of the more informal versions. Later on, however, having the option to be called James as an adult adds to the respect the name possesses. Famous Jameses include James Taylor, James Stewart, James Cagney, James Mason, and Jimi Hendrix. Variations: *Jacques, Jaime, Jaimey, Jaimie, Jaimito, Jamey, Jamie, Jayme, Jaymes, Jaymie, Jim, Jimi, Jimmey, Jimmie, Jimmy.*

JAMESON (English) Son of James. Variations: *Jamieson, Jamison.*

JARED (Hebrew) Descend. Jared, with its many variants, has been very popular since the mid-'60s, when it first began to appear with some regularity. Jared, however, was around as a common name in Puritan America, although it fell into a kind of black hole. Variations: *Jarad, Jarid, Jarod, Jarrad, Jarred, Jerad, Jered, Jerod, Jerrad, Jerrod, Jerryd, Yarden, Yared.*

JARETH (African-American) Newly created. Variations: *Jarreth, Jerth.*

JARON (Hebrew) To shout. Variations: *Gerron, Jaran, Jaren, Jarin, Jarran, Jarren, Jarron, Jeran, Jeren, Jeron, Jerrin, Jerron.*

JARRETT (English) Brave with a spear. Variations: *Jarret, Jarrete.*

JARVIS (German). Honorable. Variation: *Jervis.*

JASON (Hebrew) God is my salvation. Jason Priestley, Jason Robards, and a variety of other TV and Hollywood stars combined to turn Jason into one of the hottest names of the '70s and '80s. Names that start with the letter "J" constitute a sizable percentage of names today, and when Jason first began to catch on, it represented a fresh new approach to "J" names. Today, Jason is still popular, but it can border on overuse in some areas of the country; your selecting a form of Jason with a different spelling will help your son to stand apart. Variations: *Jace, Jacen, Jaison, Jase, Jasen, Jayce, Jaycen, Jaysen, Jayson.*

JASPER (English) Wealthy one. Variation: *Jaspar.*

JAY (Latin) Blue jay. Jay Gould, Jay Leno, and the wealthy Jay Gatsby from F. Scott Fitzgerald's novel *The Great Gatsby* are just three of the famous men with this name who have pierced the public consciousness. Parents like Jay as a choice for their sons because it's a simple name, yet still conveys a bit of a sophisticated image, probably from the Gatsby connection. Variations: *Jae, Jai, Jave, Jaye, Jeays, Jeyes.*

JEDIDIAH (Hebrew) Beloved of God. Variations: *Jed, Jedd, Jedediah, Jedidia, Yedidia, Yedidiah, Yedidya.*

JEFFREY (German) Peace. Jeffrey was one of the most popular names in the United States in the 1970s, but like many names that are strongly tied with a particular point in time, Jeffrey is declining in popularity today. When parents do choose it, they tend to select one of its more unusual spellings. Jeffrey and its variations beginning with "G" have been extremely popular throughout Europe for most of this millennium. Variations: *Geoff, Geoffrey, Geoffry, Gioffredo, Jeff, Jefferies, Jeffery, Jeffries, Jeffry, Jefry.*

JEREMY (Hebrew) The Lord exalts. Jeremy has been a popular name among American parents in the last couple of decades. Famous Jeremys include actor Jeremy Irons and a frog in one of Beatrix Potter's books named Jeremy Fisher. However, like its counterpart Jason, Jeremy has become a bit too popular for some, who decide to opt for one of the many variants available. Variations: *Jem, Jemmie, Jemmy, Jeramee, Jeramey, Jeramie, Jere, Jereme, Jeremey, Jeremi, Jeremia, Jeremias, Jeremie, Jerimiah, Jeromy, Jerr, Jerrie, Jerry.*

JERMAINE (German) German. Variations: *Jermain, Jermane, Jermayne.*

JEROME (Greek) Sacred name. Name of a saint. Variations: *Jeron, Jerone, Jerrome.*

JERRELL (African-American) Newly created. Variations: *Gerrell, Jarell, Jarrel, Jarrell, Jeriel, Jerriel, Jerul.*

JESSE (Hebrew) God exists. Jesse Jackson, Jesse James, and Jesse Owens are the most popular people with this name, and even though it has been thought of more as a girls' name in recent years, at its peak in the '70s, it was extremely popular for boys. Like a lot of other names that begin with the letter "J," Jesse is great for all ages: little kids, teenagers, young fathers, and then even grandfathers. Jesse has staying power, and is hip to boot. Variations: *Jesiah, Jess, Jessey, Jessie, Jessy.*

JETT (English) Airplane.

JOACHIM (Hebrew) God will determine. Variations: *Joaquim, Joaquin.*

JOEL (Hebrew) God is Lord.

JOERGEN (Scandinavian) Farmer.

JOHN (Hebrew) God is good. If you count all of the variations, spellings, and the language usages around the world, it's possible that more boys are named John than any other name. John cuts across all categories: in religion, there's John the Baptist and St. John the Divine; in movies, it seemed for a while in the 1950s, there was no other name to give to the lead male character (Johnny Angel, Johnny Guitar, Johnny Cool); and in entertainment, there's John Wayne, Johnny Carson, Johnny Depp, and Johnny Cash, and then Johnny Weissmuller—an Olympic gold medalist swimmer in 1924. With this prestige and a wide variety of Johns to choose from, it's a good bet that John in one or more of its forms will never be out of style. Variations: *Jack, Jackie, Jacky, Joao, Jock, Jockel, Jocko, Johan, Johann, Johannes, Johnie, Johnnie, Johnny, Jon, Jonam, Jone, Jonelis, Jonnie, Jonny, Jonukas, Jonutis, Jovan, Jovanus, Jovi, Jovin, Jovito, Jovon, Juan, Juanito.*

JONAH (Hebrew) Dove. Biblical book. Variations: *Jonas, Yonah, Yonas, Yunus.*

JONATHAN (Hebrew) Gift from God. In the Bible, Jonathan was King Saul's oldest son and was best known as King David's best friend. Parents have liked Jonathan because it is based on a classic name—John—but is more distinctive. Robert Wagner's mystery-loving Jonathan Hart on the '80s TV show *Hart to Hart* has probably contributed to today's image of Jonathan as warm, intelligent, and sexy. Other Jonathans include Jonathan Winters and Jonathan Swift. Variations: *Johnathan, Johnathen, Johnathon, Jon, Jonathen, Jonathon, Jonnie, Jonny, Jonothon.*

JORDAN (Hebrew) To descend. Jordan is a unisex name as well as an occasional last name, which has helped to make it as popular as it is. During the Crusades, the name caught on when soldiers brought water from the River Jordan back home with them to baptize their children. Variations: *Jorden, Jordy, Jori, Jorrin.*

JOSEPH (Hebrew) God will increase. Joseph is perhaps best known as Mary's husband, and therefore a kind of stepfather to Jesus Christ. This fact, and its many varieties in America and around the world, may be the reason why the name has never fallen out of style. Amazingly enough, Joseph has been on the top ten list of boys' names in New York for almost a hundred years, longer than any other name for either boys or girls. Famous Josephs have included Franz Joseph Haydn, Mormon founder Joseph Smith, and novelist Joseph Conrad. Variations: *Jodi, Jodie, Jody, Jose, Josecito, Josef, Joselito, Josephe, Josephus, Josip.*

JOSHUA (Hebrew) God is my salvation. Joshua was the leader of the Jews after Moses, and a book in the Bible is named for him. However, Joshua has only started to become popular since the 1960s, although other Biblical names have been used for centuries. Variations: *Josh, Joshuah.*

JOSIAH (Hebrew) God supports. Variations: *Josia, Josias, Josua.*

JUDE (Hebrew) Praise God. Variations: *Juda, Judah, Judas, Judd, Judson.*

JULIAN (Latin) Version of Julius. Saint. Variations: *Julien, Julion, Julyan.*

JUNIOR (English) Young.

KADEEM (African-American) Newly created.

KAHIL (Turkish) Young. Kahil is a name that is popular in many different countries, not just Turkey. In Hebrew, it means perfect; in Greece, it means beautiful. Up until the 1970s the form of the name we had most often seen was Cahil, the English version of this name. However, African-American families have made this name more popular in the United States. Variations: *Cahil, Kahlil, Kaleel, Khaleel, Khalil.*

KAI (Hawaiian) Sea.

KAMAL (Arabic) Perfect. Like many of the other Arabic and Turkish names for boys that begin with "K," Kamal is becoming more popular in this country, especially among African-American families. Variations: *Kameel, Kamil.*

KANE (Welsh) Beautiful; (Japanese) Golden. In America, Kane is becoming more popular for both boys and girls. One very hot variation has been introduced by superstar actor, Keanu Reeves. Variations: *Kain, Kaine, Kayne, Keanu.*

KAREEM (Arabic) Generous. In this country basketball star Kareem Abdul-Jabbar is the most famous man around with this name today. Its definition, generous, is one of the ninety-nine qualities ascribed to God in the Koran. Variations: *Karim, Karime.*

KARL (German) Man. Variations: *Karlen, Karlens, Karlin.*

KASPAR (Persian) Protector of wealth. Variation: *Kasper.*

KEATON (English) Hawk nest. Variations: *Keeton, Keiton, Keyton.*

KEEGAN (Irish) Small and passionate. Besides being a perfect name for a little boy who's always getting into trouble, Keegan is also considered to be the astrological sign of fire, which includes Sagittarius, Leo, and Aries. Variations: *Kagen, Keagan, Keegen, Kegan.*

KEELEY (Irish) Handsome. Variations: *Kealey, Kealy, Keelie, Keely.*

KEITH (Scottish) Forest. Keith was cool in the '70s when both a Rolling Stone and a Partridge had the name.

KELLY (Irish) Warrior. Not too long ago, Kelly was a name given in equal measure to both boys and girls. But today, a boy with the name of Kelly is a rare thing indeed. Variations: *Kelley, Kellie.*

KELSEY (English) Island. Variations: *Kelsie, Kelsy.*

KENDALL (English) Last name. Valley of the river Kent. Variations: *Kendal, Kendell.*

KENNEDY (Irish) Helmet head; ugly head. In the '60s, Kennedy was a name given to boys to honor the esteemed family from Massachusetts. In the '90s, Kennedy is more often given to girls in tribute to the MTV deejay. Go figure. Variations: *Canaday, Canady, Kenneday.*

KENNETH (Irish) Handsome; sprung from fire. Helped along by the macho image of Barbie's boyfriend Ken, this name was the epitome of masculinity through the '50s and '60s. Today, however, it conjures up images of medieval England and the Knights of the Round Table due to its appearance in a novel by Sir Walter Scott. Variations: *Ken, Kendall, Kenney, Kennie, Kennith, Kenny, Kenyon.*

KENT (English) County in England.

KERRY (Irish) County in Ireland. Variations: *Kerrey, Kerrie.*

KERWIN (Irish) Dark. Variations: *Kerwen, Kerwinn, Kerwyn, Kirwin.*

KESHON (African-American) Version of Sean. Variations: *Ke Sean, Ke Shon, Kesean.*

KEVIN (Irish) Handsome Today, Kevin, traditionally a name given to Irish Catholic boys, is used in a more multidenominational fashion than before, a trait that has been helped along by the fame of actors Kevin Kline, Kevin Bacon, and Kevin Costner. Their reputations belie the fact that the name originated with a saint in the seventh century A.D. who headed a monastery in Dublin. Even today, however, Saint Kevin is the patron saint of Dublin. Variations: *Kavan, Kev, Kevan, Keven, Kevon, Kevyn.*

KIRBY (English) Village of the church. Variations: *Kerbey, Kerbi, Kerbie, Kirbey, Kirbie.*

KIRK (Scandinavian: Norwegian) Church. Kirk was once an extremely appealing name, owing to the success of Michael's father, Kirk Douglas. Variations: *Kerk, Kirke.*

KITO (African: Swahili) Jewel.

KLAUS (German) Victorious people. Short for Nicholas. I don't think this name is going to be on the top ten list anytime soon, what with such personalities as Klaus Barbie, Claus von Bulow, and the ubiquitous Santa all boasting this name. Variations: *Claes, Claus, Clause, Klaas, Klaes.*

KNOWLES (English) Grassy hill. Variations: *Knolls, Nowles.*

KNOX (English) Hills.

KNUTE (Scandinavian: Danish) Knot.

KOJO (African: Ghanian) Born on Monday.

KWAN (Korean) Powerful.

KYLE (Scottish) Narrow land. When I was at the beach last summer, there must have been at least four little boys under the age of five with the name of Kyle running around. Though Kyle is also a popular choice for girls these days, the name for boys has made it into the top twenty most popular names of the '90s. In Hebrew, it means crowned with laurel. Since the name is so newly popular, expect it to be prominent for the next five to ten years. Variations: *Kiel, Kile, Ky, Kyele, Kyler.*
KYROS (Greek) Master.

LA VONN (African-American) The small one. Variations: *La Vaun, La Voun.*
LAMBERT (German) Bright land. Variations: *Lambard, Lampard; (*Scandinavian) Famous land. Variation: *Lammert.*
LANGSTON (English) Long town. Variations: *Langsden, Langsdon.*
LASZLO (Hungarian) Famous leader. Variations: *Laslo, Lazuli.*
LAWRENCE (English) Crowned with laurel. The name Lawrence has been popular with great regularity since it first emerged in the third century A.D.; Saint Lawrence was a martyr. Throughout the ages, this name has made regular appearances in the work of Shakespeare and in other literature, including *Lawrence of Arabia.* Lawrence was a very popular name in the '40s and '50s, but even back then parents were actively considering variations of the name, which is how we ended up with Lorne Green, Lorne Michaels, and Lorenzo Lamas. Today, parents are once again choosing the name Lawrence for their sons. Variations: *Larry, Laurance, Laurence, Laurencio, Laurens, Laurent, Laurenz, Laurie, Lauris, Laurus, Lawrance, Lawrey, Lawrie, Lawry, Loren, Lorence, Lorencz, Lorens, Lorenzo, Lorin, Lorry, Lowrance.*
LAWSON (English) Son of Lawrence.
LAWTON (English) Town on a hill. Variation: *Laughton.*
LEE (English) Meadow. It seems that the name Lee has always been hugely popular, both as a first and last name and as a good name for both boys and girls. Today, parents who see the simple spelling of Lee as a bit too run-of-the-mill are frequently choosing Leigh. Or, more frequently, they are tacking it on to the end of another boys' name, creating names like Lynnlee and Huntleigh. Lee Marvin, Lee Iaccoca, and even Lee Harvey Oswald have all contributed to the visibility of this name. Variation: *Leigh.*
LEIF (Scandinavian: Norwegian) Beloved. Leif is a great choice for parents who like the name Lee but who need something a little bit more exciting. Famous Leifs have included Leif Garrett and Leaf Phoenix, brother of the late River. Variations: *Leaf, Lief.*
LEIGHTON (English) Town by the meadow. Variations: *Layton, Leyton.*
LENNOX (Scottish) Many elm trees. Depending upon how you spell this name, it could have the feel of fine china—Lenox—or of a bull in a china shop—Lennox. Variation: *Lenox.*
LEON (Greek) Lion. Variations: *Leo, Leonas, Leone, Leonek, Leonidas, Leosko.*
LEONARD (German) Bold as a lion. Leonard owes most of its present visibility to popular culture. Leonardo is one of the Mutant Ninja Turtles, a group of hugely popular cartoon characters. The young actor Leonardo di Caprio has had leading roles in several recent movies, including *What's Eating Gilbert Grape?* and *Romeo and Juliet.* In fact, given the name's positive and somewhat exotic connotations, Leonard might be making a comeback. Nevertheless, several men who were named Leonard promptly gave up the name once they got into the entertainment field, including Tony Randall and Roy Rogers. Variations: *Len, Lenard, Lennard, Lenny, Leonardo, Leonek, Leonhard, Leonhards, Leonid, Leontes, Lienard, Linek, Lon, Lonnie, Lonny.*
LEROY (French) The king. Variations: *Le Roy, LeeRoy, Leeroy, LeRoi, Leroi, LeRoy.*
LESLIE (Scottish) Low meadow. One famous Leslie who held onto his name is the actor Leslie Howard; one who let go of it was Bob Hope. He had to or else he would have been known as Less Hope! Variations: *Les, Leslea, Lesley, Lesly, Lezly.*
LESTER (English) Last name. Area in Britain, Leicester. Like its cousin Leslie, Lester has gone way out of fashion. The most famous Lester in recent years has been the character Les Nessman on the old sitcom *WKRP in Cincinnati.* Variation: *Les.*
LEVI (Hebrew) Attached. Variations: *Levey, Levin, Levon, Levy.*

LEYLAND (English) Uncultivated land.

LINCOLN (English) Today, Lincoln is more likely to be used as Linc after the character on the TV series *Mod Squad*. Variations: *Linc, Link*.

LINDELL (English) Valley of the linden trees. Variations: *Lindall, Lindel, Lyndall, Lyndell*.

LINDSAY (English) Island of linden trees. Variations: *Lindsee, Lindsey, Lindsy, Linsay, Linsey, Lyndsay, Lyndsey*.

LINFORD (English) Ford of linden trees. Variation: *Lynford*.

LIONEL (Latin) Little lion. Variations: *Leonel, Lionell, Lionello, Lonell, Lonnell*.

LIVINGSTON (English) Leif's settlement. Singer Livingston Taylor is perhaps the best-known Livingston around. The name itself is rarely used, but presents a good choice for parents who are looking for a name that is distinctive and just a bit different, but still commands respect. Variation: *Livingstone*.

LLOYD (Welsh) Gray or sacred. Variation: *Loyd*.

LOGAN (Irish) Hollow in a meadow. Logan is one of those names that manages to convey a wealth of different connotations, all of them positive. What comes to mind? Swift, smart, sexy, and just a bit intriguing.

LORNE (Scottish) Area in Scotland. Variation: *Lorn*.

LOUDON (German) A low valley. Variations: *Louden, Lowden, Lowdon*.

LOUIS (French) Famous warrior. Louis is an old and highly esteemed French name. Dating from the sixth century A.D., Louis has been the name of no fewer than eighteen kings in France, a great jazz trumpeter, and my own father. Today, Louis is on the verge of making a comeback. It is that kind of traditional yet non-boring name that might just appeal to parents today. Variations: *Lew, Lewe, Lotario, Lothair, Lothar, Lothario, Lou, Luigi, Luis*.

LOWELL (English) Young wolf. Variation: *Lowel*.

LUCAS (English) An area in southern Italy. Lucas is cool. It is a very popular name today, partially because it makes a great name for a little boy toddling around and a teenager who grows six inches a year as well as for a sensitive, handsome adult who you'd be proud to call your son. Lucas conveys a sense of intrigue, and it's on the verge of becoming more frequently chosen,

even for girls. Luke, another version of the name, is also very popular, though it seems to be on the downswing while Lucas has not yet peaked. Variations: *Loukas, Luc, Lukas, Luke*.

LUCIUS (Latin) Light. Variations: *Luca, Lucan, Lucca, Luce, Lucian, Luciano, Lucias, Lucien, Lucio*.

LUDWIG (German) Famous soldier.

LUTHER (German) Army people. Luther has been popular in the past as a middle name, probably owing to Martin Luther King. The visibility of singer Luther Vandross, however, may make this name more popular as a first name in the next few years.

LYLE (French) The island. Lyle is one those wonderful, lazy names that conjures up long summer afternoons on the porch when it's too hot to do anything but drink a glass of lemonade. Singer Lyle Lovett only encourages this image and probably also the name's usage in coming years. Variations: *Lisle, Ly, Lyall, Lyell, Lysle*.

LYNDEN (English) Hill with lime trees. Variations: *Linden, Lyndon, Lynne*.

LYSANDER (Greek) Liberator. Variation: *Lisandro*.

MAC (Scottish) Son of. Variation: *Mack*.

MACAULAY (Scottish) Son of the moral one.

MACBRIDE (Irish) Son of Saint Brigid. Variations: *Macbryde, McBride*.

MACDONALD (Scottish) Son of Donald. The Macdonalds were a powerful Scottish clan. Variations: *MacDonald, McDonald*.

MACGOWAN (Irish) Son of the blacksmith. Variations: *MacGowan, Magowan, McGowan*.

MACKENZIE (Irish) Son of a wise leader. Variations: *Mack, MacKenzie, Mackey, Mackie, McKenzie*.

MACKINLEY (Irish) Learned ruler. Variations: *MacKinley, McKinley*.

MADDOX (Welsh) Generous. Variations: *Maddock, Madock, Madox*.

MADISON (English) Son of the mighty warrior. Whether it's an avenue, a president, or a baby name, Madison is an up-and-comer, for both girls and boys. Variations: *Maddie, Maddison, Maddy, Madisson*.

MADU (African: Nigerian) People.

MAGUIRE (Irish) Son of the beige man. Variations: *MacGuire, McGuire, McGwire*.

MAKOTO (Japanese) Honesty.

MALCOLM (English) A servant. Malcolm is currently popular although it used to be about the nerdiest name that any kid could have. Its burgeoning popularity has probably been helped along by Malcolm X, Malcolm-Jamal Warner from the *Cosby* show, and even the late publisher Malcolm Forbes. Variations: *Malcolum, Malcom, Malkolm.*

MALLORY (French) Sad. Variations: *Mallery, Mallorie, Malory.*

MANDELA (African-American) Name of the South African president.

MANFRED (English) Man of peace. Variations: *Manafred, Manafryd, Manfrid, Manfried, Mannfred, Mannfryd.*

MANLEY (English) Man's meadow. Variations: *Manlea, Manleigh, Manly.*

MANSFIELD (English) Field by a river. One couple conceived their youngest in Stowe, Vermont, and named him in honor of Mount Mansfield.

MANSUR (Arabic) Divine assistance. Variation: *Mansour.*

MARCUS (Latin) Warlike. Marcus is one of the more popular names that African-American parents have been giving their sons these days. Variations: *Marco, Marcos.*

MARIO (Italian) Roman clan name.

MARK (English) Warlike. No one could really put their finger on why this name became so suddenly popular in the early '60s. In 1976, of course, Olympic swimmer Mark Spitz and his victories set off a whole new wave of babies named Mark, but it didn't seem to last as long as the first wave. Before these two recent waves, the most famous Marks were Mark Antony, Saint Mark, and the writer Samuel Clemens, who is known by his pen name, Mark Twain. Today, parents who are partial to the name tend to choose one of the variations listed here and not its original incarnation. Variations: *Marc, Marco, Marko, Markos.*

MARSHALL (French) One who cares for horses. Because this name conveys such an in-charge tone, perhaps people in the military will prefer it for their kids, but for the rest of us, expect it to be quite an unusual choice. Variations: *Marschal, Marsh, Marshal.*

MARTIN (Latin) Warlike. Martin was always much more popular as a last name than a first name, except of course in the case of the Reverend Martin Luther King, Jr., who ironically was first christened with the name Michael. The feminine forms of Martin—Martina and Martine—seem to be more popular today than the male version. Most parents who use the name for their sons today tend to use it as a middle name. Variations: *Mart, Martan, Martel, Marten, Martey, Martie, Martinas, Martiniano, Martinka, Martino, Martinos, Martins, Marto, Marton, Marty, Martyn, Mertin.*

MARVIN (English) Mariner. Variations: *Marv, Marvyn.*

MASON (French) Stone carver or worker. Variations: *Mace, Masson.*

MATTHEW (Hebrew) Gift of the Lord. Matthew has been a very popular name, both 2,000 years ago and today. Though one of its offshoots—Hugh—may have fallen into disfavor recently owing to a popular British actor's dalliances, this should not affect the wild popularity of Matthew anytime soon. Why? Matthew is a more interesting name than many of the other traditional Biblical names, for instance, John and James, but it is also immensely helped by the multitudes of attractive Hollywood men with the name. There's Matthew Broderick, Matthew Modine, and Matt Dillon. And if Matthew doesn't strike your fancy, there are many variations for you to choose from to inject a little spice into your son's name. Variations: *Mateo, Mateus, Mathe, Mathew, Mathia, Mathias, Mathieu, Matias, Matt, Matteo, Matthaus, Matthia, Matthias, Mattias, Matty.*

MAURICE (Latin) Dark-skinned. Variations: *Maurey, Mauricio, Maurie, Mauris, Maurise, Maurizio, Maury, Morey, Morice, Morie, Moris, Moriss, Morrice, Morrie, Morris, Morriss, Morry.*

MAXIMILIAN (Latin) Greatest. Variations: *Maksim, Maksimka, Maksum, Massimiliano, Massimo, Max, Maxi, Maxie, Maxim, Maxime, Maximilano, Maximiliano, Maximillian, Maximino, Maximo, Maximos, Maxy.*

MAXWELL (Scottish) Marcus's well. Twenty years ago who could have ever foreseen the vast popularity of the name Max today? Parents who are choosing this name for their sons invariably give them the full name of Maxwell but refer to them as Max. Max is probably cool because it has an "x" in it, which follows the lead of the many radio stations in the early '90s that changed their call letters so that at least one of the letters would be an "x." In this case, and in the case of the name Max, the "x" does not refer to a movie that you need to be eighteen or over to see, but a trend that is very hot that shows no signs of burning out anytime soon. Variation: *Max.*

MAYER (Latin) Larger. Variations: *Mayor, Meier, Meir, Meirer, Meuer, Myer.*

MAYNARD (English) Hard strength. Variations: *Maynhard, Meinhard, Menard.*

MELVIN (Irish) Great chief. Although other clearly nerdy names have become popular today, even an actor with Mel Gibson's appeal doesn't seem to be popularizing this name—notice that he goes by the short form. Variations: *Malvin, Malvinn, Malvon, Malvonn, Mel, Melvern, Melvyn, Melwin, Melwinn.*

MENACHEM (Hebrew) Comforting. Variations: *Menahem, Mendel.*

MEREDITH (Welsh) Great leader. Variations: *Meredyth, Merideth, Meridith.*

MERLIN (English) Falcon. Merlin actually originated as a name for girls, but the name gradually gravitated to common use for males. While actress Merle Oberon is the most famous female of this name, the name and its variations are mostly claimed by male celebrities: Merle Haggard and Merlin Olsen. Variations: *Marlin, Marlon, Merle, Merlen, Merlinn, Merlyn, Merlynn.*

MERRILL (English) Bright as the sea. Masculine version of Murie. Variations: *Meril, Merill, Merrel, Merrell, Merril, Meryl.*

MESHACH (Hebrew) Unknown definition.

MICHAEL (Hebrew) Who is like God? Along with Mohammed and John, Michael could be one of the most popular boys' names in the world in any language. The reasons? Famous Michaels get lots of press, both good and bad, and as a result, the name is always out there. In addition, the name is liberally scattered through both the Old and New Testaments as well as throughout the Koran. Today's famous Michaels include Michael Millken, Michael J. Fox, Michael Jackson, Michael Jordan, and Michael Douglas, plus others with variations of the name: Mickey Rourke, Mickey Rooney, and Mick Jagger. Michael has been at the top of the names list in this country for over four decades. Variations: *Makis, Micah, Micha, Michail, Michak, Michal, Michalek, Michau, Micheal, Michel, Michele, Mick, Mickel, Mickey, Mickie, Micky, Miguel, Mihail, Mihailo, Mihkel, Mikaek, Mikael, Mikala, Mike, Mikelis, Mikey, Mikhail, Mikhalis, Mikhos, Mikkel, Mikko, Mischa, Misha, Mitch, Mitchel, Mitchell.*

MILO (German) Generous.

MILTON (English) Mill town.

MOHAMMED (Arabic) Greatly praised. If Michael is the most popular name in the United States and many European countries, then Mohammed and its numerous variations is probably the most popular name in Muslim countries, if not actually the world. Mohammed is the name of the prophet of Islam, and the popularity of the name could possibly be explained by an old Muslim proverb: If you have a hundred sons, give them all the name of Mohammed. The name is also becoming hugely popular among African-Americans. The most famous recent bearer of this name, obviously, is the great fighter Mohammed Ali. Variations: *Ahmad, Amad, Amed, Hamdrem, Hamdum, Hamid, Hammad, Hammed, Humayd, Mahmed, Mahmoud, Mahmud, Mehemet, Mehmet, Mohamad, Mohamed, Mohamet, Mohammad, Muhammad.*

MONTEL (English) Unknown definition. As with his counterpart named Arsenio, talk-show host Montel Williams probably provided most Americans with their first exposure to his name. However, as is the case with any unusual name that is exposed by a celebrity, you should be on the lookout for a rash of Montels over the next few years.

MORGAN (Welsh) Great and bright. Variations: *Morgen, Morrgan.*

MOSES (Hebrew) Arrived by water. Variations: *Moise, Moises, Moisey, Mose, Mosese, Mosha, Moshe, Moss, Moyse, Moze, Mozes.*

MURDOCH (Scottish) Sailor. Variations: *Murdo, Murdock, Murtagh.*

MURRAY (Scottish) Mariner. Murray is another one of those great last-names-as-first-names that is perfectly posed for rejuvenation. Somewhat popular during the '40s and '50s, Murray has fallen out of favor and has since been used mostly as a middle name. Be the first on your block to use it as a first name. Variations: *Murrey, Murry.*

MYERS (English) One who lives in a swamp. Variation: *Myer.*

MYRON (Greek) Aromatic oil. Variations: *Miron, Myreon.*

NAJIB (Arabic) Smart. Variations: *Nagib, Najeeb.*

NATHAN (Hebrew) Gift from God. The real name of the late, great comedian George Burns was Nathan, and though the name might seem really stodgy or old-fashioned, it is actually very popular today. Not only is it in the top hundred boys' names of the 1990s, but it was also on the top hundred list back in George Burns's day. Nathan was the name of a prophet who appeared in the Old Testament book of II Samuel, and it's been around ever since. Nathan is a pretty common name in Great Britain and Australia, as well as in the United States. Famous Nathans who kept their names include Nathaniel Hawthorne and Nat King Cole. Variations: *Nat, Natan, Nataniele, Nate, Nathanial, Nathaniel, Nathen, Nathon, Natt, Natty.*

NAVEED (Hindu) Good thoughts.

NEHRU (East Indian) Canal.

NEIL (Irish) Champion. Neil is an easygoing name; its original spelling is Niall. Famous Neils include Neil Simon, Neil Sedaka, and Neil Young. Variations: *Neal, Neale, Neall, Nealle, Nealon, Neile, Neill, Neille, Neils, Nels, Niadh, Nial, Niall, Nialle, Niel, Niels, Nigel, Niles, Nilo.*

NELSON (English) Son of Neil. The former vice-president Nelson Rockefeller probably didn't have the effect of enhancing the popularity of the name Nelson, but it is beginning to gain some ground these days. Other Nelsons include Nelson Mandela and singer Nelson Eddey. Variations: *Nealson, Neilson, Nilson, Nilsson.*

NEVILLE (French) New town. Variations: *Nevil, Nevile, Nevill, Nevyle.*

NEWELL (English) New hall. Variations: *Newall, Newel, Newhall.*

NEWTON (English) New town.

NICHOLAS (Greek) People of victory. Nicholas has been hot for about the last two decades. Nicholas was first mentioned in the Book of Acts, and the Biblical figure was followed by Saint Nicholas, who is considered to be the patron saint of children (and eventually transmogrified into Santa Claus). Why is Nicholas so popular? It just sounds like a folksy, friendly name that will serve a boy well from toddlerhood all the way through to grampahood. Whether it's little Nicky or Grampa Nick, Nicholas fits no matter what the age. Famous Nicholases, besides Santa Claus, include the

protagonist of *Nicholas Nickleby* by Dickens and Nicholson Baker. Though some feel the name is too popular, most parents who choose the name for their sons won't agree. Variations: *Nic, Niccolo, Nichol, Nick, Nickolas, Nickolaus, Nicky, Nicol, Nicolaas, Nicolai, Nicolas, Nikita, Nikki, Nikky, Niklas, Niklos, Niko, Nikolai, Nikolais, Nikolas, Nikolaus, Nikolo, Nikolos, Nikos, Nikula.*

NIGEL (Irish) Champion. Variation of Neil. Variations: *Nigal, Nigiel, Nigil.*

NISHAD (Hindu) Seventh note of a scale.

NOAH (Hebrew) Rest. Every little kid knows who Noah is, and so do an increasing number of parents who are choosing this name for their baby boys. Of course, any child with this name should expect the requisite ribbing: where's your Ark? Variations: *Noach, Noak, Noe, Noi, Noy.*

NOAM (Hebrew) Delight.

NOEL (French) Christmas. Variations: *Natal, Natale, Nowel, Nowell.*

NOLAN (Irish) Little proud one. Variations: *Noland, Nolen, Nolin, Nollan, Nuallan.*

NORMAN (English) Northerner. The name Norman originated from the French tribe in Normandy which is most famous for invading England in the year 1066. Despite its strong, warlike history, today Norman mostly conjures up the image of a small, frail boy with big glasses who is always getting beat up out on the playground. Despite his personality, the novelist Norman Mailer has not done much to reverse this image. Neither has Norman Bates in *Psycho*. Variations: *Norm, Normand, Normando, Normen, Normie.*

NORRIS (English) Northerner. Alternative spellings: Noris, Norreys, Norrie, Norriss, Norry.

NORTON (English) Northern town.

NURI (Arabic) Light. Variations: *Noori, Nur, Nuria, Nuriel, Nury.*

OAKLEY (English) Meadow of oak trees. Variations: *Oaklee, Oakleigh, Oakly.*

OBADIAH (Hebrew) Servant of God. Obadiah has the potential to catch on among parents who would like to give their baby boys a name from the Bible that is just a bit different. One of its nicknames, Obie, is close to Opie, the character played by an extremely young Ron

Howard back in the wholesome days of TV sitcoms. Variations: *Obadias, Obe, Obed, Obediah, Obie, Ovadiach, Ovadiah.*

OBERON (German) Noble and bearlike. Variations: *Auberon, Auberron.*

OBI (African: Nigerian) Heart.

OCTAVIUS (Latin) Eighth child. Variations: *Octave, Octavian, Octavien, Octavio, Octavo, Ottavio.*

OGDEN (English) Valley of oak trees. Variations: *Ogdan, Ogdon.*

OLAF (Scandinavian) Forefather. Olaf is a very common name in Norway. There have been many other ethnic names that have become part of the American culture, but Olaf doesn't seem as if it will ever totally fit in. What comes to my mind is that the name is just too close to the word oaf. And so despite its esteemed background—Olaf served as the name of no fewer than five Norwegian kings—it will probably never be a popular name here. Variations: *Olaff, Olav, Olave, Olen, Olin, Olof, Olov, Olyn.*

OLEG (Russian) Holy. The chance of Oleg's reaching the top hundred names list in this country is just a little less remote than the chances for Olaf, primarily because of Oleg's association with the designer Oleg Cassini. Variation: *Olezka.*

OLIVER (Latin) Olive tree. Variations: *Oliverio, Olivero, Olivier, Olivor, Olley, Ollie, Olliver, Ollivor.*

OMAR (Hebrew) Eloquent. Omar Sharif, General Omar Bradley, and poet Omar Khayyam have all lent exposure to this name. Despite the lack of a public figure with this name today, some parents are beginning to consider this name for their own sons. Variations: *Omarr, Omer.*

OREN (Hebrew) Ash tree. Variations: *Orin, Orrin.*

ORION (Greek) Son of fire or light; sunrise. Mythological son of Poseidon.

ORLANDO (Italian) Famous land. Variations: *Ordando, Orland, Orlande, Orlo.*

ORRICK (English) Old oak tree. Variation: *Orric.*

ORSON (Latin) Bearlike. Orson Welles—whose real first name was George—put this name on the map. Today the name seems to be making a comeback, probably in deference to the late great actor from *Citizen Kane.* Variations: *Orsen, Orsin, Orsini, Orsino.*

ORTON (English) Shore town.

ORVILLE (French) Golden town. Variations: *Orv, Orval, Orvell, Orvelle, Orvil.*

OSAKWE (African: Nigerian) God agrees.

OSCAR (English) Divine spear. Back when Oscar the Grouch first arrived on the scene, Jack Klugman was starring as Oscar Madison in *The Odd Couple.* The reputations that both of these Oscars had back then tended to discourage parents from choosing the name for their own kids. Today, however, Oscar is considered to be cool, and actually a way to poke fun at our earlier associations with the name. The great success of Steven Spielberg's movie *Schindler's List,* about Oskar Schindler, will probably do a lot to enhance the name. Other famous Oscars have included Oscar Wilde, Oscar Hammerstein, and Oscar de la Renta. Variations: *Oskar, Osker, Ossie.*

OSMAN (Polish) God protects.

OSWALD (English) Divine power. Variations: *Ossie, Osvald, Oswaldo, Oswall, Oswell.*

OTIS (English) Son of Otto.

OTTO (German) Wealthy. Otto is so out on a limb that there are some people who consider it to be a cutting-edge name to give their sons. Otto is popular all over the world, including in Hungary, Germany, Sweden, and Russia. Variations: *Odo, Otello, Othello, Otho, Othon, Oto, Ottomar.*

OWEN (Welsh) Well born. Owen could easily be considered a second cousin to the name Evan. Some parents consider Owen to be a better name than Evan these days, since the latter is a bit overused. Variations: *Owain, Owin.*

OXFORD (English) Oxen crossing a river.

PADDY (Irish) Nickname for Patrick. Variations: *Paddey, Paddie.*

PAGE (French) Intern. Variation: *Paige.*

PALMER (English) Carrying palm branches. Palmer is one of those mild-mannered last names that is quickly catching on as a popular first name for both boys and girls. Look for Palmer to make gentle inroads into the top hundred names for boys. Variations: *Pallmer, Palmar.*

PARIS (English) The city. Variation: *Parris.*

PARKER (English) Park keeper. Though actress Parker Posey has recently leapt onto the Hollywood scene with a great flourish, Parker actually started out as a popular boys' name during the 1800s in this country. The most famous male Parker was of course Parker Stevenson, who played in the *Hardy Boys* TV show. Variations: *Park, Parke, Parkes, Parks.*

PARNELL (French) Little Peter. Variations: *Parkin, Parnel, Parrnell.*

PARRISH (English) County; church area. Variation: *Parish.*

PASCAL (French) Easter child. Variations: *Pascale, Pascalle, Paschal, Pascoe, Pascow, Pasqual, Pasquale.*

PATRICK (Irish) Noble man. Today, parents who have absolutely no ethnic connection to Ireland are choosing the name Patrick for their sons. Saint Patrick, the patron saint of Ireland, has been popular all over the world for the last two centuries. There are a slew of famous Patricks in this country, including Pat Boone, Patrick O'Neil, Patrick Ewing, and Patrick Swayze. Parents who like the name but who want something just a little bit different for their own sons are choosing one of the many variations of the name. Variations: *Paddey, Paddie, Paddy, Padraic, Padraig, Padruig, Pat, Patek, Patric, Patrice, Patricio, Patricius, Patrik, Patrizio, Patrizius, Patryk.*

PATTON (English) Soldier's town. Variations: *Paten, Patin, Paton, Patten, Pattin.*

PAUL (Latin) Small. Most of the little kids running around lately with the name Paul have actually been given one of the name's more exotic varieties, of which there are many to choose from. Paul was big in the '60s, which could be solely due to the lead Beatle, Paul McCartney. Variations: *Pablo, Pal, Pali, Palika, Pall, Paolo, Pasha, Pashenka, Pashka, Paska, Paulin, Paulino, Paulis, Paulo, Pauls, Paulus, Pauly, Pavel, Pavils, Pavlicek, Pavlik, Pavlo, Pavlousek, Pawel, Pawl, Pol, Poul.*

PAXTON (English) Peaceful town. Variations: *Packston, Pax, Paxon, Paxten.*

PAYNE (Latin) Countryman. Variation: *Paine.*

PEARSON (English) Son of Piers. Variation: *Pierson.*

PELEKE (Hawaiian) Wise counselor. Variation: *Ferede.*

PEMBROKE (Irish) Cliff. Variation: *Pembrook.*

PERCY (English) Valley prisoner. Variations: *Pearce, Pearcey, Pearcy, Percey.*

PERRY (English) Traveler.

PETER (Greek) Rock. Peter is a common, friendly name that seems to be one of the oldest names around. It appears in the Bible as a saint's name, in a much-loved children's book, and in nursery rhymes—Peter Rabbit, Peter Piper—as well as onstage and in the movies: consider Peter O'Toole, Peter Sellers, and Peter Ustinov. Though it was popular as a Biblical name up until the sixteenth century, Peter fell out of favor until almost the early part of the twentieth century in both the United States and Europe. Peter has never been a trendy name; it's rock-solid like its definition. Variations: *Pearce, Pears, Pearson, Pearsson, Peat, Peder, Pedro, Peers, Peet, Peeter, Peirce, Petey, Petie, Petras, Petro, Petronio, Petros, Petter, Pierce, Piero, Pierre, Pierrot, Pierrson, Piers, Pierson, Piet, Pieter, Pietro, Piotr, Pyotr.*

PEYTON (English) Soldier's estate. Variation: *Payton.*

PHELAN (Irish) Wolf.

PHILIP (Greek) Lover of horses. In recent times, Philip has a bit of a regal feel to it, owing to Britain's Prince Philip. Philip was also one of the original twelve apostles in the Bible, and though the name was pretty popular in this country in the '60s, it seems that Philip is more common as a last name these days. The name Philip strikes many people as an exclusively French name; however, it is found in the languages of most European countries. Besides the prince, the Philip that many Americans are most familiar with is Phil Donahue. Variations: *Felipe, Felipino, Fil, Filib, Filip, Filipo, Filippo, Fillipek, Fillipp, Fillips, Phil, Philippel, Phill, Phillip, Phillipe, Phillipos, Phillipp, Phillippe, Phillips, Pilib, Pippy.*

PHINEAS (Hebrew) Oracle. Variation: *Pinchas.*

PHOENIX (Greek) Immortal. Variation: *Phenix.*

PICKFORD (English) Ford at a peak.

PITNEY (English) Island of a headstrong man. Variation: *Pittney.*

PLACIDO (Spanish) Peaceful. Singer Placido Domingo has added some degree of visibility to this name, and it might make the short list for parents who are looking for specifically Italian names for their sons. Variations: *Placid, Placidus, Placyd, Placydo.*

PORTER (Latin) Gatekeeper.

POWELL (English) Last name. General Colin Powell has brought this name to the forefront. There's no telling what the future for Powell as a first name will be if the general ever decides to enter politics, but it's safe to say that more parents would consider it for a possible first name for their sons. Variation: *Powel*.

PRENTICE (English) Apprentice. Variations: *Pren, Prent, Prentis, Prentiss*.

PRESCOTT (English) Priest's cottage. Variations: *Prescot, Prestcot, Prestcott*.

PRESTON (English) Priest's town. Preston seems to be one of those names that has great potential, but it still retains a bit of prissiness that keeps many parents from considering it for their sons.

PRICE (Welsh) The son of an ardent man. Variation: *Pryce*.

PRINCE (Latin) Prince. Variations: *Prinz, Prinze*.

PRYOR (Latin) Leader of the monastery. Variation: *Prior*.

PUTNAM (English) One who lives near a pond.

QUENTIN (Latin) Fifth. Names with "*x*"s and "*z*"s in them seem to be pretty popular right now and you would expect the same thing to be true of names with "*q*"s in them. Quentin is probably the leading candidate for the most common name that begins with a "Q," especially since actor and director Quentin Tarantino hit the bigtime with his movie *Pulp Fiction*. Variations: *Quent, Quenten, Quenton, Quint, Quinten, Quintin, Quinton, Quito*.

QUIGLEY (Irish) One with messy hair.

QUILLAN (Irish) Cub. Variation: *Quillen*.

QUIMBY (Norse) A woman's house. Variations: *Quenby, Quim, Quin, Quinby*.

QUINCY (French) The estate of the fifth son. Famous Quincys in recent years include the composer and singer Quincy Jones as well as the TV medical examiner Quincy played by actor Jack Klugman. Variation: *Quincey*.

QUINLAN (Irish) Strong man. Variations: *Quindlen, Quinley, Quinlin, Quinly*.

QUINN (Irish) Wise. Variation: *Quin*.

QUINTO (Spanish) Home ruler. Variation: *Quiqui*.

RACHIM (Hebrew) Compassion. Variations: *Racham, Rachmiel, Raham, Rahim*.

RADCLIFF (English) Red cliff. The name Radcliff has a tweedy, uppercrust sound to it. Mothers who might choose Radcliff may be thinking about their alma mater, Radcliffe. Variations: *Radcliffe, Radclyffe*.

RAFI (Arabic) Exalted.

RALEIGH (English) Deer meadow. Variations: *Rawleigh, Rawley, Rawly*.

RALPH (English) Wolf-counselor. Ralph Kramden is probably the first Ralph that comes to mind for most of us because reruns of *The Honeymooners* have been influential for decades. Variations: *Ralphie, Raoul, Raul, Raulas, Raulo, Rolf, Rolph*.

RANDOLPH (English) Wolf with a shield. One of the variations for Randolph, Randy, has become more popular as a given name than the original. Variations: *Randal, Randall, Randel, Randell, Randey, Randie, Randil, Randle, Randol, Randolf, Randy*.

RAOUL (French) Variation of Ralph. Variation: *Raul*.

RAPHAEL (Hebrew) God has healed. Contrary to popular opinion, Raphael is not a variation of Ralph, but a name that has stood on its own ever since Biblical times. One famous Raphael was the great painter; however, most kids and parents these days are more familiar with Raphael, the Teenage Mutant Ninja Turtle. Variations: *Rafael, Rafel, Rafello, Raffaello*.

RASHID (Turkish) Righteous. Variations: *Rasheed, Rasheid, Rasheyd*.

RAYMOND (German) Counselor and protector. Raymond began to catch on in the United States only in the mid-nineteenth century, before becoming one of the most popular names for boys in 1900. Famous Rays include Raymond Burr, the character that Dustin Hoffman played in the movie *Rainman*, Raymond Chandler, and Raymond Carver. Saint Raymond is considered to be the patron saint of lawyers, so if you don't particularly care for attorneys, better not choose that name for your son. Variations: *Raimondo, Raimund, Raimunde, Raimundo, Rajmund, Ramon, Ramond, Ramone, Ray, Rayment, Raymonde, Raymondo, Raymund, Raymunde, Raymundo, Reimond*.

REDMOND (Irish) Counselor. Variation of Raymond. Variations: *Radmond, Radmund, Redmund*.

REECE (Welsh) Fiery, zealous. Variations: *Rees, Reese, Rhys*.

REGINALD (English) Strong counselor. Reginald is almost never used as a proper name except when it stands in as the formal version of the much more popular Reggie. Famous Reggies include Reggie Jackson and Reggie White, but more often than not, famous men who were born with the name Reggie or Reginald have changed their names for ones they consider to be more suitable—like Rex Harrison and Elton John. Variations: *Reg, Reggie, Reginalt.*

REMINGTON (English) Family of ravens. Variations: *Rem, Remee, Remi, Remie, Remmy.*

RENNY (Irish) Small and mighty.

REUBEN (Hebrew) Behold a son. Most people consider the name Reuben only in the context of a heaping corned beef sandwich. However, Reuben is showing signs of bubbling up, especially among parents who are looking for a name with tradition and spirit; the Biblical Reuben founded one of the tribes of Israel. Who knows if this name will catch on? Think of the singer Ruben Blades and the Partridge family manager named Reuben Kincaid. Variations: *Reuban, Reubin, Reuven, Reuvin, Rube, Ruben, Rubin, Rubu.*

REX (Latin) King.

REYNOLD (English) Powerful adviser. Variations: *Ranald, Renald, Renaldo, Renauld, Renault, Reynaldo, Reynaldos, Reynolds, Rinaldo.*

RICHARD (German) Strong ruler. For much of this century, the name Richard gave the impression of a noble Englishman who was sent to this country to teach us some manners. This impression is probably due to the vast influx of noted British actors who began to make their way to Hollywood around the middle of the century. These men include Richard Burton, Richard Chamberlain, Richard Attenborough, and Richard Todd, among others. In the mid-1970s, however, Richard took a nosedive on the popularity charts of new baby boys, the same time that Richard M. Nixon left office. Variations: *Dic, Dick, Dickie, Dicky, Ricard, Ricardo, Riccardo, Ricciardo, Rich, Richardo, Richards, Richart, Richerd, Richi, Richie, Rick, Rickard, Rickert, Rickey, Rickie, Ricky, Rico, Rihards, Riki, Riks, Riocard, Riqui, Risa, Ritch, Ritchard, Ritcherd, Ritchie, Ritchy, Rostik, Rostislav, Rostya, Ryszard.*

RICHMOND (French) Lush mountain.

RIDGLEY (English) Meadow on a ridge. Variations: *Ridgeleigh, Ridgeley, Ridglea, Ridglee, Ridgleigh.*

RIDLEY (English) Red meadow. Variations: *Riddley, Ridlea, Ridleigh, Ridly.*

RILEY (Irish) Brave. Riley seems to be a good candidate for becoming more popular as a name for boys in the United States, since it is Irish and is traditionally thought of as a last name. Variations: *Reilly, Ryley.*

RIORDAN (Irish) Minstrel. Variations: *Rearden, Reardon.*

RIPLEY (English) Shouting man's meadow. Variations: *Ripleigh, Riply, Ripp.*

ROBERT (English) Bright fame. Robert is one of the most popular names in the world, especially here in the United States. It has endless variations in every language, and one theory holds that so many men were named Robert from the time of the Middle Ages up until today that many variants were necessary so that people could distinguish one Robert from another. Famous Roberts include Robert Kennedy, Robbie Robertson, Robert Taylor, Robert Wagner, Robert Young, Robert Redford, and Robert de Niro. Variations: *Bob, Bobbey, Bobbie, Bobby, Riobard, Rob, Robb, Robbi, Robbie, Robbin, Robby, Robbyn, Rober, Robers, Roberto, Roberts, Robi, Robin, Robinet, Robyn, Rubert, Ruberto, Rudbert, Ruperto, Ruprecht.*

RODERICK (German) Famous ruler. Actor Roddy McDowell and singer Rod Stewart have brought attention to this name, but Rod and Roderick have always been more popular in Britain than in this country. Variations: *Rod, Rodd, Roddie, Roddy, Roderic, Roderich, Roderigo, Rodique, Rodrich, Rodrick, Rodrigo, Rodrique, Rurich, Rurik.*

RODMAN (English) Famous man.

RODNEY (English) Island clearing. Variations: *Rodnee, Rodnie, Rodny.*

ROGER (German) Renowned spearman. There have been plenty of famous Rogers throughout the last couple of decades, including Roger Moore, Roger Daltree, and even Roger Rabbit. Variations: *Rodger, Rogelio, Rogerio, Rogerios, Rogers, Ruggerio, Ruggero, Rutger, Ruttger.*

ROLAND (German) Famous land. Shakespeare used the name Roland in his play *As You Like It*, and in three others. In Britain today a variation of Roland—Rollo—is very popular right now; here in the United States, Rollo is a type of chocolate candy. Variations: *Rolle, Rolli, Rollie, Rollin, Rollins, Rollo, Rollon, Rolly, Rolo, Rolon, Row, Rowe, Rowland, Rowlands, Rowlandson.*

ROMAN (Latin) One from Rome. Variations: *Romain, Romano, Romanos, Romulo, Romulos, Romulus.*

RONALD (English) Powerful adviser. As American politics go, so, frequently, go popular baby names. This certainly was the case with the growing visibility of Ronald in the early '80s. Variations: *Ranald, Ron, Ronn, Ronney, Ronni, Ronnie, Ronny.*

ROOSEVELT (Dutch) Field of roses.

ROSARIO (Portuguese) The rosary.

ROSCOE (Scandinavian) Deer forest.

ROSS (Scottish) Cape. Variations: *Rosse, Rossie, Rossy.*

ROWAN (Irish) Red. Variation: *Rowen.*

ROY (Irish) Red. Roy was a very popular boys' name in the '50s because of the cowboy singer Roy Rogers. In these days when parents prefer a baby name with lots of possibilities, Roy presents only one: Roy. Variation: *Roi.*

ROYCE (American) Roy's son. Variations: *Roice, Royse.*

RUDOLPH (German) Famous wolf. If you want your kid to spend the first ten Decembers of his life with his peers asking him where his red nose is, then you can go ahead and name your son Rudolph. The great Russian dancer, Rudolf Nureyev, unfortunately has done nothing to help redeem this name. Variations: *Rodolfo, Rodolph, Rodolphe, Rolf, Rolfe, Rolle, Rollo, Rolph, Rolphe, Rudey, Rudi, Rudie, Rudolf, Rudolfo, Rudolpho, Rudolphus, Rudy.*

RUFUS (Latin) Red-haired. Variations: *Ruffus, Rufo, Rufous.*

RUPERT (German) Bright fame. Variation of Robert. Variations: *Ruperto, Ruprecht.*

RUSH (English) Red-haired. And, some might say, bigmouthed. Ten years ago, it's a good bet that ninety-nine out of a hundred Americans had never heard of this name. As much as his fans say they admire him, there hasn't been a stampede to name a baby after Mr. Limbaugh.

RUSSELL (French) Red-haired. Variations: *Rus, Russ, Russel.*

RUSTY (French) Red-haired. Variation: *Rustie.*

RYAN (Irish) Last name. The growth in popularity of Ryan seemed to coincide with both the celebrity of Ryan O'Neill and American women's desire for the sensitive American man. Ryan is not a name you'd think of for a bully. But again, a big reason for its popularity is that it is an Irish name and a last name all

rolled into one, and most names today that fit this description can count on some degree of popularity. Variations: *Ryne, Ryon, Ryun.*

RYLAND (English) Land of rye. Variation: *Ryeland.*

RYSZARD (Polish) Brave ruler. Variant of Richard.

SABIR (Arabic) Patient. Variation: *Sabri.*

SADIKI (African: Swahili) Faithful.

SAEED (African: Swahili) Happy.

SAID (Arabic) Happy. Variations: *Saeed, Saied, Saiyid, Sayeed, Sayid, Syed.*

SALVATORE (Latin) Savior. Variations: *Sal, Salvador, Salvator.*

SAMIR (Arabic) Entertainer.

SAMUEL (Hebrew) God listens. Though Samuel has tended to be somewhat popular over the last 100 years or so, it seems that it has fallen in and out of favor. Right now, Sam is popular, perhaps owing to the success of playwright Sam Shepard and the history of the TV show *Cheers*, in which Sam Malone tended bar. Sam is just-another-guy name that should continue to be popular through the rest of this decade and beyond. Variations: *Sam, Sammie, Sammy, Samouel, Samuele, Samuello.*

SANBORN (English) Sandy river. Variations: *Sanborne, Sanbourn, Sanburn, Sanburne, Sandborn, Sandbourne.*

SANTIAGO (Spanish) Saint.

SAUL (Hebrew) Asked for. If the parents of Beatle Paul McCartney had given their son the original name of Paul the Apostle, then all those girls back in the '60s would have been yelling "Saul! Saul!" Novelist Saul Bellow is probably the most famous celebrity with this name.

SAWYER (English) Woodworker. Variations: *Sayer, Sayers, Sayre, Sayres.*

SCHUYLER (Dutch) Shield. Variations: *Schuylar, Skuyler, Skylar, Skyler.*

SCOTT (English) One from Scotland. Along with all those Scottie dogs in the '60s, not to mention the Scottish kilt craze that we had to live through, the popularity of the name Scott was a good indication of America's fascination with the British isles, even thirty years ago. Scott has always been an all-American name, belying its roots. Famous Scotts from the States include F. Scott Fitzgerald and Francis Scott Key, for whom

Fitzgerald was named. Today, the name still makes the rounds, but it could show signs of moving up once the phrase "Beam me up, Scottie," disappears from everyday use. Variations: *Scot, Scottie, Scotto, Scotty.*

SEAN (Irish) God is good. Variation of John. During the last decade or so, Sean also began to become popular as a girls' name, albeit with different spellings, most frequently Shawn. Today, Sean is still a pretty hip name for boy babies—perhaps actors Sean Penn and Sean Connery have something to do with it. Variations: *Seann, Shaine, Shane, Shaughn, Shaun, Shawn, Shayn, Shayne.*

SEBASTIAN (Latin) One from Sebastia, an ancient Roman city. Like Sean, Sebastian is a really cool name, although it doesn't get one-tenth of the play today that Sean does. This is changing, however; the name does seem to be popping up with greater frequency. Variations: *Seb, Sebastien, Sebbie.*

SERGE (Latin) Servant. Variations: *Serg, Sergei, Sergey, Sergi, Sergie, Sergio, Sergius.*

SETH (Hebrew) To appoint. Of the popular names today, Seth is unusual because it really has no nicknames or variations. Perhaps the sound of the name is still distinctive enough. Seth was the third son of Adam and Eve and was born after the death of his older siblings, Cain and Abel. It's interesting to note that in the past, the name Seth was frequently given to a newborn son after his parents had already lost a child. Today, Seth has no morbid association. It's just a neat name.

SEYMOUR (French) From St. Maur, a village in France. Seymour actually has quite haughty roots, but you'd never know it by the associations that most of us make with the name: that of an elderly, retired gentleman who likes to come up with new names for his grandchildren-to-be. Variations: *Seamor, Seamore, Seamour, Si, Sy.*

SHAFER (Hebrew) Handsome.

SHALOM (Hebrew) Peace. Variation: *Sholom.*

SHAMIR (Hebrew) Flint. Variation: *Shamur.*

SHANNON (Irish) Old. Shannon was once solely a name for boys, but sometime in the early 1940s, parents began to choose it for their girls as well. Today, Shannon appears much more frequently among girls than boys, perhaps helped along by the proliferation of girls' names that begin with "Sh." Variations: *Shannan, Shannen.*

SHAQUILLE (African-American) Newly created.

SHARIF (Hindu) Respected. Variations: *Shareef, Shereef, Sherif.*

SHELBY (English) Village on the ledge. Shelby seems to be a name with real possibilities, an acceptable alternative to an outdated name like Sheldon. However, as a name that begins with the letters "Sh," it may continue to be used more for girls than for boys. Variations: *Shelbey, Shelbie.*

SHEPHERD (English) Sheepherder. Variations: *Shep, Shepard, Shephard, Shepp, Sheppard, Shepperd.*

SHERWOOD (English) Shining forest. Variations: *Sherwoode, Shurwood.*

SHILOH (Hebrew) Unknown definition. Variation: *Shilo.*

SIDNEY (English) One from Sidney, a town in France. Sidney was once quite the aristocratic name; however, a slow and gradual adoption of the name by girls (with a "y" in place of the "i") has made this name a rarity for young boys today. Variations: *Sid, Siddie, Sidon, Sidonio, Syd, Sydney.*

SIMON (Hebrew) God hears. Simon is gaining ground today among parents who see an almost French distinction in the name. Variations: *Simeon, Simion, Simm, Simms, Simone, Symms, Symon.*

SNOWDEN (English) Snowy mountain. Variation: *Snowdon.*

SOCRATES (Greek) Named for the Greek philosopher. Variations: *Socritis, Sokrates.*

SOLOMON (Hebrew) Peaceable. One of the most obviously Old Testament names around, Solomon seems to be be making headway among parents who are looking for a Biblical name that is also somewhat hip. Variations: *Salamen, Salamon, Salamun, Salaun, Salman, Salmon, Salom, Salomo, Salomon, Salomone, Selim, Shelomoh, Shlomo, Sol, Solaman, Sollie, Solly, Soloman, Solomo, Solomonas, Solomone.*

SPALDING (English) Divided field. Before the famed monologuist Spalding Gray first became well known in the '80s, the common association most of us had with the name Spalding had to do with a tennis ball. Variation: *Spaulding.*

SPENCER (English) Seller of goods. Spencer is on the upswing in this country, and not only because actor Spencer Tracy continues to permeate the American consciousness through his movies with Katharine Hepburn, which are frequently rerun on cable channels. The 1980s detective TV show *Spenser: For Hire* also helped to make this name more visible. But the simple fact of the matter is that this name is just real cool. Look for it to become more popular through the rest of the '90s and into the twenty-first century. Variations: *Spence, Spense, Spenser.*

STANLEY (English) Stony meadow. Back in its day—which was around the middle of the nineteenth century—Stanley was quite a noble name. The most famous Stanley we know is the comic actor Stan Laurel, the better half of Laurel and Hardy. Variations: *Stan, Stanlea, Stanlee, Stanleigh, Stanly.*

STAVROS (Greek) Crowned.

STEADMAN (English) One who lives on a farm. Variations: *Steadmann, Stedman.*

STEPHEN (Greek) Crowned. Stephen holds the distinction of being the name of the first Christian on record; and its history has served as a built-in boost in any country where Christianity is practiced. The different variations of the name each provide clearly distinct feels. For instance, Steve Garvey and Steve McQueen have a somewhat swaggering personality, while Stephen Sondheim, Stephen King, and Steven Spielberg convey a more artistic image. The less formal version "Stevie" is claimed by two well-known musicians: Stevie Wonder and Stevie Ray Vaughan. Nowadays, Stephen with a "ph" is used less often than Steven with a "v." Though the name is not as popular as it once was, it is still used with some regularity, and it will be with us for quite some time. Variations: *Stefan, Stefano, Stefanos, Stefans, Steffan, Steffel, Steffen, Stefos, Stepa, Stepan, Stepanek, Stepek, Stephan, Stephane, Stephanos, Stephanus, Stephens, Stephenson, Stepka, Stepousek, Stevan, Steve, Steven, Stevenson, Stevie.*

STEWART (English) Steward. Variations: *Stew, Steward, Stu, Stuart.*

SULLIVAN (Irish) Black-eyed. With its last name origins and Irish roots, the stage is set for Sullivan to become more popularly used. Variations: *Sullavan, Sullevan, Sulliven.*

SUMANTRA (Hindu) Good advice.

SUTTON (English) Southern town.

SYLVESTER (Latin) Forested. From Sylvester Stallone to Sylvester the Cat all the way to Sylvester the disco singer from the '70s, this name is a veritable grab-bag of images and associations. Variations: *Silvester, Silvestre, Silvestro, Sly.*

TAGGART (Irish) Son of a priest.

TALBOT (English) Last name. Variations: *Talbert, Talbott, Tallbot, Tallbott.*

TANAY (Hindu) Son.

TANNER (English) One who tans leather. There are a slew of last names beginning with "T" that are currently very popular for use as a first names for boys. Tanner is one of a group that includes Tucker, Taylor, and Travis. Tanner is beginning to show strength, so don't be surprised if this name ends up on the top fifty or hundred names for the decade. Variations: *Tan, Tanier, Tann, Tanney, Tannie, Tanny.*

TATE (English) Happy. Variations: *Tait, Taitt, Tayte.*

TAYLOR (English) Tailor. Taylor is really gaining ground for both boys and girls in this country but there are signs that it will soon become the sole property of girls. Boys will have to switch to Tyler or another popular last name as first name that begins with "T." Variations: *Tailer, Tailor, Tayler, Taylour.*

TEMPLETON (English) Town near the temple. Variations: *Temple, Templeten.*

TENNESEE (Native American: Cherokee) The state.

TERENCE (Latin) Roman clan name. Twenty and thirty years ago, boys called Terry had Terence as their real names. Today, Terence has become somewhat of a relic since parents have been brave enough to name their sons Terry from the start. Terry is yet another instance of a name that started out being exclusively male, crossed over to become popular for both boys and girls, and then in the end, began to be associated almost exclusively with girls. Variations: *Tarrance, Terencio, Terrance, Terrence, Terrey, Terri, Terry.*

TERRILL (German) Follower of Thor. Variations: *Terrall, Terrel, Terrell, Terryl, Terryll, Tirrell, Tyrrell.*

THADDEUS (Aramaic) Brave. Variations: *Taddeo, Tadeo, Tadio, Thad, Thaddaus.*

THANOS (Greek) Royal. Variation: *Thanasis.*

THATCHER (English) Roof thatcher. Variations: *Thacher, Thatch, Thaxter.*

THEODORE (Greek) Gift from God. Variations: *Teador, Ted, Tedd, Teddey, Teddie, Teddy, Tedor, Teodor, Teodoro, Theo, Theodor.*

THEOPHILUS (Greek) Loved by God. Variations: *Teofil, Theophile.*

THOMAS (Aramaic) Twin. Saint Thomas was the impetus for this name as it started to become popular around the time of the Middle Ages. Today, Thomas is popular all over the world, and is one of the names that parents in this country are looking to in order to instill a sense of history and tradition in their own sons. Variations: *Tam, Tameas, Thom, Thoma, Thompson, Thomson, Thumas, Thumo, Tom, Tomas, Tomaso, Tomasso, Tomaz, Tomcio, Tomek, Tomelis, Tomi, Tomie, Tomislaw, Tomm, Tommy, Tomsen, Tomson, Toomas, Tuomas, Tuomo.*

THORNTON (English) Thorny town.

THURSTON (Scandinavian) Thor's stone. Variations: *Thorstan, Thorstein, Thorsteinn, Thorsten, Thurstain, Thurstan, Thursten, Torstein, Torsten, Torston.*

TIERNAN (Irish) Little lord. Variations: *Tierney, Tighearnach, Tighearnan.*

TIMOTHY (Greek) Honoring God. Any name that rhymes with Jimmy—like Timmy does—is a great name for a kid. Variations: *Tim, Timmothy, Timmy, Timo, Timofeo, Timon, Timoteo, Timothe, Timotheo, Timotheus, Timothey, Tymmothy, Tymothy.*

TITUS (Latin) Unknown definition. Variations: *Tito, Titos.*

TODD (English) Fox. Variation: *Tod.*

TONY (Latin) Nickname for Anthony that has evolved into its own freestanding name. Variations: *Toney, Tonie.*

TRACY (French) Area in France. Variations: *Trace, Tracey, Treacy.*

TRAVIS (French) Toll-taker. No one knows for sure why this name has suddenly become popular in the last ten or fifteen years, except for the fact that it is a last name that begins with the letter "T," which accounts for many of the newly popular boys' names. Travis sounds like it originates in Britain, but it is actually French; it appears infrequently in Britain. One famous celebrity with the name is Travis Tritt. Variations: *Traver, Travers, Travus, Travys.*

TRENT (Latin) Rushing waters. Variations: *Trenten, Trentin, Trenton.*

TREVOR (Welsh) Large homestead. Since Trevor seems to be cut from the same cloth as Travis, you'd think it would be nearly as popular. This is not the case, however, so feel free to use it and think of it as unique. Variations: *Trefor, Trev, Trevar, Trever, Trevis.*

TREY (English) Three.

TRISTAN (Welsh) Famous Welsh folklore character. Variations: *Tris, Tristam.*

TURNER (English) Woodworker.

TWAIN (English) Split in two. Variations: *Twaine, Twayn.*

TYLER (English) Tile maker. Tyler is an extremely popular name in the '90s for both boys and girls, though it is more widely used for boys. If you already have a child in nursery school, there's a good chance that one or more of the boys in your child's class is named Tyler. Parents like the name because it is both formal and casual. Variations: *Ty, Tylar.*

TYRONE (Irish) Land of Owen. Variations: *Tiron, Tirone, Ty, Tyron.*

TYSON (English) Firebrand. Variations: *Tieson, Tison, Tysen.*

TZACH (Hebrew) Clean. Variations: *Tzachai, Tzachar.*

UDELL (English) Yew grove. Variations: *Dell, Eudel, Udall, Udel.*

ULYSSES (Latin) Wrathful. Variation of Odysseus. Variations: *Ulises, Ulisse.*

UMBERTO (Italian) Famous German. Variation of Humbert.

UPTON (English) Hill town.

URI (Hebrew) God's light. Variations: *Uria, Uriah, Urias, Urie, Uriel.*

VAIL (English) City in Colorado. Variations: *Vaile, Vale, Vayle.*

VALENTINE (Latin) Strong. Variations: *Val, Valentin, Valentino, Valentyn.*

VALMIKI (Hindu) Ant hill.

VANCE (English) Swampland. Variations: *Van, Vancelo, Vann.*

VANDYKE (Dutch) From the dyke. Variation: *Van Dyck.*

VANYA (Russian) God is good. Variation of John. Variations: *Vanek, Vanka.*

VARICK (German) Defending ruler. Variation: *Varrick.*

VAUGHN (Welsh) Small. Perhaps the most famous man with the name Vaughn was the British composer Ralph Vaughan Williams. Even though the name is of Welsh origin, in the middle of this century, the name was much more popular in the United States than overseas. It's a great name, and not used nearly enough today. Variation: *Vaughan.*

VERNON (French) Alder tree. Variations: *Vern, Verne.*

VICTOR (Latin) Conqueror. Owing to its definition, Victor was one of the most popular names during the time of the Romans. It fell out of favor throughout most of the Middle Ages, until it became popular in Britain again in the early part of this century. In this country, two famous Victors were Victor Borge and Victor Mature. Variations: *Vic, Vick, Victoir, Victorien, Victorino, Victorio, Viktor, Vitenka, Vitor, Vittore, Vittorio, Vittorios.*

VINCENT (Latin) To conquer. Vincent has always been a popular name throughout the ages, however today, some people equate Vincent solely with the nicknames Vinnie and Vince. Famous Vincents have included Vincent Price and Vincent van Gogh, and although the name today seems a bit dated, it's an attractive name that parents-to-be should consider more often. Variations: *Vikent, Vikenti, Vikesha, Vin, Vince, Vincente, Vincenz, Vincenzio, Vincenzo, Vinci, Vinco, Vinn, Vinnie, Vinny.*

VIRGIL (Latin) Roman clan name. The name Virgil conjures up one of two distinct reactions from people: it's either the name for a refined, tall, thin British gentleman or a back-country hillbilly from the south. Though the name seems to be making somewhat of a comeback, it'll be hard to overcome these two ingrained associations. Variations: *Vergil, Virgilio.*

VITO (Latin) Alive. Variations: *Vital, Vitale, Vitalis.*

VITUS (French) Forest. Variation: *Vitya.*

VLADIMIR (Slavic) Famous prince. Variations: *Vlad, Vladamir, Vladimeer, Vladko, Vladlen.*

WADE (English) To cross a river. Wade is one of those short, compact names that seem to command respect without inviting teasing. Margaret Mitchell used the name in her novel *Gone with the Wind.*

WADSWORTH (English) Village near a river crossing. Variation: *Waddsworth.*

WAGNER (German) Wagon maker. Variation: *Waggoner.*

WAITE (English) Watchman. Variations: *Waits, Wayte.*

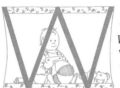

WALDEN (English) Forested valley. Walden is an attractive choice for parents today, because it falls into the category of nature names as well as last name as first name. Some parents will choose it out of deference to Henry David Thoreau and Walden Pond, while others will select it because of its fine upstanding manner and tone. Variation: *Waldon.*

WALDO (German) Strong.

WALKER (English) One who walks on cloth. Last name.

WALTER (German) Ruler of the people. Though to some ears Walter may sound a bit outdated, it seems to be rapidly gaining ground among parents-to-be as a name that is at once dignified and folksy. Though obviously the name isn't used as frequently as it was in the '30s and '40s, the far-reaching reputation of journalist Walter Cronkite has given this name a moral, honest feel to it. Other famous Walters include Walter Pidgeon, Walt Disney, and poet Walt Whitman. Today, African-American families are choosing the name Walter more frequently than their white counterparts. Variations: *Walt, Walther, Waltr, Watkin.*

WALTON (English) Walled town.

WARREN (German) Protector friend. Actor Warren Beatty has injected the name with a reputation of sex appeal and worldliness. Another famous American Warren was the president Warren Harding. Variations: *Warrin, Warriner.*

WASHINGTON (English) Town of smart men.

WAYNE (English) Wagon maker. Version of Wainwright. Variations: *Wain, Wainwright, Wayn, Waynwright.*

WEBSTER (English) Weaver. Variations: *Web, Webb, Weber.*

WENDELL (German) Wanderer. Variations: *Wendel, Wendle.*

WESLEY (English) Western meadow. Wesley first gained prominence as a religious last name, as two brothers, John and Charles Wesley, were the founders of the Methodist church in England. Parents who belonged to the church soon began to use the brothers' last name for their newborn sons' first names as a tribute to them. Today, Wesley is not among the most popular of names, but it could definitely be a sleeper. Variations: *Wes, Wesly, Wessley, Westleigh, Westley.*

WESTON (English) Western town. Variations: *Westen, Westin.*

WHARTON (English) Town on a river bank. Clearly some alums from the Wharton Business School in Philadelphia might want to name their sons Wharton because, after all, the skills acquired with the education at the famous business school are going to come in handy when it comes to supporting said baby. Though Wharton is more commonly used as a last name, it is beginning to show signs of acknowledgment as a first name. Variation: *Warton.*

WHEATLEY (English) Wheat field. Variations: *Wheatlea, Wheatleigh, Wheatlie, Wheatly.*

WHEELER (English) Wheel maker.

WHITCOMB (English) White valley. Variation: *Whitcombe.*

WHITELAW (English) White hill. Variation: *Whitlaw.*

WHITFIELD (English) White field.

WHITLOCK (English) White lock of hair.

WHITNEY (English) White island.

WILBUR (German) Brilliant. Though Wilbur means brilliant, it might be difficult to convince more parents of this definition since most of them will probably associate the name Wilbur with a man who is dumb enough to spend whole days talking to a horse, since Mr. Ed did such a great job of trilling the name. Variations: *Wilber, Wilbert, Wilburt, Willbur.*

WILEY (English) Water meadow. Variations: *Willey, Wylie.*

WILLIAM (German) Constant protector. William is one of the most popular names throughout English-speaking countries. There are a slew of famous Williams, including Prince William, William Shakespeare, Billy Idol, Willem Dafoe, Will Smith, William Faulkner, William Holden, and Willem De Kooning; four American presidents, several kings, and plenty of knights. William is as popular today in this country as it was in the 1040s. Currently, African-American parents appear to be choosing this name for their sons more frequently than white parents are. Although there are a myriad of variations of the name, the traditional William is most common as both a given name and the everyday name that parents use

to refer to their sons. Variations: *Bill, Billie, Billy, Guillaume, Guillaums, Guillermo, Vas, Vasilak, Vasilious, Vaska, Vassos, Vila, Vildo, Vilek, Vilem, Vilhelm, Vili, Viliam, Vilkl, Ville, Vilmos, Vilous, Will, Willem, Willi, Williamson, Willie, Willil, Willis, Willy, Wilson, Wilhelm.*

WILSON (English) Son of Will. Variation: *Willson.*

WINSTON (English) Friend's town. One woman named her sons Benson and Winston; can you guess why? Of course, she and her husband were both smokers and while she smoked Benson and Hedges, he favored Winstons. Fortunately, they stopped smoking shortly after the birth of Winston, and it's likely that the children's very names served as a reinforcement for the couple to stay off of cigarettes. Variations: *Winsten, Winstone, Winstonn, Winton, Wynstan, Wynston.*

WOLFGANG (German) Wolf fight. Wolfgang Puck—the famous chef—has brought new visibility to this name. Wolf and Wolfie are great nicknames for the name as long as you tell your son not to bite.

WOODROW (English) Row in the woods. Variations: *Wood, Woody.*

WYATT (French) Little fighter. If you name your son Wyatt, the immediate reaction from both adults and children will be to think of a cowboy. Variations: *Wiatt, Wyat.*

WYNN (English) Friend. Variations: *Win, Winn, Wynne.*

XAVIER (English) New house. In a game of word association, the name Xavier will bring one of two reactions to most people's minds. It will either be the Cuban musician Xavier Cugat or, if they grew up in Catholic school, the ubiquitous Saint Francis Xavier. Although first names with an "x" in them are pretty popular these days, most parents like the letter to be in the middle of the name somewhere and not announcing its presence right up front. Xavier is still more popular as a middle name. Variations: *Saverio, Xaver.*

XENOS (Greek) Guest. Variations: *Xeno, Zenos.*

YAKIM (Hebrew) God develops. Variation: *Jakim.*

YALE (English) Up on the hill.

YANCY (Native American) Englishman. Variations: *Yance, Yancey, Yantsey.*

YANNIS (Greek) God is good. Variation of John. Variations: *Yannakis, Yanni, Yiannis.*

YARDLEY (English) Enclosed meadow. The name Yardley evokes images of a fancy kind of English soap, or a town in Pennsylvania. Variations: *Yardlea, Yardlee, Yardleigh, Yardly.*

YATES (English) Gates. Variation: *Yeats.*

YEHUDI (Hebrew) Praise. The virtuoso violinist Yehudi Menuhin has made many Americans familiar with this name. Variations: *Yechudi, Yechudil, Yehuda, Yehudah.*

YERIK (Russian) God is exalted. Variation of Jeremiah. Variation: *Yeremey.*

YO (Chinese) Bright.

YONG (Chinese) Brave.

YORK (English) Yew tree. Variations: *Yorick, Yorke, Yorrick.*

YOSEF (Hebrew) God increases. Variations: *Yoseff, Yosif, Yousef, Yusef, Yusif, Yusuf, Yuzef.*

YOSHI (Japanese) Quiet.

YULE (English) Christmas.

YUMA (Native American) Son of the chief.

YUSUF (Arabic) God will increase. Variations: *Youssef, Yousuf, Yusef, Yusif, Yussef.*

YVES (French) Yew wood. Designer Yves St. Laurent brings glamor and fashion to this high-class French name, though its definition points to lowlier pursuits. Yvonne, the feminine version of Yves, has always been more popular than the male form of the name. Variation: *Yvon.*

ZACHARIAH (Hebrew) The Lord has remembered. Zachariah and its many variations is one of the more popular names around today, probably because it has that Biblical connotation as well as the trendy lightning-rod letter "Z." Little Zacharys are all over the place these days, and all the little boys with the name who are digging in the sandbox at the playground have done a lot to demystify this name. Variations: *Zacaria, Zacarias, Zach, Zacharia, Zacharias, Zacharie, Zachary, Zachery, Zack,*

Zackariah, Zackerias, Zackery, Zak, Zakarias, Zakarie, Zako, Zeke.

ZAFAR (Arabic) To win. Variation: *Zafir.*

ZAHID (Arabic) Strict.

ZAHIR (Hebrew) Bright. Variations: *Zaheer, Zahur.*

ZALE (Greek) Strength from the sea. Variation: *Zayle.*

ZAMIR (Hebrew) Song.

ZANE (English) God is good. Variation of John. Zane is a great name with the potential to become even bigger than Zachary. The recent popularity of this name can be traced to the writer Zane Grey, who chose it as a suitable substitute for his real name, Pearl. In fact, he took the name from one of his great-grandfathers, Ebenezer Zane, who founded the town of Zanesville in Ohio. Variations: *Zain, Zayne.*

ZARED (Hebrew) Trap.

ZEBULON (Hebrew) To exalt. Variations: *Zebulen, Zebulun.*

ZEDEKIAH (Hebrew) God is just. Variations: *Tzedekia, Tzidkiya, Zed, Zedechiah, Zedekia, Zedekias.*

ZEHARIAH (Hebrew) Light of God. Variations: *Zeharia, Zeharya.*

ZEKE (Hebrew) The strength of God. Zeke got its start as a nickname for Ezekiel, and gradually came into its own as an independent name. For parents who like this name, it may be best to use the original as a given name, so your son can have some variety.

ZEPHANIAH (Hebrew) Protection. Variations: *Zeph, Zephan.*

ZEUS (Greek) Living. King of the gods. Variations: *Zeno, Zenon, Zinon.*

ZINDEL (Hebrew) Protector of mankind. Variation of Alexander. A lot of kids might think that the name Zindel is actually pretty cool, due to the fact that a popular children's author is named Paul Zindel. An advantage of this name is that if your kid decides that later on he doesn't care for it, he can go to its original root, Alexander, and select another one of that name's many variations. Variation: *Zindil.*

ZOWIE (Greek) Life.

Girls Names

ABEY (Native American: Omaha) Leaf.

ABIGAIL (Hebrew) Father's joy. Abigail is one of those wonderful girls' names that conjures up images of colonial days in America. It has been in and out of fashion, but is currently enjoying a renaissance. In the Bible, Abigail was the name of King David's wife, but in this country more people are familiar with the name through the advice columnist Abigail Van Buren (more commonly known as Dear Abby). Abigail also figures strongly in politics in this country as the name of the wife of President John Adams as well as the mother of President John Quincy Adams. Abigail should continue to become more popular through the end of this decade and beyond. Variations: *Abagael, Abagail, Abagale, Abbey, Abbi, Abbie, Abbigael, Abbigail, Abbigale, Abby, Abbye, Abbygael, Abbygail, Abbygale, Abigale, Abigayle, Avigail.*

ADORA (Latin) Much adored. Variations: *Adoree, Adoria, Adorlee, Dora, Dori, Dorie, Dorrie.*

ADRIANE (German) Black earth. This pretty name is growing in popularity. Adriane should appeal to parents who are looking for a pretty name that stands out. Variations: *Adriana, Adriane, Adrianna, Adriannah, Adrianne, Adrien, Adriena, Adrienah, Adrienne.*

AGATHA (Greek) Good. Agatha is the patron saint of firefighters and nurses, but except for fans of mystery writer Agatha Christie, most new parents will crinkle up their noses at the suggestion of using this name for their young daughters. Of course, this situation could change, but someone has to be first. Variations: *Aga, Agace, Agacia, Agafia, Agasha, Agata, Agate, Agathe, Agathi, Agatta, Ageneti, Aggi, Aggie, Aggy, Akeneki.*

AISHA (Arabic) Life. This has become a popular name in the last two decades for African-American girls and for those who follow the Arabic religion, since Aisha was Mohammed's favorite wife. Perhaps the first time that many Americans heard of this name was through Stevie Wonder's song "Isn't She Lovely," which he wrote to honor his daughter Aisha. Variations: *Aishah, Aisia, Aisiah, Asha, Ashah, Ashia, Ashiah, Asia, Asiah, Ayeesa, Ayeesah, Ayeesha, Ayeeshah, Ayeisa.*

AKIBA (African) Unknown definition.

ALEXANDRA (Greek) One who defends. Feminine version of Alexander. Alexandra and its many varia-tions have always seemed to have an elitist, upper-crust aura to them. In the '80s, the visibility of Alexandra et al. was undoubtedly encouraged by Joan Collins's character Alexa on the TV show *Dynasty* as well as Billy Joel and Christy Brinkley's choice for their daughter, Alexa. The name has also been long associated with the royalty, including Great Britain's Queen Victoria, whose real name was Alexandrina, and Princess Alexandra of Denmark. Variations: *Alejandrina, Aleka, Aleksasha, Aleksey, Aleksi, Alesia, Aleska, Alessandra, Alessa, Alessi, Alex, Alexa, Alexanderia, Alexanderina, Alexena, Alexene, Alexi, Alexia, Alexie, Alexina, Alexiou, Alexis.*

ALICIA (English, Hispanic, Swedish) Truthful. Alicia and its variations are very popular today among parents who want lush, beautiful names for their daughters. Actress Jodie Foster's real name is actually Alicia. Alicia and its variants are regularly in the top twenty lists of names for girls, and will undoubtedly continue to become more and more popular. Variations: *Alesha, Alesia, Alisha, Alissa, Alycia, Alysha, Alyshia, Alysia, Ilysha.*

ALISON (German) Diminutive version of Alice. Today, the name Alison has a most interesting distinction. It is the second most popular name that mothers who have completed four years of college and beyond choose for their daughters. Alison is a feminine name that doesn't go overboard. Variations: *Alisann, Alisanne, Alisoun, Alisun, Allcen, Allcenne, Allicen, Allicenne, Allie, Allisann, Allisanne, Allison, Allisoun, Ally, Allysann, Allysanne, Allyson, Alyeann, Alysanne, Alyson.*

ALTHEA (Greek) With the potential to heal. Althea is a breathy, feminine name. The most famous example was the great tennis player of the 50s, Althea Gibson. Variations: *Altha, Althaia, Altheta, Althia.*

ANGELA (Greek) Messenger of God, angel. Actresses Angela Lansbury, Angie Dickenson, and Anjelica Huston have given us three different variations of the name. Variations: *Aingeal, Ange, Angel, Angele, Angelene, Angelia, Angelica, Angelika, Angelina, Angeline, Angelique, Angelita, Angie, Angiola, Anjelica, Anngilla.*

ANN (English) Grace. Ann, along with its many variations, was one of the most commonly used names—as either a first or middle name—until the craze for unusual names first hit in the late 1960s. It's interesting that its two major spellings—Ann and Anne—have gone back and forth in popularity. For instance, from 1900 to 1950, Ann was the most popular form. However, in 1950, after Princess Anne was named, that version became more popular than Ann, ten times over. Variations: *Ana, Anita, Anitra, Anitte, Anna, Annah, Anne, Annie, Annita, Annitra, Annitta, Hannah, Hannelore.*

APRIL (English) Named for the month. Many parents choose the name April for their daughters who are born during the month, but that seems just a little too obvious. Variations: *Abrial, Abril, Aprilete, Aprilette, Aprili, Aprille, Apryl, Averil, Avril.*

ARABELLA (English) In prayer. Variations: *Arabel, Arabela, Arbell, Arbella, Bel, Bella, Belle, Orabella, Orbella.*

ARIANA (Welsh) Silver. Variations: *Ariane, Arianie, Arianna, Arianne.*

ARIEL (Hebrew) Lioness of God. The name Ariel burst onto the scene in the early '90s when the Disney movie *The Little Mermaid* hit. Ariel was previously known as a water sprite as well as a male sprite in Shakespeare's *Tempest.* Ariel also appears as the title of one of Sylvia Plath's works, and these various sources provide a wide array of inspiration. Variations: *Aeriel, Aeriela, Ari, Ariela, Ariella, Arielle, Ariellel.*

ASHLEY (English) Ash tree. Ashley started out as a boys' name, with Ashley Wilkes from *Gone With the Wind* popularizing the name. But from that point on, Ashley seemed destined to be a girls' name, possibly because of the sensitivity of the Margaret Mitchell character. Today, giving a boy the name Ashley would almost certainly set him up for a daily dose of ridicule, since Ashley is about the most popular girls' name in the United States. Variations: *Ashely, Ashla, Ashlan, Ashlea, Ashlee, Ashleigh, Ashlie, Ashly, Ashton.*

AUDREY (English) Nobility and strength. Of course, the late actress Audrey Hepburn was responsible for making this name a popular choice through the end of the 1950s. Today, it's not as popular, but it's one of those great old-fashioned names that is due for a comeback. Variations: *Audey, Audi, Audie, Audra, Audre, Audree, Audreen, Audri, Audria, Audrie, Audry, Audrye, Audy.*

AUGUSTA (Latin) Majestic. Feminine version of August and Augustus. Variations: *Agusta, Augustia, Augustina, Augustine, Augustyna, Augustyne, Austina, Austine, Austyna, Austyne.*

AURORA (Latin) Roman goddess of dawn. Variation: *Aurore.*

AVERY (English) Elf advisor. Even though the TV character Murphy Brown named her son Avery, the exposure no doubt helped and increased usage of the name among girl babies. While it was given this initial boost, Avery fits the baby-naming trends of the '90s perfectly, since it is unisex as well as a last name.

AYESHA (Persian) Small girl.

AZARIA (Hebrew) Helped by God. Variations: *Azariah, Azelia.*

BAILEY (English) Bailiff. Bailey has become a popular name for both boys and girls in the last decade. Certainly, with the popularity of writer and NPR commentator, Bailey White, telling her stories about life in the South, this name should become more widely used for girls. Variations: *Bailee, Baylee, Bayley, Baylie.*

BARBARA (Greek) Foreign. Barbara was once one of the most popular names for girls. However, its usage has dropped off dramatically as parents today associate the name with their parents' generation. Popular Barbaras have included Barbara Bush, Barbara Stanwyck, and Barbra Streisand. As part of its legacy, however, Barbara has left behind lots of variations on a theme: *Babb, Babbett, Babbette, Babe, Babett, Babette, Babita, Babs, Barb, Barbary, Barbe, Barbette, Barbey, Barbi, Barbie, Barbra, Barby, Basha, Basia, Vaoka, Varenka, Varina, Varinka, Varka, Varvara, Varya, Vava.*

BASIA (Hebrew) Daughter of God. Variations: *Basha, Basya.*

BEATRICE (Latin) She brings joy. Beatrice was popularized through Dante's work *The Divine Comedy* and in the Shakespeare play *Much Ado About Nothing*, but the Beatrice that most American kids know is Beatrix Potter, who wrote the first stories about Peter Rabbit. Variations: *Bea, Beatrisa, Beatrise, Beatrix, Beatriz, Beattie, Bebe, Bee, Beitris, Beitriss.*

BERNADETTE (French) Brave as a bear. Feminine version of Bernard. Bernadette is a pretty name and should be used more often than it is. Actress Bernadette Peters is perhaps the most famous Bernadette around. Variations: *Berna, Bernadene, Bernadett, Bernadina, Bernadine, Bernarda, Bernardina, Bernardine, Bernetta, Bernette, Berni, Bernie, Bernita, Berny.*

BETHANY (English) House of poverty; a Biblical village near Jerusalem. As we all seem a bit Tiffanyed out, Bethany has been starting to appear a little bit more often as a close enough substitute. Variations: *Bethanee, Bethani, Bethanie, BethAnn, Bethann, Bethanne, Bethannie, Bethanny.*

BIANCA (Italian) White. Variations: *Beanka, Biancha, Bionca, Bionka, Blanca, Blancha.*

BLAIR (English) A flat piece of land. In the 1950s, Blair was a commonly used name for Waspy boys training to fill their father's gray flannel suits. In the '70s and '80s, Blair turned into a girls' name, although it still connotes the same social class. Variations: *Blaire, Blayre.*

BREANA (Celtic) Strong. Feminine version of Brian. Variations: *Breann, Breanna, Breanne, Briana, Briane, Briann, Brianna, Brianne, Briona, Bryanna, Bryanne.*

BRIDGET (Irish) Strength. Bridget sounds like a good Catholic-girl kind of name. Actress Meredith Baxter Birney played a Bridget in the '70s TV show *Bridget Loves Bernie.* Variations: *Birgit, Birgitt, Birgitte, Breeda, Brid, Bride, Bridgett, Bridgette, Bridgitte, Brigantia, Brighid, Brigid, Brigid, Brigida, Brigit, Brigitt, Brigitta, Brigitte, Brygida, Brygitka.*

BRITTANY (English) Feminine version of Britain. This is one of the most popular names for girls since the mid-1980s. In the '90s, it appears that girls' names with three syllables that end in the letter "y" and have at least one "n" in them are destined for the top ten list. Brittany falls into this category. Variations: *Brinnee, Britany, Britney, Britni, Brittan, Brittaney, Brittani, Brittania, Brittanie, Brittannia, Britteny, Brittni, Brittnie, Brittny.*

BRONWYN (Welsh) Pure of breast. Variation: *Bronwen.*

BROOKE (English) One who lives by a brook. Actress and child model Brooke Shields started the trend of baby girls named Brooke back in the '70s. Variation: *Brook.*

CAITLIN (Irish) Pure. Caitlin, created by the combination of Katherine and Lynn, has become a very popular name in the 1990s. Caitlin first became widely known in the United States in the early '80s, and it probably zoomed onto the top ten lists because it was derived from a popular, familiar name that was spelled in a fashion that was exotic to American eyes. Variations: *Caitilin, Caitlan, Caitlion, Caitlon, Caitlyn, Caitlynne, Catlin, Kaitlin, Kaitlyn, Kaitlynn, Kaitlynne, Katelin, Katelynn.*

CAMILLE (French) Assistant in the church. The name Camille used to have an aura of despair about it based on the tragic figure played by Greta Garbo in the movie of the same name. Enough time has passed, however, to make the name an attractive choice for a daughter in the '90s. Variations: *Cam, Cama, Camala, Cami, Camila, Camile, Camilia, Camilla, Cammi, Cammie, Cammy, Cammylle, Camyla, Kamila, Kamilka.*

CAROLINE (German) Woman. Feminine version of Carl, as well as Charles in diminutive form. Caroline always sounded more regal than just plain Carol, which may explain why Caroline is used more commonly today. Though Caroline could have received the same fate as Carol, several highly visible Carolines have served to redeem the name. First there was Caroline Kennedy; then came Princess Caroline of Monaco. And some parents are adding yet another regal spin on the name with one of the following Variations: *Carolenia, Carolin, Carolina, Carolyn, Carolynn, Carolynne, Karolin, Karolina, Karoline, Karolyn, Karolyna, Karolyne, Karolynn, Karolynne.*

CASEY (Irish) Observant. Also common as a boys' name. Out of all the boys' names that become popular as girls' names, Casey may actually be one of the few that remain popular in both camps. Casey is a great name to take a girl from babyhood all the way through life. It's also a classic name, and even though it's just recently become popular, it isn't likely to suffer from the same trendiness as Tiffany and Brittany. Variations: *Cacia, Casee, Casie, Cassie, Caycey, Caysey, Kacey, Kacia, Kasee, Kasie, Kaycey, Kaysey.*

CASSIDY (Gaelic) Clever. Variations: *Cassidey, Cassidi, Cassidie, Kasady, Kassidey, Kassidi, Kassidie, Kassidy.*

CATHERINE (English) Pure. Cathy-with-a-C has always been a bit more formal than Kathy-with-a-K. Catherine and all of its derivatives evoke violin lessons, afternoon tea, and gentlemen callers. The "K" form of Katherine spells tomboys, pigtails, and sleepovers. Famous Catherines include Katharine Hepburn, Saint Catherine of Alexandria, and the Catherine in the novel *Wuthering Heights.* Variations: *Catalina, Catarina, Catarine, Cateline, Catharin, Catharine, Catharyna,*

Catharyne, Cathe, Cathee, Cathelin, Cathelina, Cathelle, Catherin, Catherina, Cathi, Cathie, Cathy, Catrin, Catrina, Catrine, Catryna, Caty.

CECELIA (Latin) Blind. Feminine version of Cecil. Paul Simon's song "Cecelia" probably did more to put this name on the map than the Catholic saint of the same name. Today, variations of Cecelia, especially Cecily, seem to be more popular than the original. Variations: *C'Ceal, Cacilia, Cecely, Ceci, Cecia, Cecile, Cecilie, Cecille, Cecilyn, Cecyle, Cecylia, Ceil, Cele, Celenia, Celia, Celie, Celina, Celinda, Celine, Celinna, Celle, Cesia, Cespa, Cicely, Cicilia, Cycyl, Sessaley, Seelia, Seelie, Seely, Seslia, Sesseelya, Sessile, Sessilly, Sheelagh, Sheelah, Sheila, Sheilagh, Sheilah, Shela, Shelah, Shelia, Shiela, Sile, Sileas, Siseel, Sisely, Siselya, Sisilya, Sissela, Sissie, Sissy.*

CELESTE (Latin) Heaven. Celeste is a name that both looks great and sounds great but has never totally caught on. Parents who choose this name for their daughters will undoubtedly be complimented on their choice. Variations: *Cela, Celesse, Celesta, Celestia, Celestiel, Celestina, Celestine, Celestyn, Celestyna, Celinka, Celisse, Cesia, Inka, Selinka.*

CHANDELLE (African-American) Variations: *Chan, Chandell, Shan, Shandell, Shandelle.*

CHANTAL (French) Rocky area. Variations: *Chantale, Chantalle, Chante, Chantele, Chantelle, Shanta, Shantae, Shantal, Shantalle, Shantay, Shante, Shanteigh, Shantel, Shantell, Shantella, Shantelle, Shontal, Shontalle, Shontelle.*

CHARLA (English) Man. Feminine version of Charles. Variations: *Charlaine, Charlayne, Charlena, Charlene, Charli, Charlie, Charline, Cherlene, Cherline, Sharlayne, Sharleen, Sharlene.*

CHARLOTTE (French) Small beauty. Variant of Charles.

CHELSEA (English) Ship port. Currently a popular name: it incorporates the aura of Great Britain plus it's the name of a particular place—a region of London and of New York. President Clinton's daughter has given a huge boost to the visibility of this name today, and its popularity should continue to grow long after Clinton has left office. Variations: *Chelsa, Chelsee, Chelsey, Chelsi, Chelsie, Chelsy.*

CHERYL (English) Charity. Variations: *Cherill, Cherrill, Cherryl, Cheryle, Cheryll, Sherryll, Sheryl.*

CHEYENNE (Native American: Algonquin) Specific tribe. Cheyenne is a western place name that is bound to become more popular. Because it is more limiting than, say, Dakota (in that Cheyenne is merely a city while Dakota represents an entire region), it will probably remain somewhat on the fringes. Plus, the suicide of the most famous woman by this name—Marlon Brandon's daughter—might cause parents to shy away from it. Variations: *Cheyanna, Cheyanne, Chiana, Chianna.*

CHLOE (Greek) Young blade of grass. Today, Chloe is becoming a very popular name. Over the years, its major appearances have included many novels in the seventeenth century and, in the Bible, I Corinthians. In the '70s, Chloe began to appear with increasing frequency in Britain, and the name traveled over here in the early part of the '90s. Variations: *Clo, Cloe.*

CHRISTINE (English) Anointed one. Feminine version of Christian. Though Christine was the norm a couple of decades ago, today its variations reign. With their multiple syllables and varying endings, the variations hold much appeal for parents who are looking for a girls' name that is traditional yet still unusual. Famous Christine variations include actress Kirstie Alley, model Christie Brinkley, and the actress Kirsten Dunst from *Interview with a Vampire*. Variations: *Chris, Chrissy, Christa, Christen, Christi, Christiana, Christiane, Christiann, Christianna, Christie, Christina, Christy, Teena, Teina, Tena, Tina, Tinah.*

CLARA (English) Bright. Clara seems to be a name from the old country that has the potential for becoming widely used today, but many parents today will associate the name with the doddering Aunt Clara from the TV series *Bewitched*. Better to choose one of the many variations, except for Clarissa, because then your daughter's friends will always be asking her to explain it all. Variations: *Clair, Claire, Clairette, Clairine, Clare, Claresta, Clareta, Clarette, Clarice, Clarie, Clarinda, Clarine, Claris, Clarisa, Clarissa, Clarisse, Clarita, Claryce, Clerissa, Clerisse, Cleryce, Clerysse, Klara, Klari, Klarice, Klarissa, Klaryce, Klaryssa.*

COLETTE (French) Triumphant people. The French novelist who helped to bring this name into the public eye was actually using her last name for her pen name. Its origin is a variation of the name Nicolette. Variations: *Coletta, Collet, Collete, Collett.*

COURTNEY (English) Dweller in the court, or farm. Before singer Courtney Love came along, the image that most of us had of the name was of a privileged, upperclass girl who dutifully went from piano to ballet lessons over the course of one very crowded afternoon. Now, it seems all that has changed. Parents who once would have bestowed the name on their daughters will probably hesitate and then pass on the name today, and all because of the lead singer of the rock band Hole. In the late '80s, Courtney was one of the most popular names given to girls in this country; today it isn't even in the top fifty. Variations: *Cortney, Courtenay, Courteney, Courtnie.*

DAKOTA (English) State name; also used for boys. Dakota is currently hot, hot, hot, but that can only mean that by the end of the century the name will be on the wane. If you don't want to be seen as one who automatically goes along with the crowd, pick a state with a less popular name.

DANA (English) From Denmark. Dana is quickly becoming popular among both boys and girls, but it is more common as a girls' name. In some ways, the popularity of the name and the sex it belongs to seems to depend on which Hollywood celebrities with the name are in the majority. Despite the great visibility of actor Dana Carvey, he seems to be outnumbered by the actresses Dana Delaney, Dana Lambert, and the Dana that actress Sigourney Weaver played in the movie *Ghostbusters*. Variations: *Daina, Danay, Danaye, Dane, Danee, Danet, Danna, Dayna, Denae.*

DAPHNE (Greek) Ancient mythological nymph who was transformed into a laurel tree. Daphne first became popular in this country back in the nineteenth century when it was commonly given to women who were slaves. Although parents today of all ethnic backgrounds are choosing the name for their daughters in small numbers, Daphne remains most popular among African-American women. Variations: *Dafne, Daphney, Daphny.*

DARIA (Greek) Luxurious. Variations: *Darian, Darianna, Dariele, Darielle, Darienne, Darrelle.*

DARLENE (English) Darling. Variations: *Darla, Darleane, Darleen, Darleena, Darlena, Darlina, Darline.*

DAWN (English) Sunrise, the dawn. Dawn was a really popular name in the late '60s and early '70s

because, while it had the feel of many of the hippie names that were cool back then, it still had a long upstanding British tradition. This fact made it more acceptable among parents who knew their daughters had to get along in the real world someday. Variations: *Dawna, Dawne, Dawnelle, Dawnetta, Dawnette, Dawnielle, Dawnika, Dawnn.*

DEANDRA (African-American) Newly created name. Variations: *Deanda, Deandrea, Deandria, Deeandra, Dianda, Diandra, Diandre.*

DEBORAH (Hebrew) Bee. This name was hot in the 1960s. Today, it doesn't seem as popular. Variations: *Deb, Debbi, Debbie, Debby, Debi, Debora, Deborrah, Debra, Debrah, Devora, Devorah, Devra.*

DELIA (Greek) Visible. Variations: *Del, Delise, Delya, Delys, Delyse.*

DELILAH (Hebrew) Delicate. Delilah is perhaps best known as Samson's mistress in the Biblical book of Judges, and as the title and subject of one of the singer Tom Jones's songs. But Delilah is a feminine, lilting name that should be used more often for girls born today. Variations: *Dalila, Delila.*

DENISE (French) Lame god. Feminine version of Dennis. The name Denise has been around since the days of the Roman Empire, and it was used with some regularity through the early seventeenth century. Then it became virtually extinct until the 1950s, in the United States and overseas, where it grew to be very visible. Many parents today, however, may feel that the name is too evocative of the '50s and '60s, when it appeared as high as number fifteen on the list of top girls' names. Variations: *Denese, Deni, Denice, Deniece, Denisha, Denize, Dennise, Denyce, Denys, Denys.*

DERYN (Welsh) Bird. Variations: *Derren, Derrin, Derrine, Derron, Deryn.*

DESIREE (French) Longing. Though some people see this name as being a bit too adult to tag on a little girl, it is a pretty, feminine name. Its roots stem from Puritanical times, when Desire was the basic name. Today, Desiree seems to be used most often in African-American families, although it is being given to girls of all ethnic backgrounds. Variations: *Desarae, Desira, Desyre, Dezarae, Dezirae, Diseraye, Diziree, Dsaree.*

DEVON (English) Region in southern England. Variations: *Devan, Devana, Devanna,*

Devona, Devondra, Devonna, Devonne, Devyn, Devynn.

DEWANDA (African-American) Combination of De + Wanda.

DIANA (Latin) Divine. Roman goddess of the moon and of hunting. Diana has always been a popular name, but it has been made more widespread in the last twenty years by such high-profile Dianas as Diana Nyad, Diane Keaton, and of course, Princess Diana. The death of the princess may result in the name's becoming more widely used to commemorate her. Variations: *Dee, Diahann, Dian, Diane, Dianna, Dianne, Didi, Dyan, Dyana.*

DIONNE (Greek) Dione is a Greek mythological figure. Dionne is also the feminine version of Dennis, which in turn is formed from the name of another Greek god, Dionysus, the god of wine. Singer Dionne Warwick was the most popular Dionne around—and probably the only one—but using her name for a girl today will make it seem like 1973 all over again. Variations: *Deonne, Dion, Diona, Dione, Dionia, Dionna, Dionysia.*

DOMINIQUE (Latin) Lord. Feminine version of Dominick. The boys' name Dominick has been around since the thirteenth century; no one knows exactly when the feminine form of the name came into being. Currently it is gaining ground in popularity, and its peak seems to be a few years down the road. Variations: *Dominica, Dominika.*

DONNA (Italian) Woman of the home. The name Donna was at its peak of popularity in the '50s and '60s. The thing to do then was to combine Donna with other names, like Marie and Sue. Perhaps the Osmond parents had similar ideas in mind when they named Donny and Marie. Variations: *Dahna, Donielle, Donisha, Donetta, Donnalee, Donnalyn, DonnaMarie, Donni, Donnie, Donya.*

DOROTHY (Greek) Gift from God. Variations: *Dollie, Dolly, Dorethea, Doro, Dorotea, Dorotha, Dorothea, Dorothee, Dorothia, Dorrit, Dortha, Dorthea, Dot, Dottie, Dotty.*

EBONY (African-American) Black wood. Ebony is one of the ten most popular names that African-American parents are giving their daughters these days. Given the trend in the community to give children names that reflect the pride they have in their African-American backgrounds, Ebony is a good choice for parents who don't care for the trend of putting "La-" in front of a more common name for their daughters. Variations: *Ebbony, Eboney, Eboni, Ebonie.*

EDEN (Hebrew) Pleasure. Variations: *Eaden, Eadin, Edena, Edenia Edana, Edin.*

EDWINA (English) Rich friend. Feminine version of Edwin. Variations: *Edween, Edweena, Edwena, Edwiena, Edwuna, Edwyna.*

EILEEN (Irish) Shining, bright. Familiar version of Helen. Eileen used to be extremely popular among families of Irish heritage. Today, however, it rarely appears as a first name, and is more common as a middle name. Variations: *Aileen, Ailene, Alene, Aline, Ayleen, Eilean, Eilleen, Ilene.*

ELAINE (French) Bright, shining. Derivative of Helen. Elaine was popular as a girls' name in the 1950s, but has recently fallen out of favor. That is, until the popularity of TV's *Seinfeld* and the character Elaine. Time will tell if there is an increase in the number of girls named Elaine at the end of this century. Variations: *Alayna, Alayne, Allaine, Elaina, Elana, Elane, Elanna, Elayn, Elayne, Eleana, Elena, Eleni Alaina, Ellaina, Ellaine, Ellane, Ellayne.*

ELEANOR (English) Mercy. Derivative of Helen. Eleanor seems a commonsense type of name, based on Eleanor Roosevelt as well as the actress who played the eldest daughter on *Father Knows Best*. Though it does seems to be picking up steam recently, Eleanor is not as popular as other traditional girls' names that are being resurrected today. Variations: *Eleanore, Elenore, Eleonora, Eleonore, Elinor, Ellinor.*

ELECTRA (Greek) Shining one. A mythological figure who had her brother kill their mother and her lover in revenge for their father's murder. Variation: *Elektra.*

ELIANA (Hebrew) God has answered my prayers. Variation: *Eliane*

ELIZABETH (Hebrew) I pledge to God. As you can see by the numerous variations, if you were to add up all the derivatives of Elizabeth, you'd undoubtedly end up with the most popular girls' name in the world by far. And because of all these wonderful variations, few girls choose to go by the main root. Variations: *Alzbeta, Babette, Bess, Bessey, Bessi, Bessie, Bessy, Bet, Beta, Beth, Betina, Betine, Betka, Betsey, Betsi,*

Betsy, Bett, Betta, Bette, Betti, Bettina, Bettine, Betty, Betuska, Boski, Eilis, Elis, Elisa, Elisabet, Elisabeta, Elisabeth, Elisabetta, Elisabette, Elisaka, Elisauet, Elisaveta, Elise, Eliska, Elissa, Elisueta, Eliza, Elizabetta, Elizabette, Elliza, Elsa, Elsbet, Elsbeth, Elsbietka, Elschen, Else, Elsee, Elsi, Elsie, Elspet, Elspeth, Elyse, Elyssa, Elyza, Elzbieta, Elzunia, Isabel, Isabelita, Liazka, Lib, Libbee, Libbey, Libbi, Libbie, Libby, Libbye, Lieschen, Liese, Liesel, Lis, Lisa, Lisbet, Lisbete, Lisbeth, Lise, Lisenka, Lisettina, Lisveta, Liz, Liza, Lizabeth, Lizanka, Lizbeth, Lizka, Lizzi, Lizzie, Lizzy, Vetta, Yelisaveta, Yelizaueta, Yelizaveta, Ysabel, Zizi, ZsiZsi.

ELLEN (English) Variation of Helen that has become a full-fledged name in its own right. A few decades ago, Ellen was the type of name that parents gave to a girl from whom they expected no surprises. Today's Ellens include actresses Ellen Barkin and Ellen DeGeneres. Variations: *Elan, Elen, Elena, Eleni, Elenyl, Ellan, Ellene, Ellie, Ellon, Ellyn, Elyn, Lene, Wily.*

ELSA (Spanish) Noble. Elsa is a pretty name that has long been popular in Scandinavian as well as Hispanic countries. The name appeared in one of Wagner's operas, *Lohengrin*, and today Elsa Klensch, who stars in a TV show about fashion on CNN, has brought new life to this name. Variations: *Else, Elsie, Elsy.*

EMILY (English) Industrious. Emily is one of those names that automatically implies brains and beauty as well as a nod toward old-fashioned days. In a recent study, Emily was the name that was most often chosen for daughters of women who have completed college and have gone on to further their education. Variations: *Aimil, Amalea, Amalia, Amalie, Amelia, Amelie, Ameline, Amy, Eimile, Em, Ema, Emalee, Emalia, Emelda, Emelene, Emelia, Emelina, Emeline, Emelyn, Emelyne, Emera, Emi, Emie, Emila, Emile, Emilea, Emilia, Emilie, Emilka, Emlynne, Emma, Emmalee, Emmali, Emmaline, Emmalynn, Emele, Emmeline, Emmiline, Emylin, Emylynn, Emlyn.*

EMMA (German) Embracing all. A wonderful, Victorian-era name that conjures up images of long, wavy chestnut hair, blue eyes, and cotton petticoats. Variations: *Em, Emmi, Emmie, Emmy.*

ERICA (Scandinavian) Leader forever. Feminine version of Eric. Erica is big and has been at least since the early '70s. In addition to possessing its Scandinavian definition, Erica is also another name for the heather plant. In the mid-nineteenth century, Erica got its start in the United States with a book by novelist Edna Lyall called *We Two*. It seems somewhat surprising that this name is still so consistently popular, since it doesn't share the allure that many other traditional names boast today. However, the long-suffering Emmy nominated actress who plays Erica Kane—Susan Lucci—may be singlehandedly responsible for our continuing fascination and usage of this name. Variations: *Airica, Airika, Ayrika, Enrica, Enricka, Enrika, Ericka, Erika, Errika, Eyrica.*

ERIN (Gaelic) Nickname for Ireland; also used occasionally as a boy's name; translates to western island. The ironic thing about Erin is that it is primarily an Americanized version of Ireland; it is not to be found in Ireland at all. And since the trend today, in the United States, is to search for Irish names that are truly Irish, Erin just may be left out in the cold. Variations: *Erene, Ereni, Eri, Erina, Erinn, Eryn.*

ESMERELDA (Spanish) Emerald. Variations: *Emerant, Emeraude, Esma, Esmaralda, Esmarelda, Esmiralda, Esmirelda, Ezmeralda.*

ESTELLE (English) Star. Variations: *Essie, Essy, Estee, Estela, Estelita, Estella, Estrelita, Estrella, Estrellita, Stelle.*

EUGENIA (Greek) Well born. Feminine version of Eugene. The wife of Pinchas Zukerman is named Eugenia, and her growing visibility, along with that of the Duke and Duchess of York's second girl may well make this name more popular in the coming years. Variations: *Eugena, Eugenie, Eugina.*

EVANGELINE (Greek) Good news. Variations: *Evangelia, Evangelina, Evangeliste.*

EVELYN (French) Hazelnut. Evelyn is a great example of a name that started out as a boys' name—but then parents started to appropriate it for their daughters, rendering the male version all but obsolete. Evelyn became popular in the first couple of decades of this century as a girls' name, and by that point the name had disappeared from general consideration as a boys' name. Novelist Evelyn Waugh is perhaps the sole reminder of this name's true origins. Variations: *Aveline, Eoelene, Eveline, Evelyne, Evelynn, Evelynne, Evlin, Evline, Evlun, Evlynn.*

FAITH (English) Faith. Faith was another one of the virtue names that the Puritans liked so much back in the seventeenth century, and it is one of the few that has survived to this day. Faith, along with Hope, sounds more practical and everyday than either Charity or Prudence. Variations: *Faithe, Faythe.*

FALLON (Irish) Related to a leader. Variation: *Falon.*

FARRAH (English) Pleasant. Variations: *Fara, Farah, Farra.*

FAWN (French) Young deer. Variations: *Faina, Fanya, Fauan, Faun, Faunia, Fawna, Fawne, Fawnia, Fawnya.*

FAY (French) Fairy. Diminutive of Faith. Variations: *Faye, Fayette.*

FELICIA (Latin) Happy; lucky. Feminine version of Felix. Felicia sounds a bit clunky and awkward by itself, but take one of its variations, like Felice or Felicity, and it is transformed into a delicate, feminine name. Felicity, in fact, is becoming more popular for girls these days since the successful *American Girl* book series features a girl from colonial times named Felicity. Variations: *Falecia, Falicia, Falicie, Falisha, Falishia, Felice, Feliciana, Felicidad, Felicienne, Felicita, Felicitas, Felicity, Felise, Felita, Feliz, Feliza.*

FEODORA (Russian) Gift from God. Feminine version of Theodore.

FIONA (Irish) Fair, white. Variations: *Fionna, Fionne.*

FINOLA (Irish) White shoulders. Variations: *Effie, Ella, Fenella, Finella, Fionnaghuala, Fionneuala, Fionnghuala, Fionnuala, Fionnula, Fionola, Fynella, Nuala.*

FLANNERY (Irish) Red hair.

FLORA (English) Flower. Flora has potential to become popular in the United States, since it is one of the more popular names in other countries, including Sweden, Britain, Germany, and Russia. Variations: *Fiora, Fiore, Fiorentina, Fiorenza, Fiori, Fleur, Fleurette, Fleurine, Flo, Flor, Florance, Florann, Floranne, Flore, Florella, Florelle, Florence, Florencia, Florentia, Florentyna, Florenze, Floretta, Florette, Flori, Floria, Floriana, Florie, Floriese, Florina, Florinda, Florine, Floris, Florrie, Florry, Floss, Flossey, Flossie.*

FRANCES (English) One who is from France. Feminine version of Francis. Frances was a perennial favorite in England through the latter half of the nineteenth century, and in this country, it reached its peak by the time the Great Depression hit. Though it has been consid-

ered to be somewhat square from that time all the way up until the '80s, Frances is beginning to take off again among parents who are looking for a traditional and classy name for their daughters. Famous Franceses include actress Frances Farmer and Courtney Love's daughter Frances Bean. Variations: *Fan, Fancy, Fania, Fannee, Fanney, Fannie, Fanny, Fanya, Fran, Franca, Francee, Franceline, Francena, Francene, Francesca, Francetta, Francette, Francey, Franchesca, Francie, Francina, Francine, Francisca, Francoise, Frank, Frankie, Franni, Frannie, Franzetta, Franziska, Paquita.*

FRANCOISE (French) Frenchman.

FREDA (German) Peaceful. Variations: *Freada, Freddi, Freddie, Freddy, Frederica, Frederique, Freeda, Freida, Frida, Frieda, Fritzi, Fryda.*

GABRIELLE (Hebrew) Heroine of God. Feminine version of Gabriel. Tennis star Gabriella Sabatini has brought new life to this name in the United States and elsewhere. Gabrielle is a wonderfully cultured name that doesn't sound as haughty as some other girls' names that have a sophisticated ring to them. This is probably owing to one of its nicknames, Gaby, which sounds anything but elitist. Gabrielle has already shown signs of cracking the top fifty list of baby names for girls in the United States; this trend should continue. Variations: *Gabbi, Gabby, Gabi, Gabriela, Gabriell, Gabriella, Gaby.*

GAIA, (Greek) Earth. Variations: *Gaioa, Gaya.*

GAIL (Hebrew) My father rejoices. Gail started out as a nickname for Abigail, back in the '40s when traditionally American names started to seem a bit stodgy and old-fashioned. Variations: *Gael, Gaile, Gale, Gayle.*

GENEVIEVE (Celtic) White; Celtic woman. Genevieve has tended to be a continental sophisticated name, undoubtedly helped along by actress Genevieve Bujold. It has never been used that frequently in this country, and therefore tends to have a neutral connotation with most people. It seems the name should be more popular than it is currently, and given our culture's fascination with Europe, this could happen. Variations: *Genavieve, Geneva, Geneve, Geneveeve, Genivieve, Gennie, Genny, Genovera, Genoveva, Gina, Janeva, Jenevieve.*

GERALDINE (French) One who rules with a spear. Feminine version of Gerald. Variations: *Ceraldina,*

Deraldene, Geralda, Geraldeen, Geralyn, Geralynne, Geri, Gerianna, Gerianne, Gerilynn, Geroldine, Gerry, Jeraldeen, Jeraldene, Jeraldine, Jeralee, Jere, Jeri, Jerilene, Jerrie, Jerrileen, Jerroldeen, Jerry.

GERIANNE (American) Gerry + Anne.

GILDA (English) Golden.

GINA (Hebrew) Garden; (Italian) Nickname for names such as Regina and Angelina; (Japanese) Silvery. Gina was one of the more popular exotic names in the United States during the '50s and '60s, which is probably solely due to the exposure of Italian actress Gina Lollobrigida. Back then, Gina was the epitome of foreign glamor and sophistication. Actress Geena Davis has popularized a new spelling of the name. Variations: *Geena, Gena, Ginat, Ginia.*

GIOVANNA (Italian) God is good. Another feminization of John.

GISELLE (English) Oath; hostage. Giselle also is a picture-perfect name for a ballerina; *Giselle* is a ballet by Gautier. Variations: *Gelsi, Gelsy, Gisela, Gisele, Gisella, Gizela, Gizella.*

GITA (Hindu) Song. Variations: *Geeta, Geetika, Gitanjau, Gitika.*

GLADYS (Welsh) Lame. Form of Claudia. About a hundred years ago Gladys was considered to be the most exotic, sexy name to come down the pike in quite some time. Variations: *Gwladus, Gwladys.*

GLENNETTE (Scottish) Narrow valley. Feminine version of Glenn.

GLORIA (Latin) Glory. There have been lots of famous Glorias over the years: Gloria Steinem, Gloria Swanson, Gloria Vanderbilt, and Gloria Estefan. Variations: *Gloree, Glori, Glorie, Glorria, Glory.*

GRACE (Latin) Grace. Grace has been around since the Middle Ages, and it has never really gone out of style. It has been especially popular recently, owing to singer Grace Slick, Grace Jones, and the late Grace Kelly and Gracie Allen. The biggest boost for parents today seems to have been the character that actress Susan Dey played on the long-running series *L.A. Law*, Grace Van Owen. Variations: *Engracie, Graca, Gracey, Graci, Gracia, Graciana, Gracie, Gracy, Gratia, Grazia, Graziella, Grazielle, Graziosa, Grazyna.*

GWENDOLYN (Welsh) Fair brow. Variations: *Guendolen, Guenna, Gwen, Gwenda, Gwendaline, Gwendia, Gwendolen, Gwendolene, Gwendolin, Gwendoline, Gwendolynn, Gwendolynne, Gwenette, Gwennie, Gwenn, Gwenna, Gwenny.*

GWYNETH (Welsh) Happiness. Both Gwyneth and Gwendolyn are popular now because people consider girls' names that begins with "Gw" to be exotic and sophisticated at the same time. But Gwyneth is probably the more popular owing to the actress Gwyneth Paltrow, the daughter of Blythe Danner. Variations: *Gwenith, Gwennyth, Gwenyth, Gwynith, Gwynn, Gwynna, Gwynne, Gwynneth.*

HA (Vietnamese) River.

HADLEY (English) Meadow of heather. Variations: *Hadlea, Hadlee, Hadleigh.*

HANNAH (Hebrew) Grace. In the Bible, Hannah was mother of the prophet Samuel, but even he couldn't have foreseen how popular his mother's name would remain two millennia later. Hannah was very popular in Britain in the seventeenth through nineteenth centuries, and also in this country in the colonial era, when Biblical names were the norm. In the United States today, Hannah is white-hot, which only means that it will seem dated by the turn of the century. The reason for this most recent renaissance? Probably Woody Allen's movie *Hannah and her Sisters*. Variations: *Hana, Hanah, Hanna, Hanne, Hannele, Hannelore, Hannie, Honna.*

HARPER (English) Harp player. Harper Lee, author of *To Kill a Mockingbird*, first popularized this traditional last-name-as-first-name for girls. Surprisingly, Harper hasn't made much progress on the most popular names list, but it should, since today it pushes all the right buttons.

HARRIET (German) Leader of the house. Feminine version of Harry. Variations: *Harrie, Harrietta, Harriette, Harriot, Harriott, Hatsie, Hatsy, Hattie, Hatty.*

HASIKA (Hindu) Laughter.

HAYLEY (English) Meadow of hay. In the '90s, Hayley is an extremely popular name for girls, but few people know that the name actually originated when child actress Hayley Mills first burst onto the scene. Before her parents took her mother's middle name for their daughter's first name, Hayley—more commonly spelled Haley—was known only as a last name. Variations:

Hailee, Hailey, Haley, Halie, Halley, Halli, Hallie, Hally, Haylee, Hayleigh, Haylie.

HEATHER (English) Flower. In this country, Heather has been popular since the '70s, but it really didn't start to take hold until the movie *Heathers* came out in the mid-'80s. Its popularity in Britain preceded the name's vogue on these shores as it peaked in England during the '50s, and it appears as though the movie did nothing to enhance the name's image over there.

HEIDI (German) Noble. Variations: *Hedie, Heida, Heide, Heidie, Hydie.*

HELEN (Greek) Light. Helen has a lengthy track record. Helen was a pivotal figure in Greek mythology as the daughter of Zeus, as well as the real-life mother of emperor Constantine the Great back in the fourth century A.D. Since the early days of the United States, Helen has gone in and out of fashion, most often alternating with its close relative, Ellen. Though Helen was not too popular in the '70s and '80s in the United States, it appears to be one of those names that's just waiting to happen. Variations: *Hela, Hele, Helena, Helene, Hellen, Helli.*

HENRIETTA (German) Leader of the home. Feminine version of Henry. Variations: *Hattie, Hatty, Hendrika, Henka, Hennie, Henrie, Henrieta, Henriette, Henrika, Hetta, Hettie.*

HIALEAH (Native American: Seminole) Beautiful pasture.

HILARY (Greek) Glad. For at least the next few decades, this name will be indelibly connected with President Clinton's wife. Variations: *Hilaria, Hilarie, Hillary, Hillery, Hilliary.*

HISA (Japanese) Everlasting. Many of the more popular names for Japanese girls and boys are meant to impart the hope for longevity to the person with the name. Hisa is one of these names. Superstitions are frequently involved in picking a name for your baby, and this ancient Japanese custom could very well catch on in this country. Hisa is a beautiful name, regardless of its meaning, which may encourage non-Japanese parents to choose it. Variations: *Hisae, Hisako, Hisayo.*

HOLLY (English) Plant. Though Holly has always been more popular in England than in the United States, it should pick up over here in coming years. First, it's a seasonal name that many parents choose for their daughters who are born close to Christmastime. Second, it's a plant name, and this category of names seems particularly poised to grow in usage in the years to come. And as a bonus, Holly Hunter is a talented, prolific actress, which never hurts when it comes to the popularity of a name. Variations: *Hollee, Holley, Holli, Hollie, Hollyann.*

HONG (Vietnamese) Pink.

HOSANNA (Greek) Cry of prayer. Variation: *Hosannie.*

HUNTER (English) Hunter.

IDA (English) Youth. Ida was a big name fifty to one hundred years ago, which brought forth the Gilbert and Sullivan opera *Princess Ida*, the gay '90s song "Ida, Sweet as Apple Cider," and the actress Ida Lupino. Although other names from that period are hot today, Ida has not made much of a comeback. Variations: *Idalene, Idalia, Idalina, Idaline, Idalya, Idalyne, Ide, Idell, Idella, Idelle, Idetta, Idette, Idia.*

IMELDA (Italian) Embracing the fight. Variation: *Imalda.*

INDIA (English) The country.

INDIGO (Latin) Dark blue.

INGA (Scandinavian) In Norse mythology, god of fertility and peace. Variations: *Ingaar, Inge, Ingo, Ingvio.*

INGRID (Scandinavian) Beautiful. Of all the feminine names from Scandinavia that begin with "Ing," Ingrid is the most widely used owing to the renown of actress Ingrid Bergman. There was a flurry of activity surrounding the name back in the '50s and '60s, but it faded until just recently and is now beginning to show signs of strength again.

IRENE (Greek) Peace. Irene has a long and rich history. One Irene became a saint in the fourth century A.D. Even before that, Irene was one of the more popular names during the Roman Empire. Its popularity continued right until the middle of the twentieth century, when it suddenly seemed to run out of steam. Today, the many variations of the name are more common than the original root. Variations: *Arina, Arinka, Eirena, Eirene, Eirini, Erena, Erene, Ereni, Errena, Irayna, Ireen, Iren, Irena, Irenea, Irenee, Irenka, Irina, Irine, Irini, Irisha, Irka, Irusya, Iryna, Orina, Orya, Oryna, Reena, Reenie, Rina, Yarina, Yaryna.*

ISABEL (Spanish) Pledge of God. Version of Elizabeth. Though Isabel seems like it might be too ethnic or too old-fashioned to be popular, the truth is that it is one of the more popular names around and still growing. Actress Isabella Rossillini has helped to bring exposure to this name. Variations: *Isa, Isabeau, Isabelita, Isabella, Isabelle, Isobel, Issi, Issie, Issy, Izabel, Izabele, Izabella, Izabelle, Izebela, Ysabel.*

ISADORA (Latin) Gift from Isis. Feminine version of Isidore. Variation: *Isidora.*

ISMAELA (Hebrew) God listens. Variations: *Isma, Mael, Maella.*

ITALIA (Latin) From Italy. Variation: *Talia.*

ITO (Japanese) Fiber.

IVANA (Slavic) God is good. Feminine version of Ivan. Variations: *Iva, Ivania, Ivanka, Ivanna, Ivannia.*

IVORY (Latin) Ivory. Ivory is as popular among African-American parents as its counterpart, Ebony, though it might be too much to name twins Ebony and Ivory. Parents in many African-American families like the name Ivory because it shows pride in their heritage, whether it alludes to the substance itself or to Africa's Ivory coast. Variations: *Ivoreen, Ivorine.*

IVY (English) Plant. Variations: *Iva, Ivey, Ivie.*

JACEY (American) Newly created, possibly from the letters "J" and "C." Variations: *Jace, Jacy.*

JACINTA (Spanish) Hyacinth. Feminine version of Jacinto. Variations: *Glacinda, Glacintha, Jacinda, Jacintha, Jacinthe, Jacinthia, Jacki, Jacky, Jacquetta, Jacqui, Jacquie, Jacynth, Jacyntha, Jacynthe.*

JACQUELINE (French) He who replaces. Feminine version of Jacob. Jacqueline's heritage is undoubtedly French, however, Jackie Kennedy's glamor and poise served to put an American spin on the name. Interestingly enough, although Jackie O is as loved as ever, the name Jacqueline is still not as popular as it was back in the '20s when it regularly hit the top fifty list. Variations: *Jacaline, Jacalyn, Jackalin, Jackalyn, Jackeline, Jackelyn, Jacketta, Jackette, Jacki, Jackie, Jacklin, Jacklyn, Jacky, Jaclyn, Jaclynn, Jacoba, Jacobette, Jacobina, Jacolyn, Jacqualine, Jacqualyn, Jacqualynn, Jacquelean, Jacquelene, Jacquelin, Jacquelyn, Jacquelyne, Jacquelynn, Jacquelynne, Jacqueta, Jacquetta, Jacquiline, Jacquline, Jacqulynn, Jaculine, Jakelyn, Jaqueline, Jaquelyn, Jaquith.*

JADE (Spanish) Jade stone. Variations: *Jada, Jadee, Jadira, Jady, Jaida, Jaide, Jayde, Jaydra.*

JAIMIE (English) One who replaces. Feminine version of James. Jaimie was first popularized as a great girls' name in the '70s because it conveys so much energy and fitness, and a bit of tomboyishness—yet a girl with this name wouldn't hesitate to get dressed up to go out to dinner. At least, that's how Lindsey Wagner portrayed the character she played in the TV series *The Bionic Woman.* Variations: *Jaime, Jaimey, Jaimi, Jaimy, Jamee, Jami, Jamie, Jayme.*

JANINE (English) God is good. Feminine version of John. Variations: *Janina, Jannine, Jeneen, Jenine.*

JASMINE (Persian) Flower. If it wasn't for the great success of the animated Disney movie *Aladdin,* Jasmine would probably have been relegated to a footnote of popular flower names that first hit around the turn of the century. But Princess Jasmine—and, to a lesser extent, actress Jasmine Guy have revived this wonderfully feminine name, and it has not yet hit its peak the second time around. Variations: *Jasmeen, Jasmin, Jasmina, Jazmin, Jazmine, Jessamine, Jessamyn, Yasiman, Yasman, Yasmine.*

JAYNE (Hindu) Victorious.

JENNA (Arabic) Little bird. Variations: *Jannarae, Jena, Jenesi, Jenn, Jennabel, Jennah, Jennalee, Jennalyn, Jennasee.*

JENNIFER (Welsh) White; smooth; soft. Actually Jennifer is a version of Guinevere. It is perhaps the best example of the kind of trendy names that exploded in popularity overnight in the mid-'70s all the way up to the early '90s before almost completely burning out. Although it is still used today, it was so popular that many parents might tend to shy away from using it today. In Britain, the name peaked earlier, hitting number six in 1950. Variations: *Genn, Gennifer, Genny, Ginnifer, Jen, Jena, Jenalee, Jenalyn, Jenarae, Jenene, Jenetta Jenita, Jennis, Jeni, Jenice, Jeniece, Jenifer, Jeniffer, Jenilee, Jenilynn, Jenise, Jenn, Jennessa, Jenni, Jennie, Jennika, Jennilyn, Jennyann, Jennylee, Jeny, Jinny.*

JERALYN (American) Combination of Jerry and Marilyn. Variations: *Jerelyn, Jerilyn, Jerilynn, Jerralyn, Jerrilyn.*

JESSICA (Hebrew) He sees. Like Jennifer, Jessica was a regular fixture on the baby name hit parade from the mid-'70s all the way through to the late '80s. It made its first appearance in the Bible in the Book of Genesis. Shakespeare also used the name in *The Merchant of Venice*, giving the name to the daughter of Shylock. Parents today who like the name but who don't want to be considered trendy are choosing other variations related to Jessica. Variations: *Jesica, Jess, Jessa, Jesse, Jesseca, Jessey, Jessi, Jessie, Jessika.*

JILL (English) Young. Shortened version of Juliana. The late actress Jill Ireland was perhaps the most famous Jill that we've seen in this country in a while. Jill is a classic name, but it doesn't seem to have enough pizzazz to hit the "most-popular" charts of the '90s. Variations: *Gil, Gill, Gyl, Gyll, Jil, Jilli, Jillie, Jilly, Jyl, Jyll.*

JOANNE (English) God is good. Variations: *Joana, Joanna, Joannah, Johanna, Johanne.*

JOCELYN (English) Unknown definition, possibly a combination of Joyce and Lynn. Variations: *Jocelin, Joceline, Jocelyne, Joci, Jocie, Josaline, Joscelin, Josceline, Joscelyn, Joseline, Joselyn, Joselyne, Josiline, Josline.*

JOELLE (French) God is Lord. Feminine version of Joel. Variations: *Joda, Joell, Joella, Joellen, oellyn, Joely.*

JOLENE (American) Jolene is a combination name, formed by using "Jo" and "lene," a popular suffix in the beginnings of the baby boom. As you can see, the variations in spelling tended to get very creative. Jolene is considered by some to be a contemporary version of Josephine. Variations: *Jolean, Joleen, Jolian, Jolin, Joline, Jolinn, Jolinne, Jolyn, Jolynn, Jolynne, Jolyon.*

JOLIE (French) Pretty. Variations: *Jolee, Joley, Joli, Joline, Joly.*

JORDAN (English) To descend. The name Jordan has a very curious background: during the Crusades, Christians who returned home brought water from the Jordan river for the express purpose of baptizing their children. As a result, many of those children were named Jordan—the boys at least. The name really didn't start to catch on for girls until the 1980s. Today, alas, Jordan is beginning to show the signs of strain that many androgynous names go through: parents are ceasing to consider the name for their sons. Variations: *Jordana, Jordon, Jordyn.*

JOSEPHINE (Hebrew) God will add. Feminine version of Joseph. Variations: *Jo, Joey, Jojo, Josefa, Josefina, Josefine, Josepha, Josephe, Josephene, Josephina, Josetta, Josette, Josey, Josi, Josie.*

JOYCE (Latin) Joyous. Joyce actually started out as a boys' name. It was the name of a saint in the seventh century A.D. This usage continued occasionally until the late Middle Ages, but Joyce started to be regularly used only during the nineteenth century. During the Flapper Era, Joyce was the third most common name for girls, which lasted through the '50s. Variations: *Joice, Joyousa.*

JUDITH (Hebrew) Jewish. Variations: *Jitka, Jucika, Judey, Judi, Judie, Judit, Judita, Judite, Juditha, Judithe, Judy, Judye, Jutka.*

JULIA (English) Young. Roman clan name. Julia is a name that, shall we say, has legs. It's popular all over the world and has been since women in ancient Rome gave the name to their babies in honor of the emperor Julius Caesar. In this century, Julia was popular from the years immediately following World War II throughout the mid-'70s, when it rested for about a decade until actress Julia Roberts burst onto the scene and made it very popular again. Parents seem to prefer Julia over the perkier Julie. Variations: *Iulia, Jula, Julcia, Julee, Juley, Juli, Juliana, Juliane, Julianna, Julianne, Julica, Julie, Julina, Juline, Julinka, Juliska, Julissa, Julka, Yula, Yulinka, Yuliya, Yulka, Yulya.*

JYOTI (Hindu) Light of the moon. Variation: *Jyotsana.*

KAI (Japanese) Forgiveness; (Hawaiian) Sea. Although most people haven't heard of Kai as the name for a girl, they may be familiar with it as a word, since it frequently occurs in many Hawaiian place names. Kai has just recently started to appear in the United States as a name for girls, most often by African-American parents, but I think that this is a name that is on its way up overall. Variations: *Kaiko, Kaiyo.*

KAITLIN (English) Combination of Kate and Lynn. Variations: *Kaitlinn, Kaitlinne, Kaitlynn, Katelin, Katelyn, Katelynne.*

KALLI (Greek) Singing lark. Variations: *Cal, Calli, Callie, Colli, Kal, Kallie, Kallu, Kally.*

KAMELIA (Hawaiian) Vineyard. Variation: *Komela.*

KARA (Latin) Dear. Kara started out life spelled the Italian way with a "C," but somehow it became more popular with a "K." In any case, Kara is both exotic and familiar and parents should start to consider it more. Variations: *Kaira, Karah, Karalee, Karalyn, Karalynn, Kari, Kariana, Karianna, Karianne, Karie, Karielle, Karrah, Karrie, Kary.*

KAREN (Scandinavian) Diminutive of Katerina. Variations: *Caren, Carin, Caryn, Karin, Karina, Karon, Kerena.*

KATHERINE (Greek) Pure. Katherine and all of its derivatives have been popular since the days of its Greek origin, when it was known as Aikaterina. Some of the most famous Katherines in this country have been Katherine Hepburn and authors Katharine Anne Porter and Katherine Mansfield. Though many parents today are favoring the more Gaelic forms of the name—like Katriona and Caitriona—Katherine itself presents a good choice simply based on all the variations you can choose from later. Variations: *Caitriona, Caren, Caron, Caryn, Caye, Kaethe, Kai, Kaila, Kait, Kaitlin, Karen, Karena, Karin, Karina, Karine, Karon, Karyn, Karyna, Karynn, Kata, Kataleen, Katalin, Katalina, Katarina, Kate, Katee, Kateke, Katerina, Katerinka, Katey, Katharin, Katharina, Katharine, Katharyn, Kathereen, Katherin, Katherina, Kathey, Kathi, Kathie, Kathleen, Kathlyn, Kathlynn, Kathren, Kathrine, Kathryn, Kathryne, Kathy, Kati, Katia, Katica, Katie, Katina, Katrina, Katrine, Katriona, Katryna, Kattrina, Katushka, Katy, Karrin, Katya, Kay, Kisan, Kit, Kitti, Kittie, Kitty, Kotinka, Kotryna, Yekaterina.*

KAYLA (English) Pure. Variation of Katherine. Kayla may have started to become popular about the same time that the name Caleb started to appear more frequently for boys. Although in definition they are not closely related, they both share a lyrical but compact sound. Once Kayla hit the American consciousness, it hit big and spread like wildfire. Today, Kayla is solidly entrenched on the top ten list for girls' names, even though it was nowhere to be seen even ten years ago. Variations: *Kaela, Kaelee, Kaelene, Kaeli, Kaeleigh, Kaelie, Kaelin, Kaelyn, Kaila, Kailan, Kailee, Kaileen, Kailene, Kailey, Kailin, Kailynne, Kalan, Kalee, Kaleigh, Kalen, Kaley, Kalie, Kalin, Kalyn, Kayana, Kayanna, Kaye, Kaylan, Kaylea, Kayleen, Kayleigh, Kaylene, Kayley, Kayli, Kaylle.*

KAYA (Native American) Wise child.

KEESHA (African-American) Newly created. Variations: *Keisha, Keshia, Kiesha.*

KELLY (Irish) Female soldier. Kelly has had multiple personalities over the last hundred years: first it was a last name, then many Irish and American parents chose it for their boys, and today it is almost exclusively a girls' name. Kelly was at its most popular in the '70s, and parents who have selected the name for their daughter since then have, more often than not, selected one of the name's expressive variations. Variations: *Kealey, Kealy, Keeley, Keelie, Keellie, Keely, Keighley, Keiley, Keilly, Keily, Kellee, Kelley, Kellia, Kellie, Kellina, Kellisa.*

KELSEY (English) Island. Although actor Kelsey Grammer has made us aware that Kelsey can also be a male name—and actually the name started out as being for boys only—Kelsey captivated many parents-to-be during the mid-to-late '80s, when Mr. Grammer was still a part-time patron on *Cheers*. Variations: *Kelcey, Kelci, Kelcie, Kelcy, Kellsie, Kelsa, Kelsea, Kelsee, Kelseigh, Kelsi, Kelsie, Kelsy.*

KENDRA (English) Origin unknown; possibly a combination of Kenneth and Sandra. Kendra is particularly popular among African-American parents today, although no one can trace where the name first appeared or what it means. Kendra first surfaced in the United States in the 1940s, and even though it sounds like it could have come from Great Britain, it didn't reach those shores until the later part of the '60s. Variations: *Kena, Kenadrea, Kendria, Kenna, Kindra, Kinna, Kyndra.*

KENISHA (African-American) Beautiful woman. Variations: *Keneisha, Keneshia, Kennesha.*

KERRY (Irish) County in Ireland. Like its counterpart, Kelly, Kerry was once a very popular name in this country. However, it seems as though its variations and creative spellings have gotten the better of it, rendering the original form almost obsolete. Like Kelly, Kerry started out as a boys' name. Variations: *Kera, Keree, Keri, Keriana, Keriann, Kerianna, Kerianne, Kerra, Kerrey, Kerri, Kerrianne, Kerrie.*

KESIA (African-American) Favorite. Variation: *Keshia.*

KIMBERLY (English) King's meadow. Kimberly was a well-used name at the turn of the century for boys, since it was a town in South Africa and many men were fighting a war there. To commemorate the battles, parents named their sons after the town. By the 1940s, Kimberly had already begun to take root as a girls' name, and it turned into one of the most popular names in the '60s and '70s. Today, however, it appears less frequently both here and in Britain. Variations: *Kim, Kimba, Kimba Lee, Kimball, Kimber, Kimberlea, Kimberlee, Kimberlei, Kimberleigh, Kimberley, Kimberli, Kimberlie, Kimberlyn, Kimbley, Kimmi, Kimmie, Kymberlee.*

KIRA (Bulgarian) Throne. Variations: *Kiran, Kirana, Kiri, Kirra.*

KIRSTEN (Scandinavian) Anointed. Feminine version of Christian. Kirsten and its variations have always seemed to be underused in this country, compared to their relatives Kristen and Christine. However, because it's been underused, Kirsten is becoming more popular than its counterparts today. Also, the visibility of the actress Kirstie Alley doesn't hurt. Variations: *Keerstin, Kersten, Kersti, Kerstie, Kerstin, Kiersten, Kierstin, Kirsta, Kirsti, Kirstie, Kirstin, Kirstine, Kirsty, Kirstyn, Kirstynn, Kyrstin.*

KITRA (Hebrew) Wreath.

KOKO (Japanese) Stork.

KRISTEN (English) Anointed. Feminine version of Christian. Kristen is stuck in the middle: not as common as Christine but not as unusual as Kirsten. The other names have been around for centuries, however, while Kristen has actually only been around in any measure since the 1960s in the United States. Kristen is one of the more popular girls' names around these days, but is not yet overused. Variations: *Krista, Kristan, Kristin, Kristina, Kristine, Kristyn, Kristyna, Krysta, Krystyna.*

KYLE (Scottish) Narrow land. Of course, by now, you can see the signs: this highly popular '90s name for boys has already started to develop a following among girls.

KYOKO (Japanese) Mirror.

LACEY (French) Last name. Some name experts consider Lacey to be the American version of Larissa. Lacey was a common French name in the nineteenth century. Variations: *Laci, Lacie, Lacy.*

LADONNA (African-American) Newly created. The uninitiated might think that Ladonna is just a cheap imitation of the famous singer's name Madonna, but in fact it is one of the more common "La" names that African-Americans have created for their daughters out of more common names. This trend began in the early 1980s, and has been wildly popular ever since. Variations: *Ladon, Ladonne, Ladonya.*

LAINE (English) Bright one. Variation of Helen. Variations: *Lainey, Lane, Layne.*

LAKEISHA (African-American) Newly created. Lakeisha is one of the most popular African-American "La" names. Compared to the other "La" names, there are numerous ways to spell this name. Lakeisha also can be traced to Ayesha, which many Muslim families chose for their daughters before the "La" trend began. Variations: *Lakecia, Lakeesha, Lakesha, Lakeshia, Laketia, Lakeysha, Lakeyshia, Lakicia, Lakiesha, Lakisha, Lakitia, Laquiesha, Laquiesha, Laquisha, Lekeesha, Lekeisha, Lekisha.*

LARISSA (Greek) Happy. Though Lara and Larissa seem to be related, they actually are derived from different roots. Larissa first began to appear in the 1960s, as did Lara, but today it is Larissa that is still around. Variations: *Laresa, Laressa, Larisa,* Laryssa.

LASHANDA (African-American) Newly created.

LATASHA (African-American) Newly created. Latasha sounds like Natasha, the name that many of us automatically associate with a female Russian spy. A lot of other people out there must like it, since Latasha has shown up in the top fifty names for African-American girls since the mid-'80s. Variation: *Latashia.*

LATOYA (African-American) Newly created. The visibility—and some say, the notoriety—of LaToya Jackson has made her first name one of the more popular "La" names around. As her reputation continues to ebb and flow, it will be interesting to see how that affects the popularity of Latoya as a baby name. Variations: *Latoia, Latoyia, Latoyla.*

LAURA (Latin) Laurel. Laura was a common name in my elementary school, but some thought it was a bit nerdy, perhaps owing to too many of the Dick van Dyke shows where Mary Tyler Moore played Dick's wife, Laura Petrie. Many parents today, however, don't agree,since Laura has appeared in the top twenty-five list of girls' names since the mid-'70s. Laura can trace its roots back to the fourteenth century in Italy, when it was spelled Lora. Laura has been equally popular both in the United States and in Britain. Variations: *Larette, Laural, Laure, Laureana, Laurel, Lauren, Laurena, Lauret, Laureta, Lauretta, Laurette, Laurie, Laurin, Lauryn, Lora, Loren, Lorena, Loret, Loreta, Loretta, Lorette, Lori, Lorin, Lorita, Lorrie, Lorrin, Lorry, Loryn.*

LEAH (Hebrew) Weary. Slowly but surely, Leah is starting to appear more frequently among baby girls born today, especially among Jewish families. Leah, in the Book of Genesis, was first used as a given name in sixteenth-century Puritan England. Variations: *Lea, Leia, Leigha, Lia, Liah.*

LEANNA (Gaelic) Flowering vine. Variations: *Leana, Leane, Leann, Leanne, Lee Ann, Lee Anne, Leeann, Leeanne, Leianna, Leigh Ann, Leighann, Leighanne, Liana, Liane, Lianne.*

LEIGH (English) Meadow. In its simpler spelling, Lee, this name has always been more popular for boys than for girls, but Leigh is beginning to gain a following. Variation: *Lee.*

LEIKO (Japanese) Proud.

LENA (English) Bright one. Variation of Helen. Variations: *Lenah, Lene, Leni, Lenia, Lina, Linah, Line.*

LESLIE (Scottish) Low meadow. Leslie has had a rich and colorful history, adapted from its original use as a last name in one of Robert Burns's poems. Burns spelled it as Lesley, but when parents began to use the name for their boys, they used the spelling of Leslie. The name remained popular among both sexes and in both spellings up until the 1940s. Today, Leslie is primarily a girls' name, although neither spelling predominates. Variations: *Leslea, Leslee, Lesley, Lesli, Lesly, Lezlee, Lezley, Lezli, Lezlie.*

LILITH (Arabic) Night demon. It's a good bet that few people would have heard of Lilith without the character Dr. Lilith Sternin, the psychiatrist played by actress Bebe Neuwirth on the TV show *Cheers*. Lilith is actually the name of the wife that Adam had before Eve. According to legend, Lilith didn't like having a man calling the shots, so she departed, turning herself into a demon instead. Variation: *Lillis.*

LILLIAN (English) Lily + Ann. Variations: *Lileana, Lilian, Liliana, Lilias, Lilika, Lillia, Lillianne, Lillyan, Lillyanna, Lilyan.*

LILY (Latin) Flower. Variations: *Lili, Lilia, Lilie, Lilli, Lillie, Lillye, Lilye.*

LINDSAY (English) Island of linden trees. Perhaps Lindsay was the reason that Linda hasn't remained more popular, even though except for sharing a few letters, the names have nothing in common. Lindsay was mostly a boys' name until the "bionic woman"—played by Lindsay Wagner—helped to bring this name to the forefront. Lindsay and its variant spellings appeared on the top ten baby name lists in the '80s, but as with all very popular names, ten or fifteen years can make a huge difference in how the name is perceived. Variations: *Lindsaye, Lindsey, Lindsi, Lindsie, Lindsy, Linsay, Linsey, Linzey, Lyndsay, Lyndsey, Lynsay, Lynsey.*

LINETTE (Welsh) Idol. Variations: *Lanette, Linet, Linetta, Linnet, Linnetta, Linnette, Lynetta, Lynette, Lynnet, Lynnette.*

LISA (English) Pledged by oath to God. Version of Elizabeth. Though I don't particularly think of my own parents as being faithful to the trends of their day, the fact that they named me Lisa is testament to how attuned they really were. In terms of popularity, Lisa was number four on the baby name hit parade in 1970, and number twelve in 1980, but today parents are clearly preferring to use one of the other derivatives of Elizabeth such as Liza or Libby. Some parents may have been swayed by Nat King Cole's number-one song, "Mona Lisa." Variations: *Leesa, Leeza, Leisa, Liesa, Liese, Lisanne, Lise, Liseta, Lisetta, Lisette, Lissa, Lissette, Liza, Lizana, Lizanne, Lizette.*

LISANDRA (Greek) Liberator. Variations: *Lissandra, Lizandra, Lizann, Lizanne, Lysandra.*

LOLA (English) Sorrow. Nickname for Dolores. Variations: *Loleta, Loletta, Lolita.*

LORELEI (German) Area in Germany. Variations: *Loralee, Loralie, Loralyn, Lorilee, Lura, Lurette, Lurleen, Lurlene, Lurline.*

LORRAINE (French) Area in France. *Saturday Night Live* actress Laraine Newman helped increase popularity for this name, but it has never really hit in the United States the way it's been used in England and Scotland. In Ireland, it was one of the most popular names for girls in the '70s. Variations: *Laraine, Lauraine, Laurraine, Lorain, Loraine, Lorayne, Lorine, Lorrayne.*

LOUISE (English) Famous soldier. Feminine version of Louis. The author of *Little Women*, Louisa May Alcott, is probably the most famous American woman with this name, perhaps causing the name to remain on the top fifty baby names list throughout the Great Depression. It is currently popular in Britain, and the name may have been given a boost here by the popular movie *Thelma and Louise*. Variations: *Aloise, Aloysia, Louisine, Louiza, Luisa, Luise.*

LUCY (English) Light. Feminine version of Lucius. Lucy is a great old name that has finally made the comeback in the '90s that it deserves. Lucia, the root for all Lucy-related names, is in turn the feminine version of an ancient Roman family name. Today, it seems that parents are choosing Lucy more often; it may become one of the hipper names associated with the '90s. Variations: *Lucetta, Lucette, Lucia, Luciana, Lucie, Lucienne, Lucilla, Lucille, Lucina, Lucinda, Lucita.*

LYDIA (Greek) Woman from Lydia, a region in ancient Greece. Variations: *Lidi, Lidia, Lidie, Lidka, Likochka, Lydiah, Lydie.*

MABEL (English) Lovable. Associated for years with housekeepers on TV, Mabel is actually starting to appear on birth certificates today as often as it did a hundred years ago, when it was a popular name in this country. Variations: *Mabelle, Mable, Maybel, Maybell, Maybelle.*

MADELINE (French) Mary Magdalen. Most parents today are familiar with the Madeleine books by the author Ludwig Bemelmans. The character that Cybil Shepherd played in the TV show *Moonlighting* a few seasons back named Maddy may be responsible for the small upward blip we see today connected with the name. Variations: *Mada, Madalaina, Maddalena, Maddi, Maddie, Madelaine, Madelayne, Madeleine, Madelena, Madelene, Madelina, Madge, Magda.*

MADISON (English) Last name.

MALLORY (French) Unfortunate. Actress Justine Bateman, who played the character Mallory in the TV show *Family Ties* back in the '80s, may have unwittingly provided the spark for the whole trend of using boys' names and/or last names as suitable attractive names for girls. Though today the name is indelibly connected with that era as well as the show, there are hundreds of like-minded names that a parent could choose from. Variations: *Malloreigh, Mallorey, Mallorie, Malorey, Malori, Malorie, Malory.*

MARCIA (Latin) Warlike. Feminine version of Mark. After *The Brady Bunch* faded from our weekly Friday dose, only to reemerge in daily rerun heaven, most parents would shudder at the thought of naming their daughters after the eldest Brady goody-two-shoes. However, as everything old becomes new again, eventually, Marcia just may start to catch on among parents. Variations: *Marce, Marcee, Marcela, Marcelia, Marcella, Marcelle, Marcena, Marcene, Marcey, Marci, Marcie, Marcina, Marcy, Marsha.*

MARGARET (English) Pearl. Margaret has very deep roots, reaching back to the third century when it was the name of a popular saint. Later on, in the eleventh century, it was so popular that it was known as the national Scottish female name. It was also very popular in England and the United States: Margaret was a consistent member of the top ten girls' names list for the better part of the first half of this century. Today, many parents are beginning to take a second look.

Variations: *Greeta, Greetje, Grere, Gret, Greta, Gretal, Gretchen, Gretel, Grethal, Grethel, Gretje, Gretl, Gretta, Groer, Maggi, Maggie, Maggy, Mair, Maire, Mairi, Mairona, Margara, Margareta, Margarethe, Margarett, Margaretta, Margarette, Margarita, Margarite, Marge, Margeret, Margerey, Margery, Margrett, Marguerette, Marguerite, Marj, Marjorie, Meagan, Meaghan, Meaghen, Meg, Megan, Megen, Meggi, Meggie, Meggy, Meghan, Meghann, Peg, Pegeen, Pegg, Peggey, Peggi, Peggie, Peggy, Reet, Reeta, Reita, Rheeta, Riet, Rieta, Ritta.*

MARIE (French) Variation of Mary. It's funny what the difference a letter will make to determine the popularity of a given name. Marie is a perfect example. While some parents consider Mary to be too Catholic and Maria to be too Hispanic, it seems that Marie has found a middle ground. French in origin, Marie was the second most popular name in the United States during the 1920s, when Flapper Era parents must have thought that it represented the best of Europe and everything it had to offer. Today in the United States, Marie is still used more frequently than Mary and Maria combined.

MARILYN (English) Combination of Mary and Lynn. Variations: *Maralin, Maralynn, Marelyn, Marilee, Marilin, Marilynne, Marralynn, Marrilin, Marrilyn, Marylin, Marylyn.*

MARIS (Latin) Star of the sea. Though many people consider the up-and-coming Maris and its variations to be derivatives of Mary, it actually comes from the Latin marine term *stella maris*, which means "star of the sea." Maris first started to appear in the United States in the 1920s, and some of the variations—Marissa, for example—began to pop up in the '50s, but it is only in the '90s that the name has taken a real foothold. Actress Marisa Tomei has been responsible for providing most of the exposure. Variations: *Marieca, Marisa, Marise, Marish, Marisha, Marissa, Marisse, Meris, Merisa, Merissa.*

MARLENE (English) Combination of Maria and Magdalene. Variations: *Marla, Marlaina, Marlaine, Marlana, Marlane, Marlayne, Marlea, Marlee, Marleen, Marleina, Marlena, Marley, Marlie, Marlina, Marlinda, Marline, Marlyn.*

MARY (Hebrew) Bitterness. The Virgin Mary. Back in the Middle Ages, you could be tried for blasphemy if you chose the name Mary for your daughter; back then, it was considered to be too sacred to use for a mere mortal. Of course, once attitudes changed, Mary quickly grew to become one of the most popular names among English-speaking countries. After the 1950s in the United States, Mary rapidly began to decline in popularity, to the point where today it is a fairly uncommon name. Famous Marys of the past include Mary Pickford, Mary Poppins, and Mary Tyler Moore. Today, without a famous face spreading the good news about Mary, don't expect it to reach its previous heights of popularity. Variations: *Maree, Marella, Marelle, Mari, Marial, Marieke, Mariel, Mariela, Mariele, Mariella, Marielle, Marika, Marike, Maryk, Maura, Moira, Moll, Mollee, Molley, Molli, Mollie, Molly, Mora, Moria, Moyra.*

MATILDA (Old German) Maiden in battle. Matilda is a wonderful, lyrical name that many American parents are finding to be a perfect match for their newborn daughters. It's expressive enough on its own, but the many different variations are also very distinctive. Variations: *Maddi, Maddie, Maddy, Mat, Matelda, Mathilda, Mathilde, Matilde, Mattie, Matty, Matusha, Matylda, Maud, Maude, Tila, Tilda, Tildie, Tildy, Tilley, Tilli, Tillie, Tilly, Tylda.*

MAUREEN (Irish) Variation of Mary. Maureen was a quintessentially Irish name that appeared to be equally popular in Ireland, Britain, and the United States, at least up until 1960, when it began to become used less frequently. Famous Maureens include Maureen O'Sullivan and Maureen O'Hara, both movie stars who seemed to go into retirement about the same time that the name began to fade. Variations: *Maurene, Maurine, Moreen, Morreen, Moureen.*

MELANIE (Greek) Dark-skinned. Variations: *Mel, Mela, Melaine, Melana, Melane, Melani, Melaniya, Melanka, Melany, Melanya, Melashka, Melasya, Melenia, Melka, Mellanie, Mellie, Melloney, Mellony, Melly, Meloni, Melonie, Melony, Milena, Milya.*

MELINDA (Latin) Honey. Variations: *Malina, Malinda, Malinde, Mallie, Mally, Mel, Meleana, Melina, Melinde, Meline, Mellinda, Melynda, Mindi, Mindie, Mindy.*

MELISSA (Greek) Bee. Today Melissa hovers around the bottom half of the top twenty-five list. The name is destined to move up the ranks slightly, owing to the success and popularity of singer Melissa Etheridge. Melissa is an ancient name that was first popular during the early Roman Empire as it was the name of the woman who nursed the mighty god Juno when he was a baby. Variations: *Melisa, Melisande, Melisandra, Melisandre, Melissande, Melissandre, Melisse, Mellisa, Mellissa.*

MENASHA (Native American: Algonquin) Island.

MERCEDES (Spanish) Mercy. Though it might be assumed that any girl named Mercedes today would be directly inspired by the luxury car, the fact is that the car received its name from the Spanish version of one of the popular ways to refer to the Virgin Mary, Our Lady of the Mercies. However, if you already have a son named Ben, don't choose this name. Variations: *Merced, Mercede.*

MEREDITH (Welsh) Great leader. Variations: *Meredithe, Merideth, Meridith, Merridith.*

MERYL (English) Bright as the sea. Actress Meryl Streep is an obvious reason why this name has become popular for girls since the early '80s. Nevertheless, parents today are more likely to choose one of the variations that sounds androgynous and resembles a last name. Of course, these two trends are responsible for many of the new girls' names out there. Variations: *Merill, Merrall, Merrel, Merrell, Merrill, Meryle, Meryll.*

MICHAELA (Hebrew) Who is like the Lord? Feminine version of Michael. Variations: *Makaela, Micaela, Mical, Michael, Michaella, Michal, Michala, Mickaula, Micki, Mickie, Micky, Mikella, Mikelle, Mychaela.*

MICHELLE (French) Who is like the Lord? More common feminine version of Michael. Michelle has been one of the few names that has been in the top ten list since the 1960s. The song "Michelle" by the Beatles can take credit for some of this popularity, as well as Michelle Pfeiffer, who grabbed the torch in the mid-'80s. Used quite frequently in African-American families today, it is beginning to see a challenge by a close relative, Michaela, and its variations that sound more androgynous to the ear. Variations: *Michele, Nichelle.*

MIDORI (Japanese) Green.

MING (Chinese) Tomorrow.

MIRABEL (Latin) Wonderful. Magazine editor Grace Mirabella has been a factor in the increasing number of parents who are looking toward Mirabel and its variations as a suitable first name for their daughters. Though it seems that every girls' name that ends in "bel" is rising on the popularity scale, Mirabel is probably the most melodious. Variations: *Mirabell, Mirabella, Mirabelle.*

MIRANDA (Latin) Admirable. Variations: *Maranda, Meranda, Mira, Myranda, Randa, Randee, Randene, Randey, Randi, Randie, Randy.*

MIYO (Japanese) Beautiful generations. Variation: *Miyoko.*

MONICA (Latin) Adviser or nun. The name Monica has a lot of energy to it; this trait is perhaps best embodied by the tennis champion Monica Seles. On the other hand, one of its variations, Monique, always sounds sultry; it's one of the best French names that you could give your daughter. Today, Monique is most popular among African-American families, who have placed it in the top fifty list of names for their daughters. Variations: *Monika, Monique.*

MORGAN (Welsh) Great and bright. Though in the past, Morgan has been more widely known as both a last name and a name for boys, actress Morgan Fairchild provided great exposure for this name. Originally, the sister of King Arthur, Morgan Le Fay, helped to create some feminine allure to the name. Variations: *Morgana, Morganne, Morgen.*

MURIEL (Irish) Bright as the sea. Though Muriel was a popular name in Britain from approximately the 1870s through to the 1930s, it has faded away ever since then. In this country, it never really got a foothold to begin with. But that could all change owing to the success of the Australian movie *Muriel's Wedding.* Variations: *Muirgheal, Murial, Muriell, Murielle.*

MYRA (Latin) Scented oil. Feminine version of Myron. Variations: *Murah, Myria, Myriah.*

NADA (Arabic) Dew at sunrise. Variation: *Nadya.*

NADIA (Russian) Hope. Variations: *Nada, Nadeen, Nadene, Nadina, Nadine, Nadiya, Nadja, Nadya, Natka.*

NANCY (Hebrew) Grace. Though its origins are Hebrew, Nancy seems more like one of the quintessentially American names. Nancy's peak in the United States occurred in the 1950s, when it placed in the top ten. It had peaked in Britain twenty years earlier. The famous Nancys that most of us know do date from that earlier period, including former First Lady Nancy Reagan and fictional detective Nancy Drew. Nancy may be on the way back up, as a result of skater Nancy Kerrigan's performance at the 1994 Winter Olympics. Variations: *Nan, Nana, Nance, Nancee, Nancey, Nanci, Nancie, Nancsi, Nanette, Nann, Nanna, Nanncey, Nanncy, Nanni, Nannie, Nanny, Nanscey, Nansee, Nansey.*

NAOMI (Hebrew) Pleasant. Naomi seems poised for newfound popularity for several reasons. It's a pretty name, it has strong Biblical overtones that appeal to many parents today, and it is also being spread by the fame of Naomi Judd and Naomi Campbell. Given this combination, Naomi should continue to flourish through the end of the '90s and well into the first decade of the twenty-first century. Variations: *Naoma, Naomia, Naomie, Neoma, Noami, Noemi, Noemie.*

NATALIE (Latin) Birthday. Though one famous Natalie that many Americans hear about is Garrison Keeler's Nattily Attired, Natalie is quietly beginning to make its mark in this country. The name was very popular in Britain from the 1960s through the mid-'80s (when it hit number fifteen on the top twenty list), but it has never been extensively used in the United States. Of course, its being associated with the singer Natalie Cole won't exactly hurt the name. Variations: *Natala,*

Natalee, Natalene, Natalia, Natalina, Nataline, Natalka, Natalya, Natelie, Nathalia, Nathalie.

NATASHA (Greek) Rebirth. Natasha is a name that has many exotic connotations associated with it. For most of us, the first Natasha we met was on the *Rocky and Bullwinkle show.* In the '70s and '80s, actress Nastassja Kinski kept the name alive, and today it's Natasha Richardson who is the preeminent example. But leaving all that aside, Natasha is just a beautiful name for a girl and later a woman. There was one famous Natasha who settled for a more American form of her name: the late Natalie Wood. Variations: *Nastasia, Nastassia, Nastassja, Nastassya, Nastasya, Natashia, Tashi, Tashia, Tasis, Tassa, Tassie.*

NELL (English) Light. Jodie Foster's recent movie entitled *Nell,* in which she played the main character, has brought this name with a Victorian flair into the American consciousness. Back around the turn of the century, when the name was first popular, the variation Nellie was more common than its root. Today, both should grow in popularity as both a first and middle name. Variations: *Nella, Nelley, Nelli, Nellie, Nelly.*

NEVADA (English) The state. Like Montana, Nevada is quickly becoming one of the more popular girls' names that are taken from a state. This trend seems to be spreading overseas as well—the name Nevada is also popularly used in Great Britain.

NICOLE (English) People of victory. Feminine version of Nicholas. Back in the first half of 1994, Nicole was enjoying a nice quiet ride up the rungs of the popularity ladder, helped along in part by actress Nicolette Sheridan. Then in June of that same year, chaos broke loose with the O. J. Simpson murder case. It's too soon to tell if the name's sudden and complete notoriety will translate to an increase in babies named Nicole these days, but time will tell if Nicole reaches its earlier heights—in 1980, it was the fourth most popular girls' name in the United States. Variations: *Nichol, Nichola, Nichole, Nicholle, Nicki, Nickola, Nickole, Nicola, Nicoleen, Nicolene, Nicoletta, Nicolette, Nicolina, Nicoline, Nicolla, Nicolle, Nikki, Nikola, Nikoletta, Nikolette.*

NINA (Spanish) Girl. Nina is an ancient name that has been around for several millennia. In Babylonian mythology, Nina was the goddess of the seas, and in the Incan culture, Nina ruled over fire. In this country, it seems as if Nina is a name that could always be just a bit more popular, and given the slight stirrings the name has had since the mid-'70s, it may well start to become more visible. Variations: *Neena, Ninelle, Ninet, Nineta, Ninete, Ninetta, Ninette, Ninita, Ninnette, Ninotchka, Nynette.*

NITA (Hindu) Friendly. Variations: *Neeta, Nitali.*

NOEL (French) Christmas. Names that reflect the seasons in some way are starting to become very popular, and Noel is no exception. Traditionally, parents named their baby boys and girls born on Christmas day with a variation of Noel, but today's parents have taken the liberty of giving the name to children who are born throughout the month of December. The variation Nowell appears to have come about because this is how the holiday is spelled in many Christmas carols. Variations: *Noela, Noelani, Noele, Noeleen, Noelene, Noeline, Noell, Noella, Noelle, Noelline, Noleen, Nowell.*

NOLA (English) White shoulder. Variations: *Nolah, Nolana.*

NORA (Greek) Light. Variation: *Norah.*

NOREEN (English) Diminutive of Nora, light. Variations: *Noreena, Norene, Norina, Norine.*

NORMA (Latin) Pattern. Though Norma was once fashionable enough to belong to several movie actresses including Norma Shearer, off the screen the name always seemed to belong to mothers and grandmothers and never little girls. Though a similar-sounding name—Martha—has caught on in the '90s in some circles, Norma doesn't seem as if it will have the same clout. Variation: *Normah.*

OCTAVIA (Latin) Eighth. Octavia is a wonderfully intriguing name. The name brings up images of reruns of the old British series *I, Claudius,* which exhibited some of the more decadent characteristics of the Roman Empire. Most everyone will admit to liking the name, but you'll have to be brave to give it to your own daughter. Variations: *Octavie, Ottavia.*

ODE (African: Nigerian) Born while traveling.

ODELE (German) Wealthy. Variations: *Oda, Odeela, Odela, Odelia, Odelinda, Odell, Odella, Odelle, Odelyn, Odila, Odile, Odilia.*

ODETTE (French) Wealthy. Variation: *Odetta.*

OLA (Polish) Protector of men; (Scandinavian) Ancestor's relic. Variations: *Olesia, Olesya.*

OLGA (Russian) Holy. The two Olgas who are perhaps best known are a saint from the tenth century and the petite gymnast Olga Korbut, who helped bring a new grace to the name in this country during the 1976 Summer Olympics. Olga is still one of the more popular names in Russia today, but it is also widely used across Europe. Variations: *Elga, Ola, Olenka, Olesya, Olia, Olina, Olka, Olli, Olly, Olunka, Oluska, Olva, Olya, Olyusha.*

OLIVIA (Latin) Olive tree. Olivia, currently very popular and hovering near the top ten list in this country, has a long and illustrious history in the arts and on TV. Though its roots are Italian, most Americans tend to think of Olivia as a very British name, associating it with Olivia De Havilland and Australian singer Olivia Newton-John. Olivia made its first appearance in literature in Shakespeare's play *Twelfth Night,* but today its popularity seems to stem from its wide usage on TV: Olivia was not only the name of the sainted mother on the '70s show *The Waltons,* but has also appeared as a character in no fewer than three soap operas. Parents like the name because it has eloquence and sophistication, and yet a down-home, almost southern feel to it. Variations: *Lioa, Lioia, Liovie, Liv, Olia, Oliva, Olive, Olivet, Olivette, Olivine, Ollie, Olva.*

OPAL (English) Gem. Some of the old-fashioned jewel names, like Opal, were pretty common around the 1900s. Today, while Ruby and Jade are quickly becoming hot names in the United States, Opal doesn't seem to be keeping up. Variations: *Opalina, Opaline.*

OPHELIA (Greek) Help. Variation: *Ofelia.*

ORIANA (Latin) Sunrise. Variations: *Oraine, Oralia, Orane, Orania, Orelda, Orelle, Oriane.*

PAGE (French) Intern. Page is a girls' name that isn't used too frequently, but when it is, it seems to command a sense of respect and power. One prominent Paige who certainly fits this definition is Paige Rense, the editor of the magazine *Architectural Digest,* who transformed the publication into one of the foremost influences in the industry. Paige also appeared as a character on the TV show *Knots Landing,* played by Nicollette Sheridan. The name Page will probably continue to be used sparingly, but when it does appear, it will always pack a punch. Variation: *Paige.*

PAMELA (Greek) Honey. Despite the omnipresence of *Baywatch* vixen Pamela Anderson Lee, the name actually has quite a number of strong literary connections. Pamela's first known usage was by author Sir Philip Sidney in his work entitled *Arcadia,* which dates from the very end of the sixteenth century. Next, it appeared in a popular novel entitled *Pamela* by another author, Samuel Richardson, in the middle of the eighteenth century. Latter-day authors who were actually christened with the name include Brits Pamela Moore and Pamela Hansford Johnson. Pamela fell into the top ten list from the '50s through the '70s, but then tended to fall off in popularity. Mrs. Lee could very well bring the name back into popular usage once again. Variations: *Pam, Pamala, Pamalia, Pamalla, Pamelia, Pamelina, Pamella, Pamilia, Pamilla, Pammela, Pammi, Pammie, Pammy.*

PARIS (English) The city. In keeping with the current trend toward naming girls after cities, states, and regions, Paris is right up there as a name for a baby girl, and some parents have even chosen this name for their daughter because it was where they believe she was conceived. Variations: *Parisa, Parris, Parrish.*

PASCALE (French) Child of Easter. Feminine version of Pascal. Variations: *Pascalette, Pascaline, Pascalle, Paschale.*

PATRICIA (English) Noble. Feminine version of Patrick. Though Patricia has a long, esteemed history dating from the sixth century, when it began to be used within the Catholic church, a surge in Patricia's popularity can clearly be distinguished from the time that one of Queen Victoria's granddaughters was given the name. From there, it basically exploded in both Great Britain and the United States. This fervor lasted until well into the '70s. As with many other formal names, even though Patricia may be the given name, it's more likely that you'll use one of Patricia's nicknames. And when parents are choosing the name today, they are leaning toward one of the more exotic variations listed here. Famous Patricias include actresses Patty Duke and Patricia Neal. Variations: *Pat, Patreece, Patreice, Patria, Patric, Patrica, Patrice, Patricka, Patrizia, Patsy, Patti, Pattie, Patty, Tricia, Trish, Trisha.*

PAULA (Latin) Small. Feminine version of Paul. Variations: *Paola, Paolina, Paule, Pauleen, Paulene, Pauletta, Paulette, Paulie, Paulina, Pauline, Paulita, Pauly, Paulyn, Pavla, Pavlina, Pavlinka, Pawlina, Pola, Polcia, Pollie, Polly.*

PEARL (Latin) Pearl. Variations: *Pearla, Pearle, Pearleen, Pearlena, Pearlette, Pearley, Pearline, Pearly, Perl, Perla, Perle, Perlette, Perley, Perlie, Perly.*

PENELOPE (Greek) Bobbin weaver. Penny is a great worldly name that dates back to the ancient Greek myth in which Penelope remained faithful to Ulysses. Today, we tend to think of Penelope as exclusively British and Penny as uniquely American, though birth registries show that the names seem to be used equally in both countries. Famous Penelopes include Penelope Leach and Penny Marshall. Variations: *Lopa, Pela, Pelcia, Pen, Penelopa, Penina, Penine, Penna, Pennelope, Penni, Penny, Pinelopi, Piptisa, Popi.*

PERRY (French) Pear tree; (Greek) Nymph of mountains. Perry started out as a boys' name that was actually a nickname for Peregrine. Parents began to consider the name for their daughters around the middle of this century, but it seems to be so rarely used by either sex that it has remained a gender-neutral name even after all these years. More parents should consider this name, which meets several of the current baby-naming trends. Variations: *Peri, Perrey, Perri, Perrie.*

PHILIPPA (Greek) Lover of horses. Feminine version of Philip. Variations: *Philipa, Philippine, Phillipina, Pippa, Pippy.*

PHYLLIS (Greek) Green tree branch. Variations: *Philis, Phillis, Philliss, Phyllys, Phylis, Phyllida, Phylliss.*

PIA (Latin) Pious.

POLLY (English) Variation of Molly, which in turn is a diminutive form of Mary, which means bitter. In the minds of most people, the name Polly will forever be connected with a cracker-eating parrot or the goody-two-shoes in the novel by author Eleanor H. Porter, *Pollyanna.* The first thing that comes to my mind is the hapless girlfriend of Underdog, sweet Polly Purebred. One way around this might be the variation Pauleigh; however, anyway you spell it, it turns out to be Polly. Variations: *Pauleigh, Pollee, Polley, Polli, Pollie, Pollyann, Pollyanna, Pollyanne.*

PORTIA (Latin) Roman clan name. Variations: *Porcha, Porscha, Porsche, Porschia, Porsha.*

PRISCILLA (English) Old. Once upon a time, Priscilla seemed to have the same kind of reputation as Polly, since it was a popular Puritan name; its most famous bearer was Priscilla Alden. Today, however, the widow of Elvis Presley, Priscilla Presley, has given new visibility to this name and singlehandedly altered its reputation from prim and proper to smart and alluring. Variations: *Precilla, Prescilla, Pricilla, Pris, Priscila, Priss, Prissie, Prissilla, Prissy, Prysilla.*

QUINN (Gaelic) Advisor. Variation: *Quincy.*

RACHEL (Hebrew) Lamb. Rachel is essentially one of the oldest names in the Bible. It has proven to be a popular name in this country ever since the Puritans first arrived in the 1600s. During the Middle Ages, however, Christians wouldn't touch the name since they considered it to be a strictly "Jewish" name. After the Puritans broke through with its more common use, it remained popular among parents who wished their daughters to eventually emulate the mother of Joseph in the Bible, and as time went on, parents from all faiths began to see the beauty in the name. In the '90s, Rachel has consistently appeared in the top twenty names list. Variations: *Rachael, Racheal, Rachele, Rachell, Rachelle, Rae, Raelene, Raquel, Raquela, Raquella, Raquelle.*

RAFAELA (Spanish) God heals. Feminine version of Raphael. Variations: *Rafa, Rafaelia, Rafaella, Rafella, Rafelle, Raffaela, Raffaele, Raphaella, Raphaelle, Refaela, Rephaela.*

RAMONA (Hindu) Wise protector. Feminine version of Raymond. Many parents casting around for a suitable name for their daughters will remember Ramona primarily as the impish character in the children's books by author Beverly Cleary.

RASHEDA (Turkish) Righteous. Feminine version of Rashid. Variations: *Rasheeda, Rasheedah, Rasheida, Rashidah.*

RAYNA (Hebrew) Song of the Lord. Variations: *Raina, Rana, Rane, Rania, Renana, Renanit, Renatia, Renatya, Renina, Rinatia, Rinatya.*

REBECCA (Hebrew) Joined together. The first Rebecca known to us was the Biblical wife of Isaac and the mother of Jacob. Other famous Rebeccas since then have been Rebecca of Sunnybrook Farm from Kate Douglas's novel, as well as another literary figure, novelist Rebecca West. Novelist Daphne Du Maurier also wrote a novel called *Rebecca,* later turned into a movie by Alfred Hitchcock. Name-watchers point to Du Maurier's book as the main influence that put Rebecca on the map back in the '40s. Variations: *Becca, Becky, Reba, Rebbecca, Rebbie, Rebeca, Rebeccah, Rebecka, Rebeckah, Rebeka, Rebekah, Rebekka, Rebekke, Rebeque, Rebi, Reby, Reyba, Rheba.*

RENÉE (French) Reborn. French names with accent marks appeared to be pretty popular during the '70s and Renée fit right in. The Latin version of Renée is Renata, and it was commonly used by people in the Roman Empire for their daughters. Somewhere between back then and the 1600s, Renata turned into Renée; Renata rarely appears anymore. Variations: *Renata, Renay, Rene, Renelle, Reney, Reni, Renia, Renie, Renni, Rennie, Renny.*

RHIANNON (Welsh) Goddess. Variations: *Rheanna, Rheanne, Rhiana, Rhiann, Rhianna, Rhiannan, Rhianon, Rhuan, Riana, Riane, Rianna, Rianne, Riannon, Riannon, Rianon, Riona.*

ROBERTA (English) Bright fame. Feminine version of Robert. Variations: *Bobbet, Bobbett, Bobbi, Bobbie, Bobby, Robbi, Robbie, Robby, Robena, Robertena, Robertha, Robertina, Robin, Robina, Robine, Robinette, Robinia, Robyn, Robyna, Rogan, Roynne.*

ROCHELLE (French) Little rock. Variations: *Rochele, Rochell, Rochella, Roshele, Roshelle.*

ROLANDA (German) Famous land. Feminine version of Roland. Before TV talk-show host Rolanda Watts came onto the national scene in the early '90s, this name was primarily known as a rarely used feminine version of Roland. As Ms. Watts grows in popularity, the name may become more common. Variations: *Rolande, Rollande, Rolonda, Rolonde.*

ROSALIND (Spanish) Pretty rose. Variations: *Rosalina, Rosalinda, Rosalinde, Rosaline, Rosalyn, Rosalynd, Rosalyne, Rosalynn, Roselind, Roselynn, Roslyn.*

ROSANNA (English) Combination of Rose and Anna. Variations: *Rosana, Rosannah, Rosanne, Roseana, Roseanna, Roseanna, Roseannah, Rosehannah, Rozanna, Rozanne.*

ROSE (Latin) Flower. Flower names have been making a comeback in the '90s, and Rose seems to be the runaway leader. It has Victorian overtones, it's elegant, and it's also becoming extremely popular as a middle name. Rose should continue to bloom through the rest of this decade and beyond. Variations: *Rosabel, Rosabell, Rosabella, Rosabelle, Rosalee, Rosaley, Rosalia, Rosalie, Rosalin, Rosella, Roselle, Rosetta, Rosette, Rosey, Rosi, Rosie, Rosita, Rosy, Ruza, Ruzena, Ruzenka, Ruzsa.*

ROSEMARY (Latin) Dew of the sea. Variations: *Rosemaree, Rosemarey, Rosemaria, Rosemarie.*

ROSSALYN (Scottish) Cape. Feminine version of Ross. Variations: *Rosslyn, Rosslynn.*

ROXANNE (Persian) Dawn. Variations: *Roxana, Roxane, Roxann, Roxanna, Roxianne, Roxie, Roxy.*

RUBY (English) Jewel. Ruby was part of the first wave of jewel names that began to hit right after the Civil War. Today, Ruby is slowly beginning to become more popular. Variations: *Rube, Rubey, Rubie, Rubye.*

RUTH (Hebrew) Companion. Variations: *Ruthe, Ruthella, Ruthelle, Ruthetta, Ruthi, Ruthie, Ruthina, Ruthine, Ruthy.*

SACHI (Japanese) Bliss. Variation: *Sachiko.*

SAMANTHA (English) His name is God. Samantha is widely considered to be the feminine version of Samuel, and though it's been around from the 1600s, when it was used mostly by black Americans, it wasn't until the TV series *Bewitched* first appeared in the 1960s that this name really took off. Samantha is still the fourth most popular girls' name in the mid-nineties. Samantha was a well-regarded but little-used name in Britain in the mid-'60s but, when *Bewitched* started airing in England, the popularity of the name soared, and Samantha turned into one of the top names for girls. Besides Samantha Stevens, another famous Samantha was Samantha Eggar, a British actress who was popular in the 60s. Variations: *Sam, Samella, Samentha, Sammantha, Sammee, Sammey, Sammi, Sammie, Sammy, Semanntha, Semantha, Simantha, Symantha.*

SARAH (Hebrew) Princess. Sarah was once primarily notable for its popularity as a name for Jewish girls, but in the '90s Sarah hovers among the most popular names for all daughters in the United States. In the Bible, Sarah was the wife of Abraham, and the name has been well-used and well-liked in both Great Baritain and the United States since Puritan times. Famous Sarahs today include Sarah Jessica Parker and Sara Gilbert. Though some fear Sarah will become overused if its popularity continues, others believe that it's destined to be a timeless classic. Variations: *Sadee, Sadie, Sadye, Saidee, Saleena, Salena, Salina, Sallee, Salley, Sallianne, Sallie, Sally, Sallyann, Sara, Sarai, Saretta, Sarette, Sari, Sarita, Saritia, Sarra.*

SAVANNAH (Spanish) Treeless. Place name. Savannah is hot. It seems that in every other movie, as well as many books, the name of the female protagonist who must jump through hoops and face seemingly insurmountable challenges all in 300 pages or 90 minutes, is named Savannah. Melinda Dillon played Savannah in the movie *The Prince of Tides,* and Whitney Houston played Savannah in the movie *Waiting to Exhale.* Variations: *Savana, Savanah, Savanna, Savonna, Sevanna.*

SCARLETT (English) Red. Variations: *Scarlet, Scarlette.*

SELA (Polynesian) Princess.

SELENA (Greek) Goddess of the moon. Many of the girls' names that begin with "S" and have lots of vowels in them are very pretty and Selena is no exception. Though Selena's first use was as a Greek goddess, the name began to become popular in the 1800s when a countess in Britain went by the name of Selina. Variations: *Celena, Celina, Celinda, Celine, Celyna, Salena, Salina, Salinah, Sela, Selene, Selina, Selinda, Seline, Sena.*

SERENA (Latin) Serene. If you'd like your daughter to be cute and a little bit mischievous, then Serena is a good name for her. Serena was alter ego to Samantha in the sitcom *Bewitched,* and Serena was always doing things to get Samantha into trouble. Variations: *Sareen, Sarena, Sarene, Sarina, Sarine, Sereena, Serenah, Serenna, Serina.*

SHALONDA (African-American) Newly created. Putting the prefix "Sha-" before the suffix of a popular name—like "Londa"—or placing it before an independent name—like "Linda"—is another popular way that African-Americans are creating new names for their daughters. Though the "La-" prefix seems to be more popular, "Sha-" presents an original, thought not entirely unfamiliar, way to create a new name.

SHANIKA (African-American) Newly created. Variations: *Shaneeka, Shaneeke, Shanicka, Shanikah, Shaniqua, Shanique, Shenika.*

SHANNON (Irish) Ancient. Though Shannon is thoroughly Irish in its origin, it has primarily only been used as a last name in that country. It first appeared as a girls' name in the United States, in fact, back in the 1930s. Britain had only started to discover the name by 1950. Bucking the tide, many parents then began to use it for their sons, but the female habit of totally assimilating a boys' name has taken over, and today Shannon is mostly thought of as a girls' name. Variations: *Shanan, Shann, Shanna, Shannah, Shannan, Shannen, Shannie, Shanon.*

SHARMAINE (English) Roman clan name. Variations: *Sharma, Sharmain, Sharman, Sharmane, Sharmayne, Sharmian, Sharmine, Sharmyn.*

SHAYLEEN (African-American) Unknown definition.

SHELBY (English) Estate on a ledge. Shelby is most commonly thought of as a name for boys and as a last name, but it is currently one of the hottest names in the mid-'90s for baby girls. Julia Roberts played a woman named Shelby in the movie *Steel Magnolias,* and the rest is history. Variations: *Shelbee, Shelbey, Shellby.*

SHELLEY (English) Meadow on a ledge. Variations: *Shellee, Shelli, Shellie, Shelly.*

SIBYL (Greek) Seer, oracle. When most people hear the name Sibyl today, they think of the woman with multiple personality disorder. More than a century earlier, however, a novel written by Benjamin Disraeli entitled *Sybil* helped to popularize the name. Actress Cybill Shepherd has also helped to add some glamor to the name in recent years. Variations: *Sibbell, Sibel, Sibell, Sibella, Sibelle, Sibilla, Sibyll, Sibylla, Sybel, Sybella, Sybelle, Sybil, Sybill, Sybilla, Sybille, Sybyl.*

SIERRA (English) Mountain. Variation: *Siera.*

SIGOURNEY (English) Unknown definition.

SIMONE (French) God listens. Feminine version of Simon. Simone may initially resemble Renée, since it was a French name that was popular in the '70s, but I think Simone has a much more timeless quality, perhaps owing to the actress Simone Signoret and the author Simone de Beauvoir. Look for the name to become more popular in the coming decade.

Variations: *Simona, Simonetta, Simonette, Simonia, Simonina, Symona, Symone.*

SKYLER (Dutch) Shelter. Variations: *Schuyler, Skye.*

SOPHIA (Greek) Wisdom. Sophia and its close relation Sophie have both zoomed onto the top ten list in the United States and Great Britain in the '90s. The names have had a great deal of exposure from celebrities, starting with the seemingly ageless Sophia Loren, continuing with the novel and movie *Sophie's Choice,* and, in the '90s, singer Sophie B. Hawkins. Sophie holds a slight edge over Sophia in popularity. Variations: *Sofi, Sofia, Soficita, Sofka, Sofya, Sophey, Sophie, Sophy, Zofe, Zofia, Zofie, Zofka, Zosha, Zosia.*

STEPHANIE (English) Crown. Feminine version of Stephen. Stephanie is turning into one of those perennially popular names. It has a timeless quality that parents like and sounds like a name that will fit the shy, retiring girl as well as the active and more outgoing daughter. Famous Stephanies include Princess Stephanie, singer/actress Stepanie Mills, and Stefanie Powers. When Stephanie first began to become popular back in the 1970s, few people would have foreseen that the name would still be hot decades later, as it regularly appears on the list of the top twenty-five names for girls. Variations: *Stefania, Stefanie, Steffi, Stepania, Stepanie, Stephana, Stephanine, Stephannie, Stephena, Stephene, Stepheney, Stephenie, Stephine, Stephne, Stephney, Stevana, Stevena, Stevey, Stevi, Stevie.*

SUMI (Japanese) Clear.

SUSAN (Hebrew) Lily. Susan today tends to appear more frequently as a middle name than as a first name, but some of its exotic variations are beginning to be used more often. Variations: *Susann, Susanna, Susannah, Susanne, Susetta, Susette, Susi, Susie, Susy, Suzan, Suzane, Suzanna, Suzannah, Suzanne, Suzetta, Suzette, Suzi, Suzie, Suzy, Zsa Zsa, Zusa, Zuza.*

SUZUKI (Japanese) Little bell tree. Variations: *Suzue, Suzuko.*

SVETLANA (Czech) Star. Variations: *Svetla, Svetlanka, Svetluse, Svetluvska.*

SYDNEY (French) Feminine version of Sidney. Saint Denis. Variations: *Sydnie, Sydny.*

SYLVIA (Latin) From the forest. Variations: *Silvana, Silvia, Silvianne, Silvie, Sylva, Sylvana, Sylvanna, Sylvee, Sylvie.*

SYONA (Hindu) Happy.

SYREETA (Arabic) Companion.

TABITHA (English) Gazelle. About the only character in the hit TV series *Bewitched* whose name hasn't caught on among baby-naming parents is the irrepressible Darren. As with Samantha and Serena, the show was singlehandedly responsible for promoting the name Tabitha into popular culture. It continues to be used quite frequently, even today, almost 30 years later. Variations: *Tabatha, Tabbitha, Tabby, Tabetha, Tabotha, Tabytha.*

TALIA (Hebrew) Dew. Talia is a sweet and unique name that its fans feel is terribly underexposed. Most of us are familiar with the name through the actress Talia Shire, who appeared in many of the *Rocky* movies. However, its history is a bit loftier: in the Old Testament, Talia was the name of one of the angels who escorted the Sun from Dawn to Dusk. Variations: *Talie, Talley, Tallie, Tally, Talora, Talya, Thalie, Thalya.*

TALLULAH (Native American: Choctaw) Leaping water. Variations: *Tallula, Talula, Talulah, Talulla.*

TARA (Irish) Hill. Of course, the most famous Tara around was the name of the estate in *Gone With the Wind.* Scarlet's home seems to have served as the catalyst for the increasing presence of this name in the United States and in England. Variations: *Tarah, Taran, Tareena, Tarena, Tarin, Tarina, Tarra, Tarrah, Tarren, Tarryn, Taryn, Taryna, Teryn.*

TASHA (Russian) Christmas. Diminutive of Natasha. Variations: *Tashina, Tashka, Tasia.*

TASHANEE (African-American) Unknown definition.

TATIANA (Russian) Ancient Slavic king. Feminine version of Tatius. Variations: *Latonya, Tahnya, Tana, Tania, Tanis, Tanka, Tannia, Tannis, Tarnia, Tarny, Tata, Tatianna, Tatyana, Tatyanna, Tonia, Tonya, Tonyah.*

TAYLOR (English) Tailor. Variations: *Tailor, Talor, Tayler.*

TEMPEST (French) Storm.

TERESA (Greek) Harvest. Teresa and all of its variations are wonderfully feminine names that are as timely today as they were back in the '60s, when they first started to become popular in the United States. Two Catholic saints made this name part of the lexicon: Saint Teresa of Avila from the sixteenth century and Saint Therese from nineteenth-century France, who was commonly referred to as a little flower. And of course, there is also Mother Theresa. Variations: *Terasa, Teree, Terese, Teresia, Teresina, Teresita, Teressa, Teri, Terie, Terise, Terrasa, Terresa, Terresia, Terri, Terrie, Terrise, Terry, Terrya, Tersa, Terza, Tess, Tessa, Tessie, Tessy, Theresa, Therese, Theressa, Thereza, Thersa, Thersea.*

TESSA (Polish) Beloved by God. Variations: *Tess, Tessia, Tessie.*

THEODORA (Greek) Gift of God. Feminine version of Theodore. Theodora has been one of those unexpectedly popular names that appear from nowhere basically overnight. It's a weighty name that also shows its fun side through its abbreviated version, Theo. Theodora has only begun to catch on, so look for more girls with this name over the next ten to fifteen years. Variations: *Teddy, Teodora, Theadora, Theda, Theodosia.*

TIFFANY (Greek) God's appearance. Modern version of Theophania. As the '80s went, so did certain baby names, and Tiffany was one of these. In the anything-goes decade of luxury, Tiffany was one of the most popular girls' names around. Even earlier, the name was especially popular with African-American parents in the '70s. Tiffany first got its start back in ancient Greece, when it was commonly given to girls who were born on January sixth, also known as the Epiphany. But in the modern era, as with many other names that seem to come out of nowhere, this one was in a movie: Audrey Hepburn in *Breakfast at Tiffany's* put this name on the map in the 1960s. Today, the name is starting to fall out of fashion. Variations: *Tifani, Tiff, Tiffaney, Tiffani, Tiffanie, Tiffiney, Tiffini, Tiffney, Tiffy.*

TOVAH (Hebrew) Pleasant. Variations: *Toba, Tobit, Tova, Tovat, Tovit.*

TRACY (English) Summer. Variation of Teresa. Tracy was one of the more popular gender-neutral names back in the '60s when it was in the middle of its transition from boys' name to girls' name. Today, other gender-neutral names are more popular, but a number of famous Tracys may renew interest in this name: Tracy Chapman, Traci Ullman, Tracy Austin. Variations: *Trace, Tracee, Tracey, Traci, Tracie, Trasey, Treacy, Treesy.*

TRICIA (English) Noble. Feminine version of Patrick. Variations: *Treasha, Trichia, Trish, Trisha.*

TRIXIE (English) She brings happiness. Variation of Beatrice. Trixie is perhaps best known as the name of Ed Norton's wife on *The Honeymooners*. Surprisingly, it is catching on as a childhood nickname for the more formal Beatrix. Variations: *Trix, Trixi, Trixy.*

TWYLA (African-American) Newly created. Variations: *Twila, Twylla.*

TYLER (English) Last name.

UMA (Hindu) Flax.

URANIA (Greek) Heavenly. Once upon a time in nineteenth-century Great Britain, there were a number of parents who thought it ought to be all the rage to name their daughters after Greek goddesses and muses. Urania, the muse of astronomy, was one of those names. A handful of parents might be tempted to use it today. Variations: *Urainia, Uraniya, Uranya.*

URSULA (Latin) Little female bear. Variations: *Ursala, Ursella, Ursola, Ursule, Ursulina, Ursuline.*

VALERIE (Latin) Strong. A popular name during the Roman Empire, Valerie tends to be underused today. Famous Valeries include Valerie Harper, Valerie Bertinelli, and Valerie Perrine. Although some parents may feel that the name sounds like a relic from the 1960s, others will feel slightly nostalgic about the name and choose it for their own daughters. Variations: *Val, Valaree, Valarey, Valaria, Valarie, Vale, Valeree, Valeria, Valeriana, Valery, Vallarie, Valleree, Vallerie, Valli, Vallie, Vally.*

VANESSA (Greek) Butterflies. Variations: *Vanesa, Vanesse, Vania, Vanna, Vannessa, Venesa, Venessa.*

VANNA (Cambodian) Golden.

VASHTI (Persian) Beautiful.

VENETTA (English) Newly created. Variations: *Veneta, Venette.*

VENUS (Latin) Roman goddess of love. Variations: *Venise, Vennice, Venusa, Venusina.*

VERA (Slavic) Faith. Vera was at its height in both the United States and Britain during the flapper days of the 1920s. Variations: *Veera, Veira, Verasha, Viera.*

VERONICA (Latin) True image. Variations: *Veranique, Vernice, Veron, Verona, Verone, Veronice, Veronicka, Veronika, Veronike, Veroniqua, Veronique.*

VICTORIA (Latin) Roman goddess of victory. Victoria is a name that has had a number of spurts in popularity since the days of the early Roman Empire, when it was one of the most frequently bestowed names for girls. It lay dormant until Queen Victoria took the throne in Britain in the 1800s, when it began to be used with some regularity until she died after the turn of the century. The name was resurrected again in the 1940s and has remained in common usage ever since. Although Victoria's nicknames were more popular in the '60s and '70s, today the full name is the most widely used. Variations: *Torey, Tori, Toria, Torie, Torrey, Torri, Torrie, Torrye, Tory, Vicki, Vickie, Vicky, Victoriana, Victorina, Victorine, Victory, Vikki, Vikky, Vitoria, Vittoria.*

VIOLET (Latin) Violet. Variations: *Viola, Violetta, Violette.*

VIRGINIA (Latin) Virgin. Variations: *Vergie, Virgy, Virginie, Vegenia, Virginai, Virgena, Virgene.*

VIVIAN (Latin) Full of life. Actress Vivien Leigh was responsible for the name's first burst of popularity in the United States in the 1940s. Ever since actress Julia Roberts played a hooker named Vivian in the movie *Pretty Woman*, the name has started to appear on birth certificates with a little bit more regularity. Variations: *Viv, Viva, Viveca, Vivecka, Viveka, Vivia, Viviana, Viviane, Vivianna, Vivianne, Vivie, Vivien, Vivienne.*

WALLIS (English) One from Wales. Feminine version of Wallace. Variations: *Wallie, Walliss, Wally, Wallys.*

WASHI (Japanese) Eagle.

WENDY (English) Wendy first appeared as the name of a character in the novel, *Peter Pan*. Variations: *Wenda, Wendee, Wendey, Wendi, Wendie, Wendye, Windy.*

WHITLEY (English) White field.

WHITNEY (English) White island. Of course, singer Whitney Houston is the primary reason why this name has rapidly traveled from being a corporate success-track name for boys in the early '80s to one of the more popular names for girls in the '90s. Although Whitney is still popular, it is beginning to be cast aside in favor of other, more cutting-edge names. Variations: *Whitnee, Whitnie, Whitny, Whittney.*

WHOOPI (French) Unknown definition.

WILHELMINA (German) Feminine version of William, Will + helmet. Variations: *Wiletta, Wilette, Wilhelmine, Willa, Willamina, Williamina.*

WILMA (German) Feminine version of William, Will + helmet. Variations: *Wilmette, Wilmina, Wylma.*

WINIFRED (Welsh) Holy peace. Winifred is a pretty name that is both delicate and powerful. The name was at its height in popularity during the nineteenth and early twentieth centuries among English and 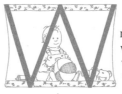 Scottish parents. Today Americans are beginning to fall for the sweet quality of the name. Look for Winifred to become more widely used in the coming years, especially with the letter "y" replacing one of the vowels in the name. Variations: *Win, Winifrede, Winifride, Winifryde, Winne, Winni, Winnie, Winny, Wyn, Wynn.*

WINTER (English) Winter.

WYNN (Welsh) Fair, white. Variations: *Winne, Wynne.*

WYNONAH (Native American) First-born. Variations: *Wenona, Wenonah, Winona, Winonah, Wynnona.*

XANTHIPPE (Greek) Wife of Socrates.

XAVIERA (English) New house. Feminine version of Xavier. The name Xaviera started out as the name of a saint from the sixteenth century. Though some parents are beginning to consider Xaviera for their daughters, an increase in usage doesn't seem too likely given the name's indelible connection to Xaviera Hollander, author of the notorious '60s book, *The Happy Hooker*. Variations: *Xavier, Xavyera.*

XENIA (Greek) Hospitable. Variations: *Xeenia, Xena.*

XIANG (Chinese) Fragrant.

XIAO-XING (Chinese) Morning star.

YAKI (Japanese) Snow. Variations: *Yukie, Yukika, Yukiko.*

YASMINE (Arabic) Flower. Though Jasmin, the name from which Yasmine is derived, is the more well-known variation of this name, Yasmine is likely to become more popular in time, simply because many parents will want to put their unique spin on what is becoming a relatively popular name. In fact, Yasmine first became popular in the United States back in the 1920s because of a play entitled *Hassan*, by playwright James Flecker, in which the female protagonist was named Yasmin. Variations: *Yasmeen, Yasmeena, Yasmena, Yasmene, Yasmin, Yasmina.*

YASU (Japanese) Calm. Variations: *Yasuko, Yasuyo.*

YEHUDIT (Hebrew) God will be praised. Variations: *Yudi, Yudit, Yudita, Yuta, Yutke.*

YELENA (Russian) Light. Variation of Helen. Variation: *Yalena.*

YENTA (Hebrew) Ruler at home. Variations: *Yente, Yentel, Yentele, Yentil.*

YETTA (English) Ruler at home Feminine diminutive version of Henry. Variation: *Yette.*

YOKO (Japanese) Child of the ocean.

YOLANDA (Greek) Purple flower. In the United States, Yolanda has long been a name that has been more popular among African-American families than white parents, but that is gradually starting to change. Yolanda first appeared as the name of a saint in thirteenth-century Spain, and later belonged to Hungarian royalty. Though some parents might feel the name is dated and too unusual to use today, it's clear that others disagree. Variations: *Eolanda, Eolande, Iolanda, Iolande, Yalanda, Yalinda, Yalonda, Yola, Yoland, Yolande, Yolane, Yolette, Yoli, Yolonda, Yulanda.*

YORI (Japanese) Honest.

YOSHIKO (Japanese) Quiet. Variations: *Yoshi, Yoshie, Yoshiyo.*

YOUNG-SOON (Korean) Tender flower.

YVETTE (French) Arrow's bow.

YVONNE (French) Yew wood. Yvonne is a name that conjures up images of black-and-white dramas from the '40s, when Yvonne was often chosen as the name of the unsuspecting tragic female heroine. Some parents today, however, may feel that the name is cool because of their exposure to the sitcom *The Munsters* starring Yvonne De Carlo. Variations: *Yvetta, Yvette, Yvone.*

ZADA (Arabic) Fortunate. Variations: *Zaida, Zayda.*

ZAHARA (Hebrew) Shine. Variations: *Zahari, Zaharit.*

ZARA (Hebrew) Dawn. In the '90s, names that have a "z," "x," or "q" in them are popular, but parents still like names that aren't totally unfamiliar. Zara fits the bill nicely, as it is close to both Tara and Sarah. It is also the name of the daughter of Princess Anne. Variations: *Zarah, Zaria.*

ZEHAVA (Hebrew) Gold. Variations: *Zahava, Zehovit, Zehuva, Zehuvit.*

ZEPHYR (Greek) Wind from the west. Variations: *Zefir, Zephira, Zephyra.*

ZERA (Hebrew) Seeds.

ZINA (English) Hospitable. Variation: *Zena.*

ZLATA (Czech) Golden. Variations: *Zlatina, Zlatinka, Zlatka, Zlatuna, Zlatunka, Zlatuse, Zlatuska.*

ZOE (Greek) Life. Zoe is perhaps the most popular "Z" name for girls in this country, and it seems to have picked up steam in the '90s. The first Zoe surfaced in the third century A.D.; she was later martyred as a saint. Today parents can choose to add an umlaut above the "e" or to leave it as-is. Parents will continue to look to Zoe for a daughter they expect to have considerable artistic talent. Variations: *Zoey, Zoie.*

ZOLA (Italian) Piece of earth.

ZONA (Latin) Belt.

ZORA (Slavic) Dawn. Variations: *Zara, Zorah, Zorra, Zorrah.*

ZURI (African: Swahili) Beautiful.

ZYTKA (Polish) Rose.

Announcing . . . Baby!

The baby has arrived, and now it's time to make the announcement. You can either call everyone immediately after the birth or mail out announcements when you get home from the hospital. The decision is yours.

Some parents compile a call list for announcing the baby's arrival. This list can be short or long, depending on whether you want to limit it to close relatives or take a "tag team" approach (in which case a designated person gets your call and then relays the news to others on your list for you).

There is a wide selection of birth announcement cards. You could order them through a business you've seen advertised in parents' magazines or on the World Wide Web. But if you do, be sure to ask for a catalog ahead of time to make certain the company is legitimate and also to choose a style. Or you could go to your local quick print shop and ask to see the catalog. Some places, such as Kinko's, have preprinted postcard stock with baby-related artwork. With these announcements, you choose what you want to say, purchase the card stock, and produce the announcements yourself on your home computer.

For those who consider themselves creatively challenged, here are a few sample announcements you could tailor to your own needs:

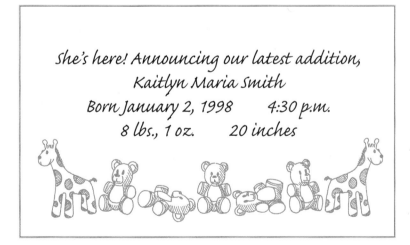

She's here! Announcing our latest addition,
Kaitlyn Maria Smith
Born January 2, 1998   4:30 p.m.
8 lbs., 1 oz.   20 inches

Oh, Joy of Joys—It's a Boy!
Please welcome our new son
Simon Alexander
Born August 22, 1998, at 12:02 a.m.
Weight: 9 lbs., 2 oz.
Length: 23 in.
Proud parents Joe and Jessica Alexander

TWICE THE FUN! TWICE THE JOY!
We've got a double package—
a girl and a boy!
Twins Michael and Maria Owens were born
July 1, 1998
Michael : 6 lbs., 1 oz., 20 in.
Maria : 5 lbs., 6 oz., 20 in.

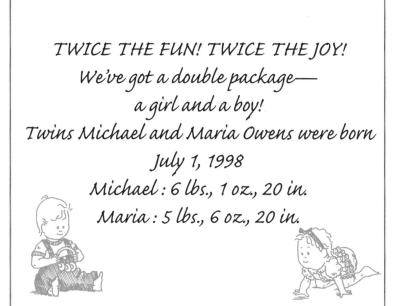

If you have other children, you might like to include them in the announcement as well; after all, it's their baby, too. Following is an example of the announcement I worked up for my daughter's birth, since I have stepchildren and my own child from a previous marriage. I had a little fun with it, because most in my inner circle know about my newspaper background.

> Akron, OH—*Madelyn Dela Yaceczko was born July 1, 1997, at 2:46 p.m. She weighed a respectable 7 lbs., 6 oz. and was 22 inches long. Maddie's mother and father were on top of the world. "We have never felt such pride," said both in a statement issued shortly after the birth. The baby has three brothers and a sister, all of whom expressed their delight at the event.*

I used this announcement not only on a printed postcard, but also for my e-mail messages to my online friends. The light, humorous approach was well received by many—no doubt it was a bit unusual for some. The point is to have as much fun as you'd like with this exciting project.

As far as other options, you could also let others know about the birth of your child by ordering a banner, billboard, or yard announcement. Banners simply announce the baby's name, birth weight, and length; some include time of birth, but you'll need a fairly large banner to include anything more than that. You can hang a banner across your front door, over your garage, or even attach it to posts and plant it in your front yard.

Billboards can be rented and placed in your front yard for a day or so after the birth. Don't be surprised, though, if passers-by honk their horns as they drive by!

A yard announcement is another popular method of getting the message out. Large, wooden storks or circus clowns bearing the birth message can, like a billboard, be rented and placed in your front yard. A lower-cost option is to make your own sign and attach balloons to it; this also leaves you with another keepsake—or something to use next time.

Another option is to leave a simple greeting on your answering machine for those who call you to find out the details. You could simply say, "You've reached the Jones household, where our newest addition arrived on Friday. She weighed 6 pounds, 2 ounces, and we've named her Ashley Kate. Leave your name and number so we can call you back—after we get her to sleep again!"

It could be that a combination of these methods of introducing your new little "star" will work best; perhaps you can call only close relatives from the hospital and then mail out announcements to those who've sent gifts or well wishes or simply expressed an interest in knowing about the baby.

For many new parents who are amazed to discover just how precious time has become, it's a combination of options that seems to do the trick. Whatever you decide to do, be sure to keep a record of it for baby (perhaps at the end of your pregnancy diary); he or she may someday want to know how you told the world about your bundle of joy.

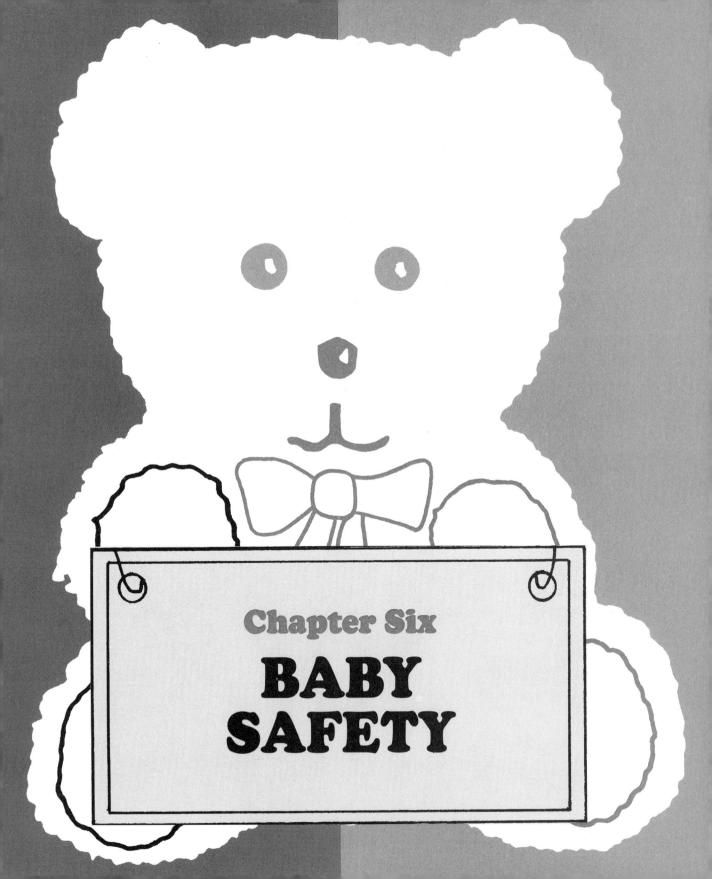

Chapter Six

BABY
SAFETY

L et's face it, when we're busy thinking about all of the wonderful days ahead in our new life as parents, the idea that
something terrible could happen is the farthest thought from
our minds. And while it isn't necessarily healthy for you to go to the
opposite extreme—to become consumed with horrible thoughts about
your baby's welfare—it is wise to prepare your house and everything
in it for the inquisitive young mind about to enter.

When it comes to baby safety tips, there is no better source
than the U.S. Government. Visit the U.S. Consumer Product Safety
Commission's Web site at http://www.cpsc.gov to get the latest information and product safety updates.

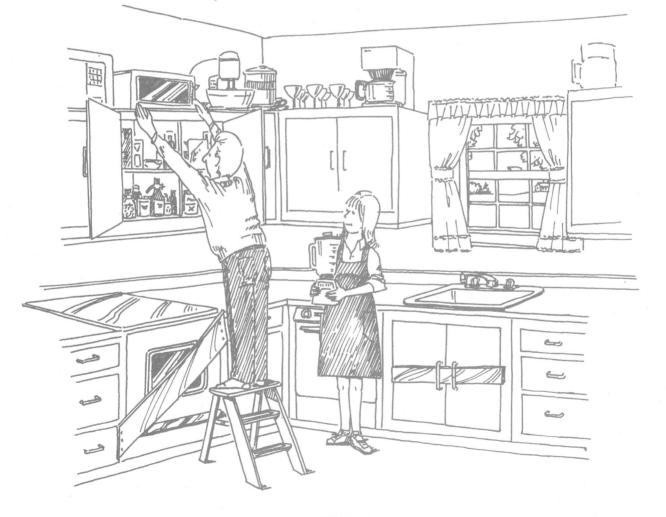

Baby-Proofing Your House

The starting point for most parents-to-be is the house itself. Cover all outlets with safety covers or plugs, and fasten latches to cabinets with dangerous items inside. Put a new battery inside your smoke detector as well. You might want to consider securing toilet lids, too, as many young children are fascinated with putting objects inside.

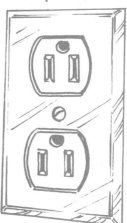

Don't leave window-blind cords hanging for baby's hands to grab onto; instead, wind them up or buy a product that does it for you. Once baby starts becoming mobile, you'd be surprised how quickly he or she begins grabbing at anything that's hanging.

In addition, use door stops to protect your baby from slamming doors, and pad sharp edges on furniture or stair rails with securely positioned foam pieces.

Finally, check your house for lead and asbestos. If you detect either substance, contact a professional to help you deal with the problem safely and effectively—and legally. Any house built before 1978 is at risk for lead paint. Although a lead-free house is optimum, be aware that it can cost as much as $30,000 to delead an old house—and the house's architectural detail may be destroyed in the process. If you can't afford to delead your older home and don't want to move, a compromise solution is checking frequently to make sure that paint is not peeling (especially on windowsills and ceilings). In general, lead paint that has been painted over with a safer paint and is intact does not pose a risk. You should avoid sanding old paint altogether from the moment you decide to get pregnant, and don't let anyone else do it either, even when you're not in the house.

Asbestos removal is also pricey but is far less than lead. Asbestos can also be encapsulated for a fraction of the cost of removing it, and many people feel that this option is safe enough for unused, unfinished basements.

Have your water tested, too; and keep distilled water on hand at all times just in case there's a problem.

Nursery Equipment Safety Checklist

Products such as cribs and high chairs must be selected with safety in mind. Parents and caretakers of babies and young children need to be aware of the many potential hazards in their environment—hazards that can occur through the misuse of products or through the use of products that have not been well designed.

The checklist that follows is intended as a guide to help you choose the safest new or secondhand nursery equipment. It also can be of help when checking over nursery equipment that is currently being used in your home or in other facilities that care for infants and young children.

Ask yourself these questions: Does your equipment have the safety features in this checklist? If not, can missing or unsafe parts be easily replaced with the proper parts? Can breaks or cracks be repaired to give more protection? Can I fix the older equipment without creating a "new" hazard?

If you answer no to any of these questions, the item is beyond help and should be discarded. If the item can be repaired, do the repair before you allow any child to use it.

Back Carriers	YES	NO
1. The carrier has a restraining strap to secure the child.	___	___
2. The leg openings are small enough to prevent the child from slipping out.	___	___
3. The leg openings are large enough to prevent chafing.	___	___
4. The frame has no pinch points in the folding mechanism.	___	___
5. The carrier has a padded covering over the metal frame near baby's face.	___	___

Do not use a back carrier until baby is four or five months old. By then, baby's neck is able to withstand jolts and not sustain an injury.

Bassinets and Cradles   YES   NO

1. The bassinet/cradle has a sturdy bottom and
   a wide base for stability.   ___   ___
2. The bassinet/cradle has a smooth surface
   (no protruding staples or other hardware that
   can injure the baby).   ___   ___
3. The legs have strong, effective locks to
   prevent folding while in use.   ___   ___
4. The mattress is firm and fits snugly.   ___   ___

*Follow the manufacturer's guidelines on the weight and size of a
baby who can safely use these products.*

Baby Bath Rings or Seats   YES   NO

1. The suction cups are securely fastened to
   the product.   ___   ___
2. The suction cups securely attach to the
   smooth surface of the tub.   ___   ___
3. The tub is filled only with enough water to
   cover baby's legs.   ___   ___
4. Baby is *never* left alone or with a sibling
   while in the bath ring, even for a moment!   ___   ___

*NEVER leave a baby unattended or with a sibling in a tub of
water. Do not rely on a bath ring to keep your baby safe.*

Carrier Seats   YES   NO

1. The carrier seat has a wide sturdy base for stability.   ___   ___
2. The carrier has nonskid feet to prevent slipping.   ___   ___
3. The supporting devices lock securely.   ___   ___
4. The carrier seat has crotch and waist straps.   ___   ___
5. The buckles or straps are easy to use.   ___   ___

Never use the carrier as a car seat.

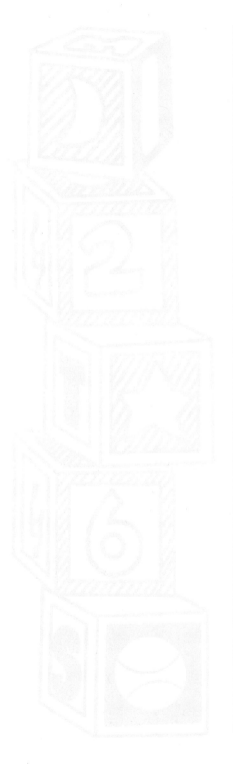

Changing Tables	YES	NO
1. The table has safety straps to prevent falls.	___	___
2 The table has drawers or shelves that are easily accessible without leaving the baby unattended.	___	___

Do not leave baby on the table unattended. Always use the straps to prevent the baby from falling.

Cribs	YES	NO
1. The slats are spaced no more than 2 inches (60 mm) apart.	___	___
2. No slats are missing or cracked.	___	___
3. The mattress fits snugly—less than two finger width between the edge of the mattress and the side of the crib.	___	___
4. The mattress support is securely attached to the headboard and footboard.	___	___
5. The corner posts are no higher than 1/16 inch (1 mm)—to prevent entanglement of clothing or other objects worn by the child.	___	___
6. There are no cutouts in the headboard or footboard that allow head entrapment.	___	___
7. Drop-side latches cannot be easily released by baby.	___	___
8. Drop-side latches securely hold sides in a raised position.	___	___
9. All screws or bolts that secure the components of the crib are present and tight.	___	___

Do not place the crib near draperies or blinds because a child could become entangled and strangle on the cords. When a child reaches 35 inches in height or can climb and/or fall over the sides, the crib should be replaced with a bed.

Crib Toys

	YES	NO
1. Toys do not have strings with loops or openings having perimeters greater than 14 inches (356 mm).	——	——
2. No strings or cords longer than 7 inches (178 mm) are dangling into the crib.	——	——
3. Crib gym has a label warning you to remove the gym from the crib when the child can push up on his or her hands and knees or reaches 5 months of age, whichever comes first.	——	——
4. The components of the toys are not small enough to be a choking hazard.	——	——

Avoid hanging toys with strings long enough to result in strangulation across the crib or on the crib corner posts. Remove the crib gym when the child is able to pull or push up on his or her hands and knees.

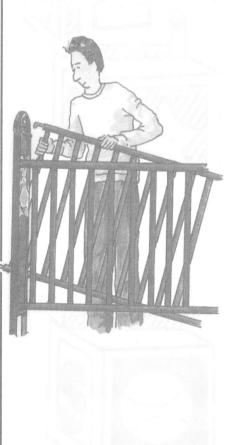

Gates and Enclosures

	YES	NO
1. Openings in gate are too small to entrap a child's head.	——	——
2. Gate has a pressure bar or some other fastener that will resist forces exerted by a child.	——	——

To avoid head entrapment, do not use accordion-style gates or expandable enclosures with large v-shaped openings along the top edge or with diamond-shaped openings within.

High Chairs

	YES	NO
1. The high chair has waist and crotch restraining straps that are independent of the tray.	——	——
2. The tray locks securely.	——	——

3. The buckle on the waist strap is easy to use. ___ ___

4. The high chair has a wide stable base. ___ ___

5. The caps or plugs on the tubing are firmly attached and cannot be pulled off and choked on by the child. ___ ___

6. If it is a folding high chair, it has an effective locking device to keep it from collapsing. ___ ___

Always use restraining straps; otherwise the child can slide under the tray and strangle.

Hook-on Chairs   YES   NO

1. The chair has a restraining strap to secure the child. ___ ___

2. The chair has a clamp that locks onto the table for added security. ___ ___

3. The caps or plugs on the tubing are firmly attached and cannot be pulled off and choked on by the child. ___ ___

4. The chair has a warning never to place the chair where the child can push off with his or her feet. ___ ___

Don't leave a child unattended in a hook-on chair.

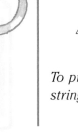

Pacifiers   YES   NO

1. There is no ribbon, string, cord, or yarn attached to the pacifier. ___ ___

2. The shield is large enough and firm enough to not fit in the child's mouth. ___ ___

3. The guard or shield has ventilation holes so the baby can breath if the shield does get into his or her mouth. ___ ___

4. The pacifier nipple has no holes or tears that might cause it to break off in baby's mouth. ___ ___

To prevent strangulation, never hang a pacifier or other items on a string around a baby's neck.

Playpens

	YES	NO
1. The drop-side mesh playpen or crib has a label warning never to leave the side in the down position.	___	___
2. The mesh has a small weave (less than a 1-inch opening).	___	___
3. The mesh has no tears, holes, or loose threads.	___	___
4. The mesh is securely attached to the top rail and the floor plate.	___	___
5. The top rail cover has no tears or holes.	___	___
6. The wooden playpen has slats spaced no more than 2 inches (60 mm) apart.	___	___
7. If staples are used in construction, they are firmly installed and none are missing or loose.	___	___

Never leave an infant in a mesh playpen or crib with the drop-side down. Even a very young infant can roll into the space between the mattress and loose mesh side and suffocate.

Rattles, Squeeze Toys, Teethers

	YES	NO
1. Rattles, squeeze toys, and teethers are too large to lodge in a baby's throat.	___	___
2. Rattles are of sturdy construction that will not break apart in use.	___	___
3. Squeeze toys do not contain a squeaker that could detach and choke a baby.	___	___

To prevent suffocation, take rattles, squeeze toys, teethers, and other toys out of the crib or playpen when the baby sleeps.

Strollers and Carriages

	YES	NO
1. The stroller/carriage has a wide base to prevent tipping.	___	___
2. The seat belt and crotch strap are securely attached to the frame.	___	___
3. The seat belt buckle is easy to use.	___	___

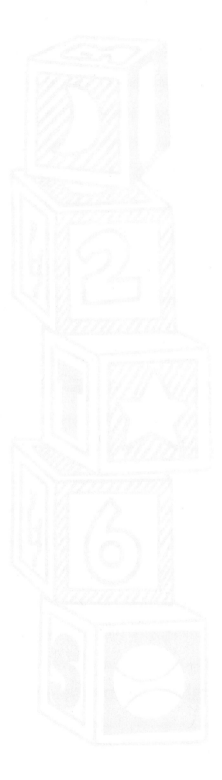

4. The brakes securely lock the wheel(s). ___ ___
5. The shopping basket is low on the back and directly over or in front of rear wheels for stability. ___ ___
6. When used in the carriage position, the leg-hold openings can be closed. ___ ___

Always secure the seat belts. Never leave a child unattended in a stroller. Keep children's hands away from pinching areas when the stroller is being folded or unfolded or the seat back is being lowered.

Toy Chests   YES   NO

1. There is no lid latch that could entrap the child within the chest. ___ ___
2. The hinged lid has a spring-loaded lid support that will support the lid in any position and will not require periodic adjustment. ___ ___
3. The chest has ventilation holes or spaces in the front or sides or under the lid. ___ ___

To avoid a head injury to a small child if you already own a toy chest or trunk with a freely falling lid, remove the lid or install a spring-loaded lid support.

Walkers   YES   NO

1. It has a wide wheel base for stability. ___ ___
2. There are covers over the coil springs to avoid finger pinching. ___ ___
3. The seat is securely attached to the frame of the walker. ___ ___
4. There are no x-frames that could pinch or amputate fingers. ___ ___

Place gates or guards at the top of all stairways or keep stairway doors closed to prevent falls. Do not use a walker as a babysitter.

* Tips and checklist courtesy of the U.S. Consumer Product Safety Commission. For more nursery equipment information, write for a free copy of *The Safe Nursery, A Buyer's Guide*, Office of Information and Public Affairs, Washington, D.C. 20207.

Used Crib Safety Tips

An unsafe used crib could be very dangerous for your baby. Each year, about fifty babies suffocate or strangle when they become trapped between broken crib parts or in cribs with older, unsafe designs. A safe crib is the best place to put your baby to sleep. Look for a crib with a certification seal showing that it meets national safety standards. If your crib does not meet these guidelines, destroy it and replace it with a safe crib.

Here are the features of a safe crib:

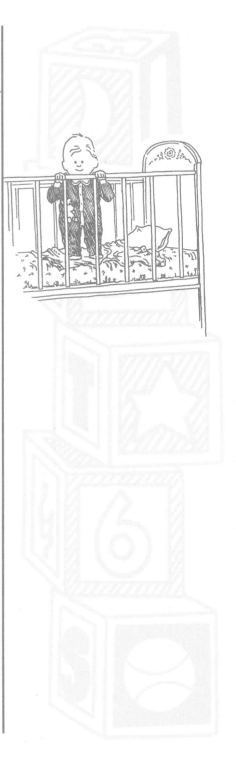

- No missing, loose, broken, or improperly installed screws, brackets, or other hardware on the crib or the mattress support
- No more than 2 3/8 inches between crib slats so a baby's body cannot fit through the slats
- A firm, snug-fitting mattress so a baby cannot get trapped between the mattress and the side of the crib
- No corner posts over 1/16 of an inch above the end panels (unless they are over 16 inches high for a canopy) so a baby cannot catch clothing and strangle
- No cutout areas on the headboard or footboard so a baby's head cannot get trapped
- A mattress support that does not easily pull apart from the corner posts so a baby cannot get trapped between mattress and crib
- No cracked or peeling paint to prevent lead poisoning
- No splinters or rough edges

For the Sake of Kids, Think Toy Safety

When buying toys choose them with care. Keep in mind the child's age, interests, and skill level. Look for quality design and construction in all toys for all ages.

- Make sure that all directions or instructions are clear—to you, and, when appropriate, to the child.
- Plastic wrappings on toys should be discarded at once before they become deadly playthings.

⚘ Be a label reader. Look for and heed age recommendations, such as *not recommended for children under three.* Look for other safety labels including *Flame retardant/Flame resistant* on fabric products and *Washable/hygienic materials* on stuffed toys and dolls.

To properly maintain toys, check them periodically for breakage and potential hazards. A damaged toy that has become dangerous should be thrown away or repaired immediately.

Wooden toys with edges that have become sharp or whose surfaces have become covered with splinters should be sanded smooth. When repainting toys and toy boxes, avoid using leftover paint, unless it has been purchased recently, since older paints may contain more lead than new paint, which is regulated by CSPA (Child Safety Protection Act). Examine all outdoor toys regularly for rust or weak parts that could become hazardous.

To store toys properly, teach children to put them safely away on shelves or in a toy chest after playing to prevent trips and falls.

⚘ Toy boxes should be checked for safety. Use a toy chest that has a lid that will stay open in any position to which it is raised and will not fall unexpectedly on a child. For extra safety, be sure there are ventilation holes for fresh air. Watch for sharp edges that could cut and hinges that could pinch or squeeze.

⚘ See that toys used outdoors are stored after play; dew can rust or damage a variety of toys and toy parts, creating hazards.

⚘ New toys intended for children under eight years of age should, by regulation, be free of sharp glass and metal edges. With use, however, older toys may break, exposing cutting edges.

⚘ Older toys can break to reveal parts small enough to be swallowed or to become lodged in a child's windpipe, ears, or nose. The law bans small parts in new toys intended for children under three. This includes removable small eyes and noses on stuffed toys and dolls and small, removable squeakers on squeeze toys.

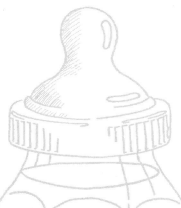

- Toy caps and some noisemaking guns and other toys can produce sounds at noise levels that can damage hearing. The law requires the following label on boxes of caps producing noise above a certain level: *WARNING—Do not fire closer than one foot to the ear. Do not use indoors.* Caps producing noise that can injure a child's hearing are banned.

- Toys with long strings or cords may be dangerous for infants and very young children. The cords may become wrapped around an infant's neck, causing strangulation. Never hang toys with long strings, cords, loops, or ribbons in cribs or playpens where children can become entangled. Remove crib gyms from the crib when the child can pull up on hands and knees; some children have strangled when they fell across crib gyms stretched across the crib.

- Broken toys may have dangerous points or prongs. Stuffed toys may have wires inside that could cut or stab if exposed. A CSPA regulation prohibits sharp points in new toys and other articles intended for use by children under eight years of age.

- Projectiles (guided missiles and similar flying toys) can be turned into weapons and can injure eyes in particular. Children should never be permitted to play with adult lawn darts or other hobby or sporting equipment that has sharp points.

All toys are not for all children. Keep toys designed for older children out of the hands of little ones. Follow labels that give age recommendations; some toys are recommended for older children because they may be hazardous in the hands of a younger child. Teach older children to help keep their toys away from younger brothers and sisters.

Protecting children from unsafe toys is the responsibility of everyone. Careful toy selection and proper supervision of children at play is still—and always will be—the best way to protect children from toy-related injuries.

Consumer Safety Commission Facts

- Effective January 1, 1995, products that are manufactured in or imported into the United States must comply with the Child Safety Protection Act (CSPA).

- Any ball with a diameter of 1.75 inches (44.4 mm) or less that is intended for use by children younger than three years of age is banned.

- Any latex balloon, or a toy or game that contains a latex balloon, shall be labeled as follows: *WARNING: Choking hazard. Children under eight years of age can choke or suffocate on uninflated or broken balloons. Adult supervision is required. Keep uninflated balloons from children and discard broken balloons immediately.*

Throw a Baby Safety Shower

Plan to select an overall theme for your baby safety shower, such as "keeping your baby safe at home." As a starting point, use the Baby Safety Checklist provided by CSPA, which presents twelve tips for keeping babies safe in the bedroom, bathroom, kitchen, and other living areas. Contact CSPA for a complete set of games and rules. You can even request multiple copies. You may want to include additional health and safety themes; for example, "choosing quality child care," "selecting safe toys and nursery equipment," or "ensuring immunizations and proper nutrition for infants and toddlers."

If you invite a small group, focus on one theme. If your group is larger and you have the space, consider broadening the scope. Bring in other partners to work with you.

For example, get the health department or local hospital to offer an immunization clinic. Or ask a local supermarket to sponsor a nutrition booth—with appropriate games and prizes.

Pick your theme early so that you can better plan your program and activities. Coordinate your work with all involved so that everyone knows what to do to make each activity successful.

Game Workshops

Games and other fun activities are an effective way to teach and reinforce safety and health messages. The games included in this section focus on the theme of keeping your baby safe at home. The games are based on the safety messages found in the Nursery Equipment Checklist at the beginning of this chapter. There is one suggested game for each area of the home: the bedroom, bathroom, kitchen, and other living areas. Adapt these games to your needs or develop new ones. Be sure you have more than enough materials for every participant to play each game.

Here is a preview of the four games that are offered in this section:

> For the bedroom: *Can You Answer This?* The game leader asks each team questions. The team that correctly answers the most questions wins the round.

For the bathroom: *Safety Sayings.* Each team calls out letters that spell a safety message. The team that first guesses the safety message wins.

For the kitchen: *Picture Safety.* One person on each team draws an image based on a particular product safety message. The team that first identifies the image and tells why it's important wins the round.

For other living areas: *Safety Bingo.* Each guest marks an answer on her bingo card for each question asked. The winner is the first to mark three answers in a row and call out "bingo!"

If you have time for only one game, play *Safety Bingo.* It includes safety tips from each area of the home, and it's easy and fun!

Bedroom Safety Game: "Can You Answer This?"

Game Tips
Before playing this game, review the relevant bedroom Baby Safety Checklist tips and reasons with shower participants. Decide whether your guests can peek at the Checklist for the answers during the game. Award points for other common-sense answers not included in the Checklist. After each game, review the Checklist again.

Materials Needed
Flip chart or blackboard, markers for scoring

Game Rules
Participants are split into two teams. The moderator asks Team A for three answers to each game question. For each correct answer, Team A gets one point. If Team A is stumped, Team B gets a chance to answer. The moderator then asks Team B one game question, and so on. When the four game questions are answered, the moderator simultaneously asks each team a bonus round question. The team that first answers the question correctly wins.

Game Questions (1 point for each correct answer)

Q: Can you name three things that describe an unsafe crib?

A: (1) missing hardware; (2) lack of sturdiness; (3) loose hardware. Also correct: mattress that doesn't fit snugly; corner posts; decorative cutouts in head or footboards; crib slats that are too far apart

Q: What are the three possible sleep positions for your baby in a crib and are they safe or unsafe?

A: (1) back (safe); (2) side (safe); (3) stomach (unsafe)

Q: Can you name three examples of soft bedding?

A: (1) pillows; (2) soft, fluffy comforters; (3) quilts. Also correct: sheepskin

Q: Can you name three things you should never place near a window with blind or curtain cords?

A: (1) crib; (2) playpen; (3) high chair. Also correct: various other pieces of children's furniture

Bonus Round Questions (2 points for each correct answer)

Q: Can you name three small objects that are choking hazards for children under three years of age?

A: Accept answers such as buttons, balloons, marbles; and grapes, peanuts, hard candy, cut-up hot dogs

Q: What are three safety concerns to look for in and on your child's toy box or toy chest?

A: Accept answers such as toys with sharp edges or points; toys that are too small; toys with detachable small parts; hinged-lid toy boxes without safety-lid supports

Q: What are three common hazards found on children's clothing?

A: Accept answers such as loose buttons, drawstrings, loose snaps, small decorations that detach

Bathroom Safety Game: "Safety Sayings"

Game Tips

Before playing this game, review the relevant bathroom Baby Safety Checklist tips and reasons with shower participants. Decide whether your guests can peek at the Checklist for the answers during the game. After each game, review the Checklist again.

Materials Needed

Flip chart or blackboard, markers

Game Rules

Participants are split into two teams. On the flip chart, draw the number of blank lines (similar to the game of hangman) corresponding to the number of letters and spaces in the safety saying. Each team in turn guesses a letter to go in the spaces; correct letters are written in the appropriate blank(s). To make the game go more quickly, you may fill in the vowels beforehand. The team that correctly guesses the most safety sayings wins.

Safety Sayings

- Keep baby safe
- Use child-safety caps
- Keep medicines locked up
- Babies and water don't mix
- Never leave children alone in water
- Check bath water temperature with wrist or elbow

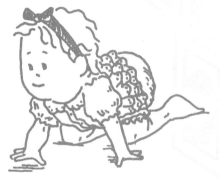

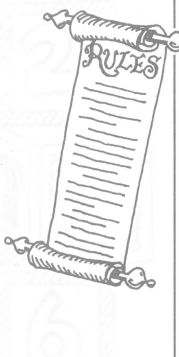

Kitchen Safety Game: "Picture Safety"

Game Tips

Before playing this game, review the relevant kitchen Baby Safety Checklist tips and reasons with shower participants. Decide whether your guests can peek at the Checklist for the answers during the game. After each game, review the Checklist again.

Materials Needed

Two flip charts, markers, 3" x 5" cards (for safety clues)

Game Rules

Participants are split into two teams. The teams sit or stand facing each other. The flip charts are positioned back-to-back between the teams. The moderator selects a safety clue card and shows it to one person from each team. When the moderator says go, each person draws a picture of the safety clue on his or her team's flip chart. The first team to guess the picture wins 5 points. The team can win 5 more points if it correctly describes how the clue is safety-related. The team with the most points wins.

Safety Clue Cards

- Cabinet safety latch: prevents children from getting into cabinets where harmful household products are kept
- Dish detergents: can be harmful if children swallow them
- High chair with safety straps: prevents children from climbing or falling out and getting injured
- Pots and pans on stoves: can burn children if they reach handles and spill hot liquid or food on themselves
- Knives: can injure children if they reach them and cut themselves
- Plastic trash bags: can cause children to suffocate if the bags get over their noses and mouths
- Matches: can burn and start fires

Other Living Areas Safety Game: "Safety Bingo"

Game Tips

Before playing this game, review the relevant Baby Safety Checklist tips and reasons, as well as the clues on the bingo cards, with your shower guests. Let your guests peek at the Checklist for the answers during the game. After each game, review the Checklist again.

Materials Needed

Bingo game cards (see the attachments section) and several "chips," buttons, small colored stick-ons, or similar item for each participant

Game Rules

This game is similar to bingo. Each participant is given a game card with pictures in each box. The moderator reads a safety clue aloud, and each participant covers the appropriate picture box on his or her bingo card. The winner is the first player who correctly covers all the boxes on his or her card in a row (across, down, or diagonally) and calls out "bingo." This game can be played many times, with the questions read in different order.

Safety Clues

Q: One of these should be on every level of the home for protection from fires.
A: Smoke detector

Q: One of these will prevent children from falling down stairs.
A: Safety gate

Q: This stops children from poking fingers and inserting objects into electrical outlets.
A: Safety plugs

Q: This round game part is a choking hazard to young children.
A: Small ball and jacks set

Q: If broken or deflated, these can be a choking hazard to young children.
A: Balloons

Q: These may look like candy to small children.
A: Medicine pills in bottles with safety caps

Q: This is the best position for babies to sleep.
A: Back or side

Q: This stops children from opening cabinet or cupboard doors in which cleaning products or medicines are stored.
A: Cabinet lock

Q: In a smoke detector, this should be changed every year.
A: Battery

Gifts and Prizes

Everyone loves receiving gifts, and your shower guests are no exception. Supermarkets, drug stores, baby stores, and specialty shops are great places to ask for contributions of gifts and prizes. Remember that your invited guests are potential customers, and merchants are always looking for ways to establish a good reputation in the community.

Try to get some donated items related to baby safety, such as cabinet locks or electric socket plugs. Also include products every parent can use: baby bath items, disposable diapers, baby food, toys, and baby clothing. Moms also may welcome special treats for themselves such as a makeover or a gift certificate from a local store.

You may want to give a prize to game winners or, even better, to all participants in the game. A "goody bag" filled with product samples, discount coupons, gift certificates, and safety literature would delight all your guests. Save your best and biggest prize for a raffle or door prize. And finish off your shower with an exciting finale!

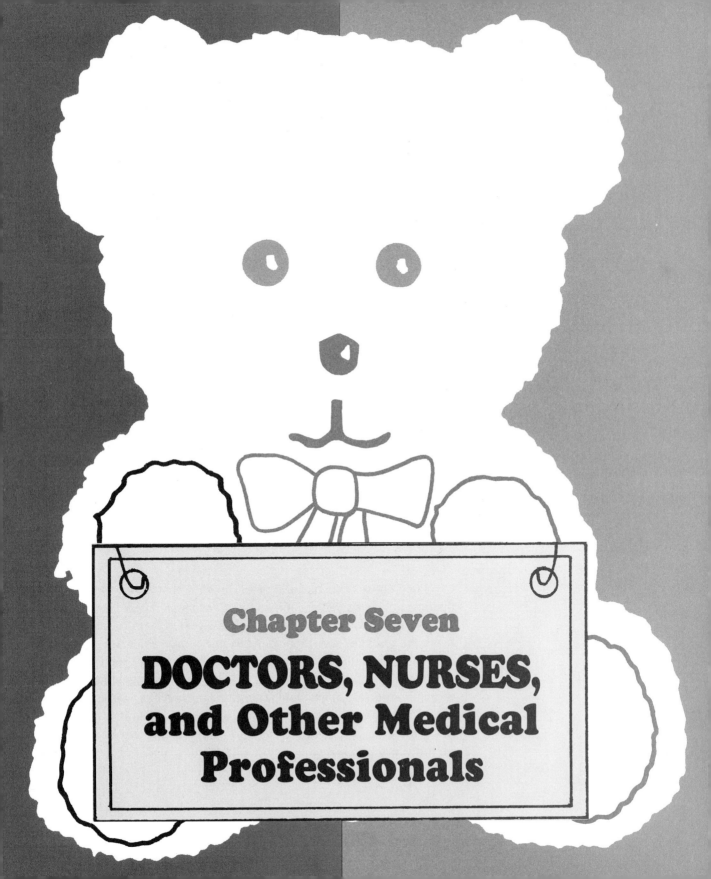

Chapter Seven

DOCTORS, NURSES, and Other Medical Professionals

Ask your obstetrician or call your local hospital to find out where and when childbirth classes are held. Some places charge a nominal fee for these classes; others offer them free of charge. Either way, you need to have some education before embarking on a birthing journey for the first time; it may be called "natural" childbirth, but for first timers there is often the feeling that nothing is going to happen naturally.

Choosing a class that suits your needs may seem like a daunting task at first; recognize that what's most important is that you ultimately feel comfortable with the teacher and the methods being presented. If you have already planned on a completely natural, unmedicated birth (and your physician has given the okay), you still need to learn about Caesarean births, because there is no guarantee that you won't have one should an emergency arise.

Most good childbirth instructors teach a little bit of all of the childbirth methods, to give first-time parents a good base from which to choose. These methods include:

- Lamaze, which stresses relaxation technique and conditioning to combat labor pain
- Grantly Dick-Read, which was the originator of the idea of including fathers and relies on a combination of relaxation technique and mental preparation to get through labor
- The Bradley method, which employs diet and exercise as a sensible way to work through the pain in a medication-free manner

Some classes take bits and pieces of each method to combine the best advice available; you can decide what will work best for you. Whatever you choose, you should sign up early in order to begin the class no later than your seventh month. You want to make sure you'll finish the course before the baby arrives. Though you may feel silly panting and blowing with a pillow up your shirt and a roomful of other couples doing the same, these types of exercises can actually help alleviate your delivery-room fears well in advance—not to mention give you and your partner something to joke about on the way to the hospital.

Partnering with Your Pediatrician

From birth to around its sixteenth birthday, your baby will be seeing a doctor of his or her own, preferably someone you've spent a lot of time in choosing. A professional you feel comfortable discussing your developing child with is tantamount to a having a healthy child.

The first step in finding a good pediatrician is to talk with other parents, your obstetrician, or your regular family doctor. You should then look in your insurance directory to make sure that the recommended physician is covered by your plan.

Next, you should call the pediatrician's office to listen for a friendly voice. If his or her staff seems rushed, or impatient, or just plain rude, hang up and call the next one on your list. Medical professionals should realize that they are representatives of the physician and practice; therefore, they should always be kind and patient with anyone on the other end of the phone—no matter who or when.

When you get a positive feeling from a receptionist or nurse's aide, you should set up an appointment to interview the pediatrician. Most will not charge you for this time with them; it should be considered a sales call, since you are in effect interviewing them for the job of caring for your little one; it is not a job you would entrust to just any name on the list.

How to Choose a Pediatrician

Once you have an appointment scheduled, jot down some questions you might like answered by the pediatrician. Always take your notes with you into the meeting; you'd be surprised how much you can forget when you're busy taking it all in.

Here are some questions that you should ask:

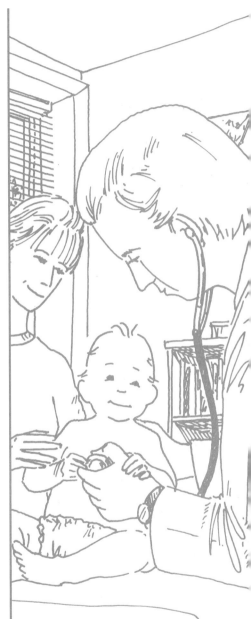

- Ask the doctor about his or her general approach to working with children. Questions such as "What do you find most fulfilling about working with youngsters?" will net you some telling answers. If the doctor says, "I most enjoy helping kids to grow, learn, and adjust to their world," you've got a good one. If, on the other hand, the response is that it was either this or become a veterinarian, continue on your search.

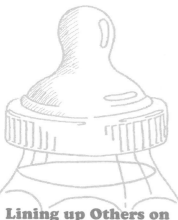

Lining up Others on Your "Team"

Be sure that in the last few weeks before your baby's birth, you line up the professionals and family members you want to help you through this new transition in your life. This group might include any or all of the following:

- **Your family.** Make sure everyone is reachable or that you have a system in place for calling everyone when it is time. Designate one or two people to make the calls for you, since you'll likely be too exhausted to do it yourself.
- **Your obstetrician.** As your due-date approaches, keep track of when your practitioner is on call and who will be covering in the event he or she is out of town when you go into labor. It can be quite a disappointment for you to think that your practitioner will be there, only to find yourself matched with someone completely new to you. Even if you can't choose a specific doctor for the delivery, at least familiarize yourself with the one you *could* have.

- Find out what the doctor's policies are, especially about whether your child will have to sit in a waiting room filled with sick kids. Ideally, there should only be a few children in the waiting area at a time—and the really sick kids (those with contagious illnesses) should be sequestered in an examining room, away from other children.
- Does your insurance cover everything the doctor orders? Finding out early in the process will help you avoid troublesome decisions later. Call your insurance company; doctors simply can't know every detail about all policies.
- What rules and regulations does the pediatrician have (if any)? One doctor I interviewed once gave me a handout three pages long—topped with the words: *I will decide what is an emergency and will call you back accordingly.* This same doctor said she would not tolerate a patient being five minutes late for an appointment; yet she evidently felt it was okay to leave me in a waiting room full of sick children for forty-five minutes. Needless to say, she didn't get another chance from me.
- What are the doctor's parental philosophies? Is the doctor a parent, too? If so, what is his or her approach to parenting? You may feel more assured calling a pediatrician who has also experienced a frantic night with a baby's temperature soaring.

Once you've chosen your pediatrician, it might be a nice gesture for you to let the doctor know why he or she was chosen. It may reinforce the positive aspects of the physician's service. For instance, if it's the doctor's responsiveness that impresses you, say it. If it's the calm, quiet atmosphere you like, mention that, too. Being as specific as you can will help the doctor keep up the good work.

What Happens at the Early Checkups?

The first visit with the pediatrician usually occurs at the hospital within hours of birth. During this visit, the doctor will examine the baby from head to toe, making sure that all of the baby's vital signs are stable and consistent with those of other newborns. The doctor will then report all of his or her findings to you in your hospital room; you will begin hearing about "percentiles" (benchmarks against other typical newborns) and how your baby measures up against others his or her age. (Overzealous parents will proudly fling these percentiles about; if you are a healthy, well-adjusted person, this practice will soon begin to greatly annoy you.)

Within a week or so after delivery, you will return to the pediatrician's office for another checkup. All of the vitals will be checked again, but you will have the chance to discuss any feeding, sleeping, or related problems with your pediatrician. Always take your notebook with you for these visits, as you will be able to look back for reference after you leave the doctor's office. Of primary concern at this time is baby's weight; if he or she has dropped a pound or more since leaving the hospital (and most babies do) but has not gained any of it back yet, the doctor may make recommendations and may ask you to return a few more times in the next two weeks for a weight check.

"Well-baby" visits need to be scheduled at 1, 3, 6, 9, 12, 15, 18, and 24 months, and here the doctor will cover everything from a brief physical to a discussion of baby's particular growth stage to track his or her physical, emotional, and motor development. You will constantly be talking about baby's eating habits. After two years of age, your child will need only an annual checkup.

Immunizations should occur at 2, 4, 6, 15, and 18 months. These immunizations protect against the following diseases: diphtheria, pertussis (whooping cough), mumps, measles, tetanus, rubella, hepatitis B, chicken pox, and haemophilus influenza type b.

Hepatitis B vaccine. This vaccine is often given to babies first at birth and then at two and six months. *Pro:* The vaccine helps protect infants at risk of developing the disease from infection passed by the mother. *Con:* Some babies, albeit a small percentage, develop minor, temporary side effects such as a rash.

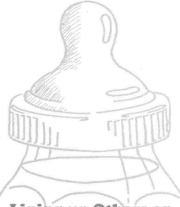

Lining up Others on Your "Team"
(continued)

- **A lactation consultant.** A few years ago, it was fairly uncommon for hospitals to have a breastfeeding consultant on staff; now, many offer such services on-site. Arrange in advance to have a lactation consultant come to your room as soon as possible after the birth, so that you can get the best help available to guide you through breastfeeding—the right way.
- **Your pediatrician.** Once you've chosen the one you'd like, you'll need to make sure that he or she does newborn visits at the hospital where you're delivering. The hospital usually contacts the pediatrician for you after you've given birth. The pediatrician will check the baby over and then come to your room to discuss the results and ask a few questions relating to family medical history.

Polio vaccine. You now have a choice between an active and an inactive polio virus immunization; this vaccine is given at 2, 4, and 18 months. *Pro:* Many parents feel more comfortable with the latter, since there is no chance of the baby actually contracting polio from the vaccine itself. *Con:* If baby has the active virus version, he or she has a 1 in 750,000 chance of contracting the disease with the first dose. Many physicians feel that is too risky. In 1996, the Centers for Disease Control and Prevention (CDC) made a new recommendation for U.S. polio immunization: to use the enhanced inactivated polio vaccine (eIPV) for the first two doses, followed by two doses of the oral (active) vaccine (OPV). You, of course, may choose to have all eIPV or all OPV.

DTP vaccine. This is the combination diphtheria-tetanus-pertussis vaccine, given at 2, 4, 6, and 18 months. *Pro:* The good news is that there is a newer-class version of this vaccine (acellular DTP, or DtaP) with fewer side effects than the old one. *Con:* There is still a significant chance baby will have an adverse reaction within hours of the shot. Watch baby carefully for signs of discomfort.

Hib vaccine. Given at 2, 4, 6, and 15 months, this one protects baby from haemophilus influenza type b. *Pro:* Baby gets protection from the disease. *Con:* Some babies show signs of discomfort afterward; report any unusually high-pitched crying or redness and swelling.

MMR vaccine. This is the measles, mumps, and rubella vaccine. *Pro:* Baby doesn't get this one until 15 months, when his or her immune system is even stronger. *Con:* Up to 15 percent of babies show adverse reactions, not immediately after the shot but within two weeks of immunization. Symptoms such as rash, fever, or swollen lymph glands could indicate a reaction; and it is best to notify your pediatrician immediately if you notice such reactions.

Perhaps the best news of all is that an all-in-one shot is currently in the final test stages and should be in use within the next two years. This shot will eliminate the need for three injections at one time; and all babies will appreciate this consideration, as will weak-stomached parents.

Building a Good Working Relationship with Your Pediatrician

Once you've established a partnership with your pediatrician, how can you keep the relationship a positive and productive one? Here are some suggestions:

- Follow the rules and policies of your pediatrician. Keep this information sheet handy, and refer to it often. Parents who expect special treatment or who think they are somehow above the rules, will ultimately turn off a pediatrician and damage their working relationship.
- Always jot down questions or thoughts for the doctor, and bring this notebook to every meeting. Write down the doctor's responses, too, so you don't have to call back later and make the doctor repeat anything that was said.
- To save the doctor time, come in with as much information as you can muster. Things like temperature, symptoms, and general behavior of the baby will provide some clues to baby's illness.
- Be willing to try what the doctor says. If he or she doesn't feel that a medication will nip the problem or that the illness must simply run its course, don't argue. If, on the other hand, you try leaving baby to fight off the problem and the symptoms get worse, do call the doctor back to try another approach.
- If you can wait until morning, do so before calling the doctor. Leave the nighttime and weekend calls for emergencies only. This is a hard concept for first-time parents, to whom everything unusual may seem like an emergency.

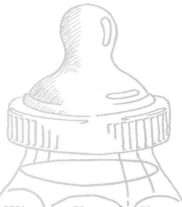

What to Keep in Your Medicine Chest

Here's a shopping list of items for you to keep in your medicine chest:

- Rubbing alcohol (mainly for cleaning thermometers)
- Syrup of Ipecac (use only if your pediatrician recommends it—in cases of accidental swallowing or poisoning)
- Hydrogen peroxide
- Sunscreen (for six-to-twelve-month-olds, especially if you live in a sunny climate)
- Flashlight (to check inside mouth if necessary)
- Decongestant for babies (use only if your pediatrician recommends it)
- Nose drops (for babies who have sinus problems)

☞ Don't use your baby's appointment as an opportunity for all of your other children to be seen by the doctor. Pediatricians agree that this one-stop-shopping approach not only takes too much of their time (affecting other scheduled appointments) but also is unfair to them. If others in your family need to be seen by the doctor, schedule a separate appointment for each.

☞ Finally, realize that part of having a healthy baby is for the baby to have a healthy you. Take care of yourself, and alert your pediatrician to any problems you might be having (such as postpartum depression, breastfeeding concerns, or even general worries about parenting). Your pediatrician can be a valuable resource for you in helping you learn more about your role as a parent.

When to Call the Doctor

First-time parents tend to worry about their baby more than veteran parents do, mainly because every new noise or cry makes them worry about illness. It's the one thing we as parents have little control over; when our little one is sick, we feel so powerless.

But it's important to remember that baby operates much like you do. There can be occasional bouts of diarrhea, some gas or tooth pain, and even crying for no real reason. Your baby might even have a constipated moment or two. None of these problems are indications of serious illness, so you need not worry if they happen occasionally or seem short lived.

But there are some times when a call to the doctor is absolutely necessary:

☞ When baby's temperature is higher than 101 degrees (rectally)
☞ When baby sleeps long or doesn't wake easily
☞ When baby is unusually fussy or irritable
☞ When baby refuses to feed well or eats only a small amount before crying in a high-pitched manner
☞ When baby isn't wetting at least one diaper every four hours or so (for a grand total of six to eight per day)

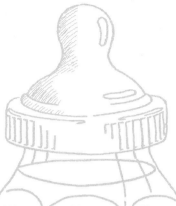

When baby vomits excessively at more than two consecutive feedings, or vomits green bile (if this occurs, call doctor immediately)

When baby has labored, distressed, or rapid breathing

If baby's color tone changes (look for blueness in the lips or fingernails or yellowish skin or eyes)

If the baby exhibits any of these symptoms and is under two months of age, you should treat it as an emergency situation and call the doctor for proper guidance.

And you might want to call the doctor (during regular office hours) for the following minor irritations:

A rash that doesn't ease with cream or air drying

Constipation, diarrhea, or a cold

A minor injury

Common Illnesses of Babyhood— and How to Deal with Them

1. **Rashes and skin irritations.** These are common problems among very young babies; everything from laundry detergent to your perfume can cause red, flaky, and itchy skin for baby. The most common culprit, however, is spillage of milk into the folds of the neck. Be sure to keep a bib on baby, and wipe the area after feeding time. Also, use a good baby cream in the affected areas two or three times per day. Eczema, or dermatitis, can occur in babies and is sometimes caused when a baby is switched from breastmilk to formula; it is, essentially, an allergic reaction. Call the doctor if you suspect your baby has eczema.

    When baby has eczema or other skin conditions, you should do the following:

    Use lots of baby cream.

    Keep baby's nails trimmed, to avoid excessive scratching.

    Give baby a bath every other day and a sponge bath in-between. Soap can further dry out already irritated skin.

What to Keep in Your Medicine Chest
(continued)

- An oral syringe (for giving the right dose of medicine)
- A rectal thermometer (rather than a possibly less accurate digital ear one that can fail or need a battery replacement at an inopportune moment)
- Antiseptic cream (to ward off infection after minor cuts and scrapes)
- Liquid pain reliever (for relief of teething pain or discomfort from immunizations)
- Heating pad
- Popsicle sticks or tongue depressors
- Cool mist vaporizer (one that doesn't make too much noise)
- Small plastic adhesive strips (bandages)

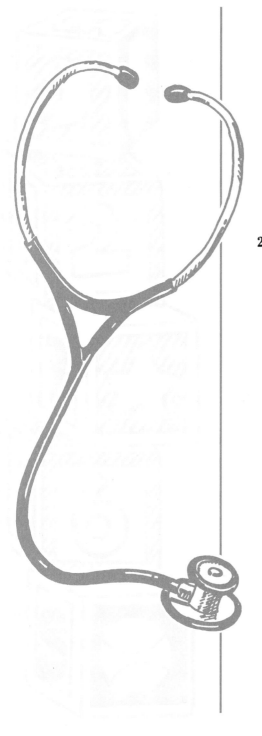

    ✂ Use a cool-mist humidifier to keep baby's environment moist.

    ✂ Avoid overdressing baby, and stay away from scratchy materials. Soft cotton outfits that leave baby's neck open to the air are preferable. Be sure to lay a cotton receiving blanket on play areas.

    ✂ Take note of any foods that seem to trigger a rash, and eliminate them from baby's diet.

    ✂ Call the doctor if the rash seems to be getting worse or if it doesn't seem to go away even after your home treatment.

2. **Fever.** The scariest thing a new parent will face is baby's first real fever. (Note: A real fever is anything over 101 degrees.) If baby has a slight temperature, you may be able to bring it down with over-the-counter baby-pain reliever. Some fevers are caused by teething pain or perhaps are a reaction to an immunization; these can usually be treated with infant pain reliever as well. However, if the fever is high, you will need to call your doctor immediately. If it's accompanied by a rash or if it seems to be hanging on for longer than a few days, call the doctor.

Here are some tips for treating baby's fever:

    ✂ Use infant pain reliever first, and then check baby's temperature again in an hour or so. If it works, administer the pain reliever every four hours as needed.

    ✂ Always use a rectal thermometer to get the most accurate temperature. You can still use the digital type for back up.

    ✂ Look for other signs of illness, such as irritability, lethargy, lack of interest in feeding, and excessive sleeping. Let your doctor know about these symptoms.

    ✂ Do not use products containing aspirin. They have been associated with Reye's syndrome, a brain disorder.

    ✂ Dress baby in light, comfortable clothing.

    ✂ To replenish fluid that is perspired out, offer as much milk, juice, or water as baby will take.

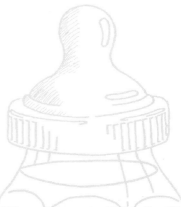

3. **The common cold.** Especially if you live in a changeable climate, your baby could be susceptible to colds throughout the fall and winter. Colds are usually passed through airborne particles or through hand-to-hand or hand-to-mouth contact with an infected person. If someone in your family has a cold, ask that person to please keep a distance from baby— and to not kiss or hold the baby until the cold has completely passed. Babies can develop a fever prior to showing full-fledged cold symptoms, such as a runny or stuffed-up nose; a cough; red, watery eyes; and lack of appetite.

   If you think baby has a cold, you should do the following:

   ⚕ Use a bulb syringe and infant nasal drops to keep nasal passages clear and open.

   ⚕ Put a pillow under the baby's mattress to keep his or her head elevated (or use a product called crib shoes to elevate the head of the crib); never place baby's head directly on a pillow, because baby can pull it over and suffocate.

   ⚕ Watch for color changes in baby's mucous. If it changes from clear to thick yellowish green, call your doctor. There may be an infection to treat as well as the cold.

   ⚕ Ask your doctor before giving baby any cold medications. Some of these are for older children and could present other problems for baby should there be an adverse reaction.

4. **Ear infections.** Middle-ear infections occur in nearly all children before they reach their second year and are more common in children who are around other kids on a regular basis (such as at a daycare). You should treat an ear infection as soon as you can, since they can be quite uncomfortable for baby and can cause delays in language development (because of hearing difficulties). Ear infections are more frequent in babies than in adults because a baby's eustachian tube is smaller than an adult's, allowing bacteria a quicker route to the middle ear. How do you know when baby has

Five Ways to Ward off Illness at Your House

1. Clean and disinfect regularly—at least once per week.

2. Rid your home of mold and other airborne virus-causing agents. Buy an air purifier, and have your basement checked for mold. Mold has been linked to sudden infant death syndrome, among other respiratory illnesses.

3. Limit the number of people who come to visit baby in the early days, and be careful who you let touch or kiss the baby.

4. Make sure everyone washes his or her hands regularly, particularly after using the restroom. Use only antibacterial soap to wash hands and dishes in; it will cut down on bacteria considerably.

5. Do laundry (especially baby's) every two to three days. Don't let baby wear soiled clothes for very long, and don't let dirty clothes (or diapers) pile up in baby's room. Spray disinfectant into diaper pails and baby hampers.

an ear infection? Usually a high-pitched cry and tugging of the ear will tell you. The more you try to lay the baby down to rest, the worse the crying becomes. Fever is also common. Finally, baby may eat less because it hurts to swallow.

Here are some tips for treating an ear infection:

- Call your doctor for his or her advice.
- If your pediatrician has recommended a prescription medication, use it exactly as indicated. Most antibiotics (amoxicillin is the most prescribed) need to be taken until completely gone.
- Hold baby upright during feeding and try letting baby sleep upright in the swing or car seat to take some pressure off the ear.
- Use baby pain reliever as directed.
- Go back to the doctor for a follow-up exam to be sure the infection is gone.

5. **Diarrhea.** The primary causes of diarrhea are a virus, bacteria, or a reaction to a new food. If baby has one or two loose stools in a day or so, there is no real cause for alarm; however, you should call the doctor if the diarrhea contains blood or if baby is dehydrated.

The following are signs of dehydration:

- Significant decrease in wet diapers (low urine output)—less than five wet diapers per day
- Dry mouth
- Sunken eyes
- Lethargy
- Tight skin

6. **Constipation.** If baby is straining or having difficulty in producing stools, the best thing you can do is try curling the baby's knees up as he or she is straining; this can help baby use gravity to push the stool out. If there is still a

Five Common Disasters That Pediatricians Believe Can Be Avoided

1. **Choking problems caused by improper toys in baby's mouth.** Make sure you have safe teething toys on hand at all times, and baby won't be as tempted.

2. **Burns.** You'd be surprised to hear how many babies get burned by a parent's hot coffee (or, worse yet, from a lit cigarette). Keep your "poisons" away from your baby; remember that baby wouldn't choose these things on his or her own. And keep the tub water warm, not hot.

3. **Injury from walkers.** More and more pediatricians are recommending that parents do away with the walkers on wheels; even my Lilly went headfirst over two small steps—and I was standing right by her at the time. They're just too unpredictable.

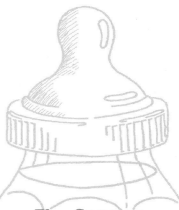

problem, you could try a tiny piece of a glycerin suppository (it would be better to ask the doctor first, however). Never give baby any kind of laxative or mineral oil, as these measures can often throw off baby's electrolyte balance and cause other problems.

7. **Vomiting.** As with diarrhea, your primary concern should be to keep your baby hydrated. Feed baby milk or water—or, better yet, an electrolyte solution—to replenish fluids more rapidly. Vomiting typically is more short lived than diarrhea but can be indicative of a more serious problem. Try to feed baby smaller amounts of food at half-hour intervals, and call your doctor. (Note: Spitting up after feeding is not considered vomiting.)

8. **Gas pain.** Your baby is crying incessantly, and nothing seems to be wrong—until you notice that baby has passed a tiny bit of gas. Where there is a little, there is usually more; so try some gas-relief drops to help baby get rid of the tummy pain. In and of itself, gas poses no real threat to baby's health; in fact, it is healthy for baby to pass as much gas as necessary.

9. **Teething pain.** It can take up to two (long) weeks for baby to cut a tooth; imagine how long baby will fuss and cry if left to fend for himself or herself! Gums will be sore, and baby will drool buckets. These are your major symptoms; now that you know what they are, how can you best help baby?

   - Give baby some pain reliever (either acetaminophen or ibuprofen; or you can try some topical pain reliever such as Anbesol).
   - Provide lots of cool teething toys for baby to gnaw on; always keep at least one in the freezer.
   - Keep a bib on baby as often as possible, and change it as frequently as it becomes wet.

Five Common Disasters That Pediatricians Believe Can Be Avoided
(continued)

4. **Poisoning.** Left alone and unsupervised, your baby could eat an entire plant in a matter of minutes. The problem is that many plants are poisonous to pets and babies. Also, be careful to keep all medications and cleaning agents out of a crawling baby's reach. It's best to keep such things locked in a cabinet.

5. **Furniture "bumps."** Get on your hands and knees and look at your home through a baby's eyes. You should make note of every sharp, pointed edge on pieces of furniture, and cover each edge with soft foam. Keep exercise equipment (and recliners) away from baby.

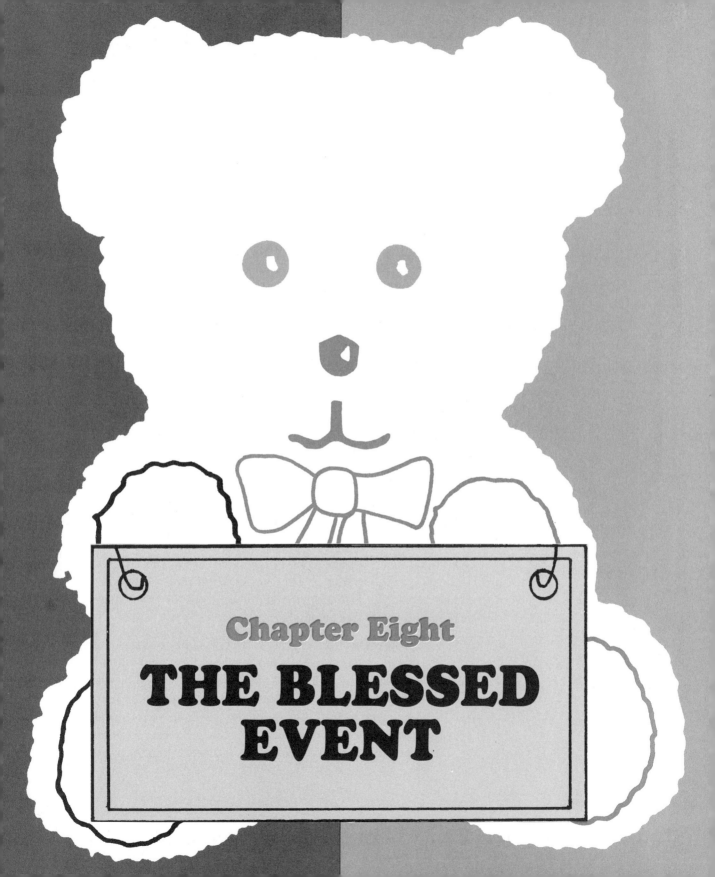

Chapter Eight

THE BLESSED EVENT

By now, you're no doubt tired of hearing all of the unsolicited comments from well-meaning friends and relatives: "Haven't you had the baby yet?" "Are you still here?" Certainly you're getting tired of carrying around your full-term baby—even if you were really excited about having it in the first place.

In the last month of pregnancy, as you await your sweet arrival, it's hard to stay positive about the whole experience. On the one hand, you have those well-meaning people constantly commenting on how "ready" you look (even weeks before you actually are—further prolonging your agony). On the other hand, you have your own feelings of anxiety and concern over everything from whether the baby's room is *really* ready to trying to imagine a pain you've never felt before (but, no doubt, have been frightened by—thanks to the stories of every other mother you know).

If you're feeling a little anxious about the details of the birth, it might help you to learn as much as you can about the stages of labor. If you're like most women I know, you already flipped to this section before reading any of the early pregnancy information—to mentally prepare yourself for the moment you've likely dreamt about since you were a little girl playing with dolls.

Birth: What Happens and How You Get Through It

You have made it this far; so take some comfort first of all in knowing that labor and delivery comprise only a small portion of the total birth experience. Do you feel better now? Okay, with this new perspective in mind, you can move on to the three stages of birth and what you can anticipate.

> ✂ **Stage One:** *Labor.* Labor itself takes three stages to accomplish its mission: *early labor* (about five to eight hours, but possibly longer if this is your first baby), which brings with it irregular contractions that open your cervix to about 4 centimeters; *active labor* (about two or three hours), which brings intensifying contractions that are closer together and open your cervix to about 8 centimeters; and *transition*

(thirty minutes to two hours), which is hard labor and opens your cervix to the 10 centimeters needed for pushing.

- **Stage Two:** *Birth of the Baby.* This is that glorious stage where you get to push the baby out of your body and into the "Everywhere." You will be totally focused on getting the baby out, and your partner may need to stay close to your head to help you stay focused. At this point, if you feel like it, you can try whatever position makes you feel most comfortable (sitting up, lying down, squatting, or a side position). As the baby moves further down in the birth canal, you will feel more and more like pushing. If your doctor says it's okay, do so. If he or she asks you to pant or blow instead, do as you are instructed, since you might have to have an episiotomy if the doctor thinks you might tear your vaginal opening. This will only take a minute to do and most doctors will perform it only if it is necessary (though you should discuss this ahead of time).

- **Stage Three:** *Afterbirth.* This is the stage where your hormones trigger delivery of the placenta, and it is either pushed out by you or removed by your doctor. The doctor will then check it over for signs of any problems and assist you in the beginning of your recovery by suturing any tears or incisions from an episiotomy. He or she will likely give you some bonding time with baby afterward and then visit you later with aftercare instructions and tips.

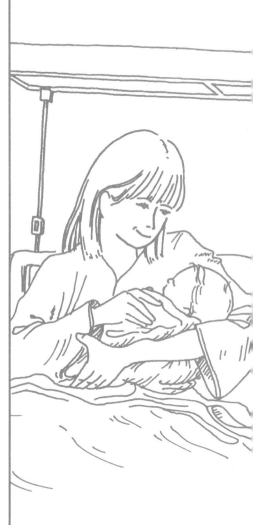

Creating the Perfect Birthing Atmosphere

The birth of your child is at once a happy and a frightening experience; and one of the best things you can do is create a positive birthing environment, one in which you feel comfortable and relaxed (okay, as relaxed as you can possibly feel in labor). Check out the birthing center at the hospital before your due date; ask what kind of things you can bring and what kind you can't. For example, you might like to bring candles and champagne for celebrating the birth, but these may be against hospital regulations. Here

are some suggestions for items that you might use to make your birthing experience a little bit more comfortable:

- Soft music on a portable CD player or cassette deck (bring several that you like, since it might take a while)
- A bottle of wine, champagne, or grape juice (check hospital rules)
- A picture of a pleasant scene to focus on during labor
- A special toy or meaningful item from one of your other children

The bottom line is, do whatever you feel will bring you the most comfort, but don't be surprised if your well-thought-out plan doesn't suit your particular mood once you're in labor. Be prepared to chuck it all if you decide you're not feeling up to it.

What If I Need a C-Section?

Caesarean sections are performed when the lives of either the baby or the mother are in jeopardy or when the baby is too large or not well positioned. If a C-section is to be performed, the mother is given a spinal or epidural and can usually be awake for the surgery. A tent is placed over her abdominal area, and her husband or partner is usually near her head. Delivery of the baby is usually within minutes, and the parents can see the baby immediately after it is removed through incisions in the abdomen and uterus. Afterward, the placenta is removed and examined, and the doctor will usually perform a check of the abdominal cavity. Once that is accomplished, the mother is stitched up and taken into the recovery room.

With both of my pregnancies, there was at least one point where a C-section was discussed; with my first child, I was actually scheduled to have one (but finally managed to go into labor and deliver naturally). Both times I had talked with other mothers who had C-sections and was usually comforted when they shattered the myths surrounding this procedure.

Myth: *The organs in the abdominal region are taken out and placed on the stomach in order to get the baby out.* In reality, the operation only takes a few minutes, with two incisions and all major organs left intact.

Myth: *You'll never be able to deliver vaginally after a C-section.* In reality, most women who want to deliver a second child after a Caesarean delivery can do so vaginally. Talk with your doctor for more complete information on VBAC (Vaginal Birth After Caesarean) deliveries.

Take the time to discuss your feelings and fears with your doctor well in advance of the possible surgery. It might be a good idea to ask the doctor exactly how the determination for a C-section is made so that you are prepared for that option and not surprised when surgery is mandated.

If your doctor should decide to perform a C-section, ask as many questions about it as you feel a need to; then try to put it all in perspective. If you had your heart set on a vaginal delivery, don't let the prospect of a C-section ruin your birthing experience. You are still a mother giving birth to her child, regardless of the way it actually happens. And the best thing you can do is put the needs of your child first, which is exactly what a C-section is about, since it is performed as a safety measure for the baby.

When recovering from a C-section, you will be encouraged to turn and move around while still in the recovery room so that your muscles don't get cramped. You should make sure that you raise the head of your hospital bed before attempting to turn your body; then place a pillow over your abdomen to keep from popping stitches when attempting to sit up. Try to move into a sitting position carefully, stretching your legs to the floor as far as you comfortably can. Then, with some help from your partner, try to stand for a few minutes. Alert your doctor to any discomfort beyond that which is expected after a C-section. Most of all, remember not to push yourself; and don't try to lift things or get out of bed by yourself until your doctor says it's okay to do so. Recovery from a C-section takes longer than for vaginal births; do line up some help in caring for baby during the first few weeks.

Birth in Other Cultures and in the Animal World

- In Greece, doulas help other women give birth, whether it's a home birth or a hospital birth.
- In Sweden, birthing women can actually check into a resort, where they give birth, have a facial and/or massage, and are basically treated like queens. This type of treatment, although pricey, should be a universal, don't you think?
- In England, women can choose from a wide variety of birthing options, from an underwater to a traditional hospital experience.
- Mother cats like to find quiet, warm, dark places to give birth. To them, birth is a very private activity; and it may also be a protective measure, since mother

Your Aftercare

Immediately after the baby is born, you will need to watch for the following signs of trouble and call your doctor immediately if you experience any:

- Discharge from your vagina that is heavier than normal, is bright red, or is foul-smelling.
- Fever or sudden rise in temperature.
- Burning on urination or difficulty in doing so.
- Soreness or irritation in your legs or in your breasts.
- Any adjustment problems that interfere with care of the baby.

Breech Baby, Breech Baby . . .

A breech baby is simply a baby who is presenting its feet first—instead of its head—toward the birth canal. Today, almost all breech babies are delivered via C-section. What if your baby is in a breech position prior to birth? Is there anything you can do to help the baby to turn?

Some experts suggest that you try getting on your hands and knees, rocking your pelvis while arching your back, to get the baby to move naturally. This does not always work, but it can sure help ease any back pain you might be experiencing.

Another option is to go to a specialist who can turn the baby through external manipulation and use of ultrasound to check baby's position. However, some doctors insist that a breech baby is in that position because it is most comfortable—that the baby, in fact, knows that it has a cord around its neck and that moving makes it tighter. And they are growing increasingly skeptical about this procedure, since a few infants have been lost because the umbilical cord was wrapped around the neck at the time of inversion—with the specialist completely unaware.

Finally, some women have used acupressure or other nontraditional methods to encourage their babies to move into birthing position. One woman I know even tried putting a radio between her knees while lying on her back, hoping the baby would turn its head in the direction of the music! Whichever method you decide to try, do consult your doctor first. Remember, the baby can still turn at the last minute—even during labor!

Induction: Why, When, and How

Some babies are just plain reluctant to be born. When a baby is more than a week beyond its due date, a physician may make the suggestion to you that the baby be induced.

When a baby is induced, the first step is often placing a prostaglandin gel on the mother's cervix to encourage dilatation. Some women spontaneously go into labor with the gel alone, while others require further medication in order to get things rolling.

If you should need more medication, pitocin is usually the drug of choice. It is given through an IV, and it usually spurs labor on within a few hours. On the downside, many women say that pitocin causes labor pains "like a runaway train," meaning fast and furious. The pains are generally more intense and closer together than in a natural labor, but the benefit is that the labor is also generally shorter with induction.

Maddie was induced and one of the main positives about that experience was that we made an "appointment" to have her—there was no rushing to the hospital and no fear of my water breaking in the mall. While I found the pain to be every bit as intense as I'd been told, it was also not intolerable. It also beat having another nineteen-hour labor (as I did with Lilly)!

Hey, Where Are They Going with My Baby?

It's the moment you've anticipated—you've finally given birth. And immediately after doing so, you expect to hold your newborn infant, just like in the movies. Suddenly, a nurse rushes to the doctor's side, and your baby gets whisked off to an incubator—where a series of tests are completed. What is the baby's coloring like? Does it have all of its fingers and toes? Can it grasp and use its reflexes? Using a rating scale called the APGAR, a neonatal nurse evaluates the baby

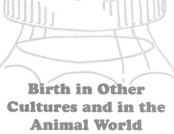

Birth in Other Cultures and in the Animal World
(continued)

cats are in a vulnerable position when giving birth. A private little spot can offer the newborn kittens shelter from outside predators.

- Birds build their nests specifically for laying eggs. Unfortunately, a relatively high percentage of eggs get stolen from birds' nests, since the mother bird cannot be in two places at once (i.e., gathering food for and protecting her young).

- Very few fathers in the animal kingdom are involved in anything past the mating stage; in fact, some fathers grow antagonistic toward their male offspring, fighting over turf when the youngster reaches maturity.

to determine its health immediately after birth; she then repeats the test one or more times in the hours to come.

This is standard procedure and nothing to be alarmed about; you should ask your doctor in advance of the birth how soon you'll be able to hold the baby; that way it won't be a disappointment to you if this is a moment you've envisioned for some time. Realize that a few minutes to make sure baby is healthy is worth all of the moments you'll have in the days to come.

Beginning a New (and Separate) Life

After nine months together, you and your baby are now embarking on separate, unique lives. And even though you had a life before baby's conception, the one you have now entered into is entirely different.

Before baby's birth, you were your own person. During your pregnancy, you were the mother-to-be. Now, you are so-and-so's mommy; we call this the "accessory-to-baby" syndrome. More and more, you will come to be known as someone's mommy before anything else. And if that's going to be a problem, you'd better adjust to it soon.

It's not so bad, really. And many women are proud to be known as a mother first. It's quite an honor—and for quite an achievement. But if you want to have a separate identity outside of your child, you'll need to decide how and where it will be. Perhaps it will mean returning to work (see the Working with Baby chapter for options) or simply joining a group such as a book club or parent's group.

Whatever you decide, know that your life will never be the same. Rather, it will be much richer and much fuller than you ever dreamed possible—now that you and baby are two separate entities.

Postpartum Issues

After the blessed event has passed and all of the guests have departed from the ceremonial "viewing of the baby," you will be left to adjust to your new life as a parent. You will suddenly be faced with a lot of situations you never had to deal with before baby came along.

First is the adjustment to being totally responsible for this new and completely dependent little life. This feeling can be overwhelming, particularly to those who were entrenched in their careers immediately prior to giving birth. Instead of daily status meetings and power lunches, you find yourself changing diapers, feeding like a milk truck, and monitoring baby's every move to make sure he or she is still okay.

It might also take a while for you and baby to get used to each other's cues. For instance, baby may cry incessantly for an hour or so before you can figure out exactly what's wrong; expect that this might happen, try not to get frustrated, and allow yourself a little time to learn baby's way of communicating. No one gets everything right the first time!

Physically, you may be feeling extremely tired from the birth experience itself, and your body will need at least four to six weeks to recuperate. Giving birth is something akin to the decathlon. Your body uses muscles you didn't even know you had to accomplish a monumental feat: bringing a new life into the world. Don't underestimate the fact that your body will take its own time to get back to normal after the birth. If you try to rush your recovery, your body could respond with negative side effects and complications, thus extending the recovery period.

Expect your emotions to run the gamut from euphoria to depression. There are plenty of ways you can deal with any stress you might be feeling:

- Write down all of your concerns and fears, and then rate them according to which seem most and which seem least rational.
- Next, write down the worst thing that could possibly happen for each item. Don't worry about judging these concerns just yet.
- Going over your list, try to write down at least two positive things or solutions to go with each worry.
- Talk about this list with your partner or a good friend. Often, writing everything down and sharing it helps alleviate the stress.

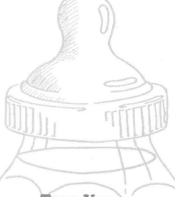

True Versus False Labor

It's probably false labor if . . .

- "Labor" pains go away after changing position or moving around.
- The contractions aren't regular, don't increase in intensity, and actually diminish after an hour or so.
- All of your pain seems to be in your lower abdomen instead of your lower back.

But it could be real labor if . . .

- Contractions seem to get stronger and intensify if you try moving around or changing activity.
- Contractions get more frequent and increasingly more painful— to the point where it's hard to speak when they're happening.
- You have pinkish or blood-streaked discharge from the vagina.
- Your water breaks. (In most cases, you will feel only a slight gush of fluid as this occurs.)
- You experience pain that seems to radiate from your lower back to your abdomen and then, possibly, down your legs.

If writing it down doesn't help, try a change of pace. Get a babysitter for a few hours and just do something for you: a massage, a facial, shopping, or even lunch alone at your favorite restaurant. Take a warm bath or cuddle up with a good book. Remember to go easy on yourself—and always make time for you.

If the stress is too much or becomes more severe (leading to depression), seek professional assistance. You should call your doctor if you experience any of the following:

- Lethargy or the inability to motivate yourself to do much except meet the baby's primary needs
- Periods of moodiness or irritability that lead to further depression
- Anxiety over the baby or in general
- Insomnia
- Difficulty concentrating or making decisions
- Crying jags or periods of sadness that do not go away easily

All of these symptoms are signs of postpartum depression (PPD), a condition that affects about 10 to 15 percent of new moms (although that number could be considerably higher, since many are afraid to tell anyone what they're experiencing). Postpartum depression is different from the more common (and shorter-lasting) "baby blues," which typically occur within days of the birth and last a maximum of two weeks. With PPD, a new mother experiences depression that cannot be alleviated without the use of antidepressants, or therapy, or, in some cases, both. Risk factors for PPD include problems with your marriage, depression or anxiety during the pregnancy (or a stressful event), lack of support from your partner or significant others, a history of premenstrual syndrome, or a previous case of PPD.

Another form of this disorder is postpartum psychosis, which affects a small percentage of the population but has symptoms of wishing to harm yourself or the baby. These thoughts are serious enough to warrant immediate attention (and intervention). Call for help if you experience such thoughts; with professional help, it is possible to overcome this disorder!

If you'd like more information about these disorders, call Depression After Delivery, a national agency that provides assistance and referrals to those who need help coping after birth. The agency's hot line number is 1-800-944-4773.

Postpartum Depression: A True Story

A few weeks after the birth of my first child, Lilly, I started feeling a little bit down in the dumps. At first, it seemed like it was more closely related to sleep deprivation—you know, that feeling of irritability that you get when you don't get enough sleep. But as a few weeks turned into a few months, I knew that something was wrong.

What started out as a need for some peace, quiet, and perhaps more sleep developed in a short period of time into irritable, PMS-like behavior and eventually into a very real depression that didn't completely subside until Lilly was nearly two years old. "What is happening?" I wondered. "This is supposed to be the happiest time of my life, and here I am lying on the couch, watching the Waltons and waiting for an organic, peaceful death." Yes, I wished for my body to shut itself off, because I didn't know how to deal with this totally foreign feeling.

I asked my doctor what was wrong, and he immediately sent me to a psychiatrist—who misdiagnosed me as manic-depressive and proceeded to put me on lithium. After a few more months of continued depression, I ditched the psychiatrist—and decided that maybe I was clinically depressed, possibly permanently so. I was at such an incredible low that my friends, who knew me to be a warm, open, and fun-loving person, were frightened by what they were seeing.

One friend called me on an extremely low day, and she gave me the number of a postpartum support group that I believe saved my life. I dialed the number, and then talked to a woman named Diane, who lived nearby and was the director of the group nearest me. She told me that she had been through this kind of depression, too; and then she listened to me for the next hour.

Diane invited me to the support group's next meeting, where I met six other women in various stages of this disorder. All of them had experienced problems similar to my own; some of them had already worked through them and were there to help those of us who were still trying to cope. The most beneficial thing for me was to know that there were others who had experienced the same thing

I was going through and that there was a good chance it would all end soon and I would be back to "normal."

The biggest problem for women with postpartum depression is that nobody wants to talk about it, except those who've been through it. Until recently, doctors have been reluctant to admit that it's anything more than the "baby blues." What was worse, just imagine trying to tell your friends and family that you're severely depressed after having this beautiful new addition to everyone's lives.

Fortunately, the subject is opening up for wider discussion. Books are available on the topic, and almost all of the parenting magazines have written about it honestly and directly.

On a happier note, going into my second pregnancy, my obstetrician and I worked out a plan for dealing with the possibility of a recurrence. We know, from a study underway at Case Western Reserve University Medical Center, that certain antidepressants, when taken as soon after birth as possible, can reduce the recurrence rate of postpartum depression significantly. And when Madelyn did arrive, I was fine, mentally and physically.

The At-Home Birth

In spite of the fact that births predominantly occur in hospitals, there are still a high number of at-home births (usually performed by midwives). These births are permitted if there are no signs of imminent danger to the mother and the baby seems to be progressing normally.

At-home births differ from hospital births in that you are free to include whomever you'd like in the process. If you'd like your whole family over to have a "welcoming" party for the baby, this option is more available to you than it would be in a hospital birth. Families who already have other children often like to include all of the children in the birth of their new sibling, and this is more easily and comfortably accomplished at an at-home birth.

As with any birth, you should prepare for the possibility of an emergency. Should any complications arise, your midwife will call an ambulance.

If you should decide to have your baby at home, take the time to plan out exactly where you'd like to give birth, and then make sure everything is kept clean in the weeks prior to your due date. Follow your midwife's instructions carefully, and then work at creating a meaningful atmosphere.

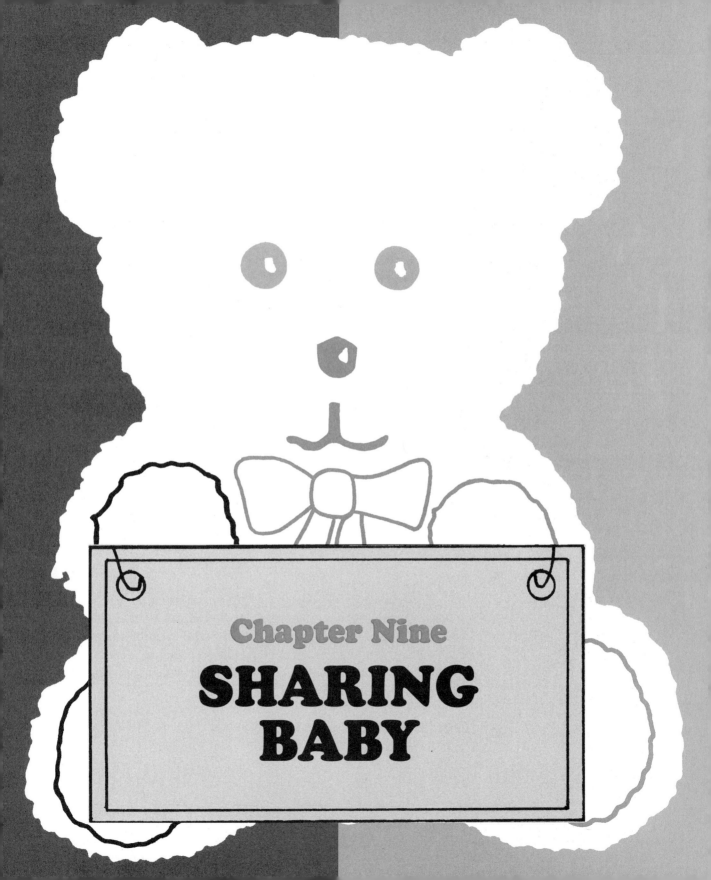

Chapter Nine

SHARING BABY

L ittle did you know in those first moments after birth that you would be bringing baby not only into your lives but also into a whole new world. You probably gave little thought to expanding your own small world to include relatives, friends, and day-care providers. But before you can consider the myriad of folks who will play a role in baby's life, you might need to take a look inward to make sure you're okay with some of the changes you're experiencing.

Adjustment Issues for New Moms

For women who have been used to running a business or working in the outside world, the prospect of spending an entire day changing diapers and breastfeeding is not exactly an easy one to adjust to. The pace is much slower, and everything takes longer than it used to. Even getting in and out of the car is more cumbersome than before, with the added diaper bag, stroller, and car seat. If you're not prepared for these kinds of changes, they can be quite a jolt.

The first six weeks after your baby's birth are consumed with new detail; every day you learn something that you didn't know before and that you were unprepared for. It's a time of trial and error—a time for you to get used to having a baby to care for and for the baby to get used to being cared for by you.

Be prepared to be tired a lot—especially in those first few weeks—and more than a little overwhelmed. The incredible sense of responsibility for this tiny little life can be scary to many new mothers.

Friends who have recently given birth have told me that this sense of responsibility was something they could never have imagined or prepared themselves for properly. They were not as worried about changing diapers and feeding the baby as they were about how they would manage to care for this tiny, needy baby from this day forward.

Your partner may be feeling some of this new responsibility, too, and may be as overwhelmed as you are. Don't be afraid to share your feelings openly with each other; you will both need each other's support during this time in your lives.

Above all else, don't be too hard on yourself, particularly if this is your first time being a mother. If you have a hard time dealing with parenting issues, seek the help of a support group for new parents or check out an online support group (see Chapter 18 for Web sites). There is help out there; you're not alone in feeling overwhelmed.

Separation Anxiety—How to Get Through It

All of us, even new parents, need time for ourselves. Many new parents simply wish for an evening out among other adults; some prefer a quiet dinner alone.

Here are some tips to ease the inevitable separation anxiety you or your baby will experience:

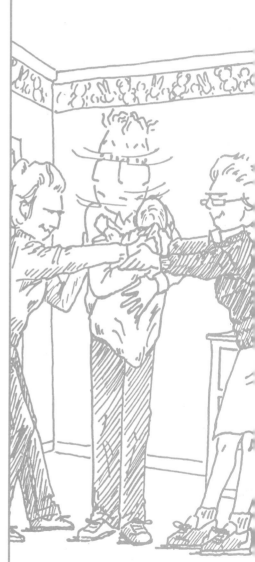

- Involve those who will care for the baby "in small doses" before leaving for a longer period of time. Have Grandma come to the house and spend time holding the baby long before you decide to leave; this way, baby and Grandma will be more comfortable with your absence.
- If you sing to the baby before naptime or bedtime, consider leaving a tape recording of your voice for the caregiver to play while you're gone.
- Have your baby sitters or caregivers come to the baby's most familiar surrounding (your home) rather than taking baby to their home. The more familiar everything is to baby, the less stress he or she will feel. Although they seem unaware, babies spend their entire first few months painstakingly making note of their new world.
- Check in with your caregiver frequently—but not too frequently. One or two calls per outing is acceptable, but you'd be a little on the manic side if you were to call every hour.

Time away from baby should not be a guilt-inducing experience but a pleasurable way of re-energizing and maybe even gaining new perspective. Don't feel as if you're a bad parent just because you need a break; in fact, the best parents know when to take time for themselves.

Information Sheet
for Baby Sitters

When you start making time for yourselves again, you'll need to leave some pertinent information at home for anyone who is babysitting your little one. Here's a list of information you might want to keep on the refrigerator door or near the phone.

We are out at _____

We will return at _____

A number you can call to reach us is _____

If you can't reach us, call _____ at _____

Baby's mealtime is _____

Baby's naptime is _____

For a snack, baby can have _____

Baby is allergic to _____

_____

Baby's bedtime is _____

Baby should _____ should not _____ have a bath before bedtime.

In case of emergency, call _____

_____

Police number: _____ Fire Department number: _____

Special instructions: _____

_____

_____

_____

_____

Building Your "Village" and Keeping It Thriving

First Lady Hilary Rodham Clinton was right on target when she wrote that it takes a village to raise a child. Even though you are the center of your baby's universe, there are others who will influence and guide your child through life: grandparents, aunts, uncles, cousins, friends, and even celebrities.

That's why you need to be as careful as possible in selecting those who will be part of your child's "inner circle." Choosing those whom you'd like to include in baby's "village" is a critical first step in baby's development, since you cannot be there every moment of every single day. This is one reason many cultures and religions encourage parents to select godparents for new babies; they are the charter members of baby's village.

In terms of family members, you really don't have much choice—family is family, after all. Still, you can choose more interaction with the family members you're close to and limit involvement with the ones you're not.

But what about those people you will rely on to help care for the baby, particularly if you are dependent on two incomes? What are your options for excellent care of your baby if you return to work? There are two primary ways to get quality care for your baby:

- **Leave baby with a relative.** Grandparents are a great choice (if they are capable and willing), but sisters, aunts, or even older siblings could work just as well. Your situation may dictate that you have more than one person on call to watch the baby.
- **Form a baby-sitting "pool" with friends and neighbors.** Particularly if you work part-time hours, you might be able to form a baby-sitting group in your neighborhood or with a group of friends. Each of you then takes a turn with the babies.

One piece of advice: Should you decide to rely on family and friends, create a contingency plan in case something unexpectedly comes up. Also, be sure to show your relatives your appreciation on a regular basis—with money, a gift, or simply a card with heartfelt thanks. A little appreciation goes a long way toward keeping everyone happy; and it can lessen any feelings of being taken for granted. Your gratitude can be every bit as rewarding as baby's smile.

How to Interview a Baby Sitter

Particularly in light of recent television-show investigations of nannies, au pairs, and baby sitters, many parents are leery to let anyone outside of family watch or take care of their children—for fear of their babies being mistreated by someone they didn't know enough about.

You will need to interview each candidate, ask for references, and make sure you feel 100 percent comfortable. Start the process as early as your fifth month of pregnancy to give yourself plenty of time to hire the right people.

Ask questions such as these:

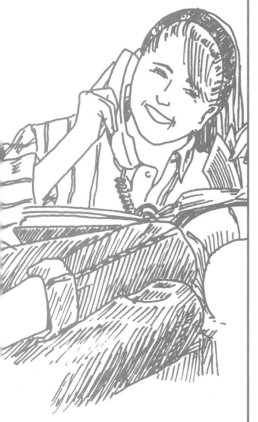

- How long have you been babysitting (or in this business)?
- Do you have references?
- What do you enjoy most about working with children? What do you enjoy least?
- Why do you think you would be a good baby sitter for my child?
- What would you do in an emergency situation?
- Is your schedule flexible?
- Is it okay if we talk to your parents (if the baby sitter is under 18)?
- Is there any equipment you like in particular?
- Do you have particular dietary requirements (for a sitter in your home)?

Remember that this is one of the most important jobs you will ever hire anyone to do. It's not out of bounds to consider running a background or police check on someone you'd like to hire. If you're looking for more than occasional baby sitting, you'll need to be even more cautious, and ask more questions. See Chapter 10 for advice on how to find a daycare situation that meets your needs.

Tips for Sibling Adjustment

The arrival of a new sibling can be a joyous occasion for a young child. But it is not without its challenges, since some children would prefer that they be the apple of Mom's (or Dad's) eye.

The hardest part for children to understand is not necessarily *that* there's a new baby coming but rather *why*: "Why do you need to have another baby, Mommy? Aren't I not good enough for you?" "Why do I have to share my room with the baby?" "Why do I have to give the baby my old clothes and toys?"

The pregnancy itself may frighten the child, especially if you're experiencing morning sickness or other less-than-desirable side effects. At the beginning of my pregnancy with Maddie, I was extremely sick—so much so that I began referring to it as my "at-any-moment" sickness. Twice I had to be hospitalized for dehydration.

My four-year-old witnessed this daily and became very concerned for my health. I reassured her that this was actually a good thing, since morning sickness has long been thought of as a means of cleansing the mother's body of impurities so that the baby can grow in a healthier environment. After weeks of fretting about Mommy's sickness, Lilly was then able to focus on something a little more positive: the healthy little baby we would have at the end of the process.

For most children, the waiting is the hardest part. Even the most excited siblings-to-be will find the nine-month wait to be painfully slow.

Here are some ways you can get your child or children more involved in the birthing process:

- **Make the pregnancy seem real from the start.** Buy or borrow books on the development of a new baby; some are geared for children under the age of ten; others can be of interest to the whole family. Use these books at story time to explain to your child the intricate process of growing a baby. Be sure to relate the pictures the child is seeing in the books to his or her own development; nothing helps a sibling-to-be understand the process more than the story of his or her own birth.

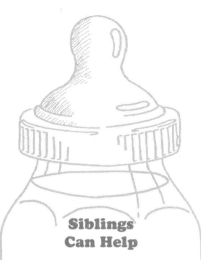

Siblings Can Help

- Fetch diapers for Mom or Dad.
- Help dress, bathe, or feed the baby.
- Help push the stroller.
- Pick out baby foods for baby to try (after six months).
- Put on the music box or lullaby tape.
- Sing to the baby.
- Play games with the baby.
- Make contributions to the baby's first-year scrapbook, either in crayon drawings or through words dictated to Mom. Or Mom could make a tape of the child's first impressions of his or her new brother or sister.
- Alert Mom to any problems. Kids love to scout for trouble spots and will usually come running to Mom with concerns ranging from "Mommy, baby is getting hungry . . . she's crying in her room" to "Baby is trying to open the cupboards!" It helps to have a little safety patrol around.

❧ **Allow your child some hands-on experience feeling the baby move.** I encouraged Lilly to rub my stomach and talk to Maddie, to tell her little sister-to-be about the fun they would have after she was born. This was also a good way to get Lilly to think about her new role in the family and what it really means to be a sister.

❧ **If you can, take your child with you to the doctor's office.** Hearing the baby's heartbeat and seeing an ultrasound are good ways to make the experience more real to your child. If your child can't attend an ultrasound for some reason, ask the doctor for a good picture to take home with you. You can explain the ultrasound process and why the picture looks the way it does; then point out the outline of the baby.

❧ **Encourage your child to ask questions, and answer them as best you can.** You should end each conversation about the baby with, "Do you have any questions or anything more you'd like to know about the baby?" This gives your child the opportunity to air any fears or concerns in a quiet, giving atmosphere. When the inevitable question arises (you know, "How did the baby get inside your tummy?"), you might do well to answer directly. For example, you might simply say, "Mommy's egg and Daddy's sperm met and started to grow a baby." You don't need to go into greater detail than that for children under eight years old. If the child presses you for detail, make a judgment call as to whether you think the child is ready for the whole story.

❧ **Involve your child in preparing the nest.** Take your child with you to buy baby clothes, diaper bags, strollers, and crib sheets. Ask whether he or she likes a particular décor for the baby's room and if there's anything he or she would like to donate to the baby. It's better to have the child feel involved in the process and to feel as though he or she has a choice in what to give baby (as opposed to your taking toys away or announcing that the siblings will have to share something). If your child does need to give up a crib or a room, make these arrangements as early as you can so that the sibling can adjust to the change. With Lilly, I gave her the bedroom furniture that had been my own as a child, and she was very touched by the "special" nature of having something of Mommy's for her very own, as well as by the idea of getting "big-girl" furniture.

SCRAPBOOK

- **Bring out your child's baby scrapbook.** He or she may wish to relive babyhood for a little while; don't be worried about this or show disapproval, since it is likely to be a quick phase your child is passing through. If your child wants to play with baby toys, it's okay. Maybe you could encourage him or her to think of ways to play with or teach the baby with these toys.

- **Tell your child what will happen at the hospital, and be honest about the new baby.** Many hospitals have classes for siblings; see if you can get into one anytime from midpregnancy on. Go over the "action plan" with your child; explain where he or she will be taken while you are giving birth. Let your child know when he or she can come to the hospital to see the baby, and be honest about what will happen when you bring the baby home from the hospital. Explain that you will be tired and that at first the baby will mostly sleep, eat, and cry. The child needs to know that the new baby will require lots of care and attention and that he or she will be a helper more than a playmate in the beginning.

- **Pack a special present for your child in your hospital bag, and give it to him or her when presenting the new baby.** Also, when guests come for the ceremonial "viewing of the baby," you might ask them to pay special attention to the new big brother or sister. Kids feel very left out when the baby is getting all of the attention— including presents. Even a small token can go a long way in making the sibling feel more comfortable.

- **Be firm and direct about your child's feelings and the way they are acted out.** If a sibling is feeling nega-

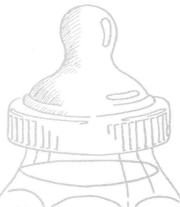

Should You Include Children in the Birth?

Some parents choose to include their other children in the birthing process, right up until the cord is cut.

If you or anyone else in your family expresses discomfort with the idea, choose another option. You could instead videotape the birth or snap select pictures for a photo scrapbook to share later.

Whatever you choose to do, decide on the plan well ahead of the actual birth. I have a friend whose father-in-law showed up in the delivery room with a video camera—much to her amazement and disbelief, since she had not opted for a filmed birth experience. Needless to say, it was a difficult situation that could have been avoided with a clearly communicated plan.

The fact is, not everyone is open to the idea that birth is a "whole family" experience; some prefer to keep it a private, personal one. Neither approach is wrong; it all boils down to the comfort levels of all involved.

tive about the baby, listen to his or her feelings in a nonjudgmental way. Try to work through these feelings by addressing the child's fears; most often, the child is afraid you won't love him or her as much as you used to. If the child begins acting out the negative feelings (by hitting or abusing the baby), seek professional help and limit contact between the two until a resolution becomes clear.

- **Set and keep a "special" time together.** Create activities that you can do together while baby is napping or otherwise occupied. If there were special things that the two of you used to do, try and preserve as many as you can to help the child feel a sense of security and continuity.

Keep in mind that your child has a lot for his or her young mind to deal with; this thought will help you keep a good perspective through your family transition. Offer your child as much individual attention as possible, and remember that you can never say "I love you" often enough.

Helping Pets Adjust to Baby

Is your pet treated like a member of the family? Do you shower your dog or cat with affection the minute you return home from work? If so, the baby's arrival will signal a definite change in the dynamics of your relationship. If Fido is used to greeting you and having a little game of Frisbee, imagine how he might feel when you start heading for baby's room first and merely pat him on the head.

The next thing you know, you have a contented baby but a pet who has begun exhibiting some annoying new habits: Suddenly your cat starts urinating on the carpet or your well-behaved dog starts chewing up your shoes. What does this bad behavior mean? In a nutshell, it means your pet is jealous.

Here are some tips to get you (and your pet) through this new transition smoothly:

- Watch any interaction between pet and infant carefully, especially if this is the first interaction of its type for both. Check for signs of aggressiveness, and if you see any, keep the

interaction limited until more time has passed and the two seem better acquainted with one another.

- Help your pet get used to the idea of a new baby in the house by letting the animal get used to the baby's scent. If he seems interested in doing so, let him sniff everything from baby's nightshirt to the rocking chair.

- Create a new "special time" with the animal, just as you might with a sibling. Your pet needs to know that he or she is still special to you, even though you have new responsibilities.

- As a good precaution, never let your pet and the baby be alone together, for any period of time. Close the baby's door during naptime or crate the animal. Some parents use baby's naptime as their "quality time" with their pet, and hardly a pet would complain about that.

- Practice regular grooming and cleanliness measures with your pet. Don't let litter boxes fill up, and check regularly for fleas. Take your animals to the groomer if you don't have time to maintain their cleanliness yourself. For hygienic purposes, anyone playing with the pet should make sure to wash his or her hands before handling the baby.

Getting into a new routine is half the battle. You can circumvent some problems by working with your pet before the baby is born. You could, for instance, involve the pet in the decorating of the baby's room, particularly by letting the pet smell every piece of furniture and perhaps by letting it sit on the baby's rocking chair. Also, before baby is born, it would be a good idea for you to take your pet to the vet for a routine checkup—just to make sure the animal is healthy.

The most important thing to keep in mind is that although there are plenty of folks who don't think that animals have feelings, they truly do. They know from the time you announce your pregnancy that change is in the air, because your attentiveness to them is affected from that moment on. As you become consumed with thoughts about the new baby, your pet may be pondering his position in the roost. Being aware of your pet's needs and tending to them in a caring, sensitive manner may be all you need to do to preserve the peace.

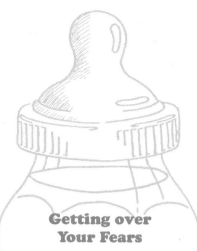

Getting over Your Fears

And just what are these fears?

- **Fear of hurting the baby.** Sometimes it starts earlier, with the fear that sex will hurt the unborn child (it will only do that in high-risk cases). Then, after the birth, a new dad is afraid to touch or hold his baby for fear that he might drop or "break" it. Both of these fears are unfounded and can be easily put to rest by asking your doctor about them ahead of time. And, if the opportunity arises, you can get in some practice by holding other people's babies.

- **The dreaded diaper.** Many new dads wonder how such a tiny little baby can produce such interesting colors and evil smells and are subsequently green faced at the prospect of handling a diaper. The nurses at the hospital and

Tips for Daddy

With all of the excitement and hoopla over the baby, it's easy for some mothers-to-be and their friends and family to forget all about dear old Dad. He's the guy who made the baby possible; yet he's rarely invited to baby showers, and few people ask him how *he's* feeling about the new baby before it's born. He can't help but feel a little bit left out.

The trouble is that with everyone scurrying around in an attempt to get mom-to-be and baby ready for the "big event," it's not easy to pick the right time to talk about your feelings. Everyone seems so preoccupied, and you certainly don't want to seem unsympathetic to their needs.

If you are a new dad or dad-to-be, you may actually have a lot on *your* mind while others think that you're uninterested. That's why, as early as possible in the pregnancy, you should start trying to figure out what questions you would like to have answered. You can start by going to as many of the obstetrician visits as possible; even if you just sit in the waiting room, there are plenty of resources available that will spark your thought process and generate the kinds of questions that would've eventually come anyway. If you choose to go into the examining room for each visit, have some of your questions ready for the doctor (who's been through this experience hundreds of times and can probably give you lots of reassurance).

Understanding your role as a father can be confusing, to say the least. Who should get more of your attention, your wife or your helpless little one? How can you balance the care of your family with your job while keeping your own stress level to a minimum? Where will all of the money come from to raise this new life and put it through college? These are typical concerns of new fathers.

Talking about your feelings as openly and directly as possible will offset any negative reactions you encounter. Ask your partner to listen without judging you or your feelings. Tell her that you simply need to express yourself and be heard. What you really need, after all, is the same thing that she does: reassurance that you can indeed be a good parent.

Most of all, relax and enjoy this exciting new stage in your life. You are going to be a major influence in your child's life, and everything will work itself out in due time. You may not realize it, but it is likely that your own father grappled with the same dilemmas, worries, and concerns that you now face; you survived, and so did he.

The most important thing you can do as a new father is communicate to your mate, your baby, and the rest of your family. Read parenting magazines to familiarize yourself with all of the issues of parenthood. Ask your father how he coped before you were born. Or talk to other new fathers you know. Ask a lot of questions; you'll feel much more confident after you hear about what other fathers have experienced. And you might get some great ideas!

How You Can Best Help—Before and After the Baby Comes

What does the mother of your child need most, and how can you anticipate those needs? Let's take it a trimester at a time:

- **First trimester (months 1 to 3).** In these first few months of pregnancy, your wife will need your emotional support as she adjusts to this exciting (yet sometimes frightening) time in her life. If she's having morning sickness, reassure her that this is only a temporary phase. If she's tired all the time, take on extra household duties and make sure she gets enough rest. What she really needs most of all is knowing that you are there for her, that you support her and love her for this beautiful, temporary sacrifice her body is making. Take an active role in reading about the baby's development, too.

- **Second trimester (months 4 to 6).** As her body changes and the baby grows, a woman needs to know she is still attractive to you. Tell her how she looks: She's not fat—she's pregnant; she's got a healthier glow than you've ever seen before. Let her know you're proud of her and the baby. Be with her as much as you can, and enjoy the time

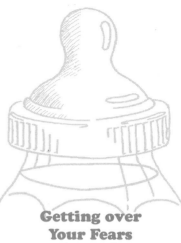

Getting over Your Fears
(continued)

Mom (if she knows how already) can help by offering to work with Dad the first few times he tries diaper changing. And after a short while, Dad will be a professional!

- **Fear of exclusion.** Some dads worry about being "shut out" of the parenting process, either by the new mom or by well-meaning relatives. Particularly if mom is breastfeeding, there doesn't seem to be much for Dad to do with baby. One solution is to give Dad a specific task, like bathing the baby, that will be his responsibility. Another is for Dad to set aside special times to take baby for a stroll around the neighborhood or to play games with baby while Mom takes a break.

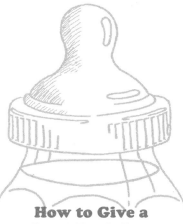

How to Give a Good Back Rub

Your pregnant partner is complaining of back pain, and you're getting frustrated because you can't seem to do it the way she would like. How can you reach the right spots in just the right way? Follow these tips:

- Start at the shoulders and work your way down, kneading and rolling rather than pinching or lightly stroking. Be careful not to rub directly on the spine, as the skin is thinner there, making even the slightest of touches seem too aggressive.
- Use rhythmic gestures, and try to keep them consistent. Don't rub longer in one spot than another unless your partner asks you to.
- Place your thumbs on the sides of the neck, curving your fingers over the top of the shoulders and kneading the muscle as gently or firmly as your partner indicates.

you have left—it'll be a long time before you're "empty-nesters" again!

- **Third trimester (months 7 to 9).** Mom-to-be may be a little uncomfortable—not to mention emotional—these last months of the pregnancy. Try to get her out of the house; go to dinner, a movie, or even for a short walk. You'll have to ask her what other things she'd like you to do, but she'll likely want to decorate the baby's room and stock it full of things for you to put together (you'll be very thankful for those handy instructions!). And—no doubt—good, strong back rubs are in order. Of course, if you're the labor coach, you'll have lots to do during that last month.

After the birth of your baby, believe it or not, you are needed even more. You can help your new family by calling everyone who needs to know about the birth (this includes shielding Mom from well-meaning folks who want to chat when she needs to rest); limiting visitors (they can make Mommy and baby very tired in the first few days); and doing housework and cooking for your family. If your wife or partner has bouts of the "baby blues," you needn't worry—these low times are brought on by hormonal changes and are normal. If she seems to grow more depressed over the next few weeks, she may have postpartum depression. Be supportive and listen to her; reassure her that you will help her get all of the help she needs, whether it's from you or her doctor. Just knowing that you are there for her and willing to help at every stage is going to go a long way in terms of adjustment and recovery.

Dealing with Your Changing Relationship

Before the baby came, you were like any other pair of young lovers, basking in the glow of your love. You went out to fancy restaurants, went sailing at the drop of a hat, and made love whenever you wanted to. What's going to happen to that wonderfully independent lifestyle now that baby's here?

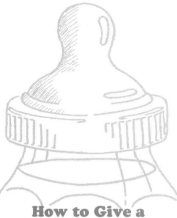

The complete turnabout that your life is taking can be very unsettling, especially for the couple used to being on the go. Now there are bottles, diapers, strollers, and naptimes to consider. There is the question of who actually has the car seat this time, where baby's pacifier is, and just why that kid is still crying after all the calming methods you've tried. It seems as though everything revolves around baby—and it does!

Now that baby is here, you might feel like you're moving in slow motion. Everything takes at least an hour longer than it used to. Your patience is tested at every turn, and it's getting harder just to talk to each other, let alone spend any meaningful moments together. What can you do to bring the intimacy back to your relationship?

First, you should always make time to talk to each other. It's easy to get bogged down in the daily details of new family management; thus, the two of you as a couple need to reserve time on a daily basis just for "catching up" with each other. It needn't be an hour; it could be accomplished in twenty minutes per day. All you need to do is be open to talking and listening to each other.

When listening to any problems your partner is experiencing, repeat back what you've heard to let her know you've understood her correctly. Many men leave this critical stage out of their communication process, only to wind up with the "you-just-don't-understand" argument. If you want to avoid a fight, it's best to respond with empathic statements such as "This must be a tough situation for you" or "I'm hearing that you aren't comfortable with the way I'm doing things." Then ask what she wants from you next. Don't be accusatory or show anger; instead, be gentle, loving, and intent on solving the problem. Work on the problem, not on your partner's personality; remember, it's about creating the family life you both want, not about winning an argument.

Show your partner how much she still means to you, and you will receive much in return. Even though her responsibilities now include someone who demands a lot of attention, you are still the man she fell in love with and the one with whom she is building this new family. You are an important part of this family's life!.

How to Give a Good Back Rub
(continued)

- Using the palm of your hand or a flattened fist, apply pressure gently to the spine, working your way up the back up to the neck. When you reach the top of her body, lightly stroke her back from top to bottom in one large sweeping motion.
- If your partner complains of dry or irritated skin, try using a medicated lotion as you massage her. This will leave her feeling totally relaxed, with skin of silk.

Stop as soon as your partner tells you that the massage is hurting her. Remember, much of her back pain is caused by the pressure of the uterus on the spine—there's a baby in there, and you must be careful not to hurt the baby or its mother with a back rub that's too aggressive.

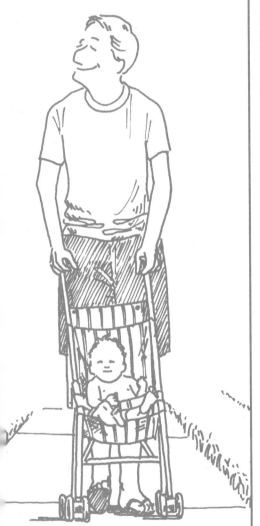

If You're a House Dad

Some nontraditional households have mothers back in the boardroom and fathers at home providing baby care after a baby is born. More and more fathers stay at home to raise their children, and although they don't provide *exactly* the same kind of care that a mother provides, they have proven that they can be equally effective parents. As surprising as it may seem, it's a growing trend—so much so that there are magazines, books, and Web sites dedicated to the "house dad."

If you should decide that you will be the primary parent to care for your new baby, here are some tips to help you get through the experience as smoothly as possible:

- **Establish a routine.** Set regular times of the day for laundry, housework, and cooking. The baby will set the schedule for feedings and diaper changes, but you can choose a time for bathing the baby and for playing games.
- **Ask for help when you need it.** Don't be afraid to call Grandma or any other knowledgeable person when you're stuck. Read any parenting magazine or book you can get your hands on. It's like I learned in News Reporting 101: What you don't know, you find out. Go for it!
- **Build connections.** Take your baby to play groups and other functions where there are other babies and their caregivers. There are networks and support systems for stay-at-home dads; check the Internet or ask other parents in your community for meeting times and places.
- **Reserve time for yourself.** You need time on your own, too. To keep your sanity, do at least two things per day that are strictly for you: Watch a sports event on TV, go out for a while after the baby's mother comes home, or take a luxury bath to unwind. You're going to relish any free moments you get and should take advantage of them without feeling any guilt. You've got an incredibly challenging job and deserve every break you can get.

Required Reading and Viewing for Dads

Fatherhood by Bill Cosby (1994). You'll laugh your way to loving your children as you read this funny and insightful book.

Modern Dad magazine.

Silas Marner by George Eliot (1861). This classic is a tale of irony and devotion. Silas loses his gold, only to discover a beautiful little yellow-haired baby girl in his home. He treasures her and raises her as his own daughter and then faces a difficult choice when the girl's biological father returns to claim her. She, of course, feels Silas was her only true father, and it's a happy ending after all.

Mr. Mom (1983, rated PG). This movie, starring Michael Keaton, shows how life changes when Dad stays home while Mom goes back into the "corporate jungle."

Parenthood (1989, rated PG) and *Father of the Bride II* (1995, rated PG). Both films star Steve Martin, and both are hilarious looks at what a long, strange trip fatherhood can be. *Father of the Bride II* focuses on Dad's coping ability in becoming a new dad again and at the same time becoming a grandfather; it's based on the classic movie *Father's Little Dividend* (1951), which starred Spencer Tracy.

Nine Months (1995, rated PG). This movie stars Hugh Grant as a yuppie who's not ready for the demands of parenthood when his girlfriend announces her pregnancy. Two very funny supporting roles by Tom Arnold and Jeff Goldblum really make this film, but it's the cameo by Robin Williams as a Russian obstetrician that is howlingly funny.

Mrs. Doubtfire (1993, rated PG). This movie puts Robin Williams in drag as a nanny to the children his ex-wife has been keeping from him. While the topics of custody and visitation (particularly when denied) are not happy ones, there is a relatively happy ending to this touching, albeit heartwrenching, film. What's most inspiring is the dad's total devotion to his children.

Kramer vs. Kramer (1979, rated PG). Okay, so it's about a single dad fighting for custody of his child . . . a little depressing on the surface; but there are plenty of touching scenes, for example, when the little boy and his father bond over French toast.

Three Men and a Baby (1987, rated PG). This comedy centers on bachelors who suddenly find themselves surrogate moms for a little girl left on their doorstep. Only one of the men is actually the father, but all three discover paternal instincts they never knew they had. The movie is based on the French film *Three Men and a Cradle* (1985). Check out the sequel, *Three Men and a Little Lady* (1990), too.

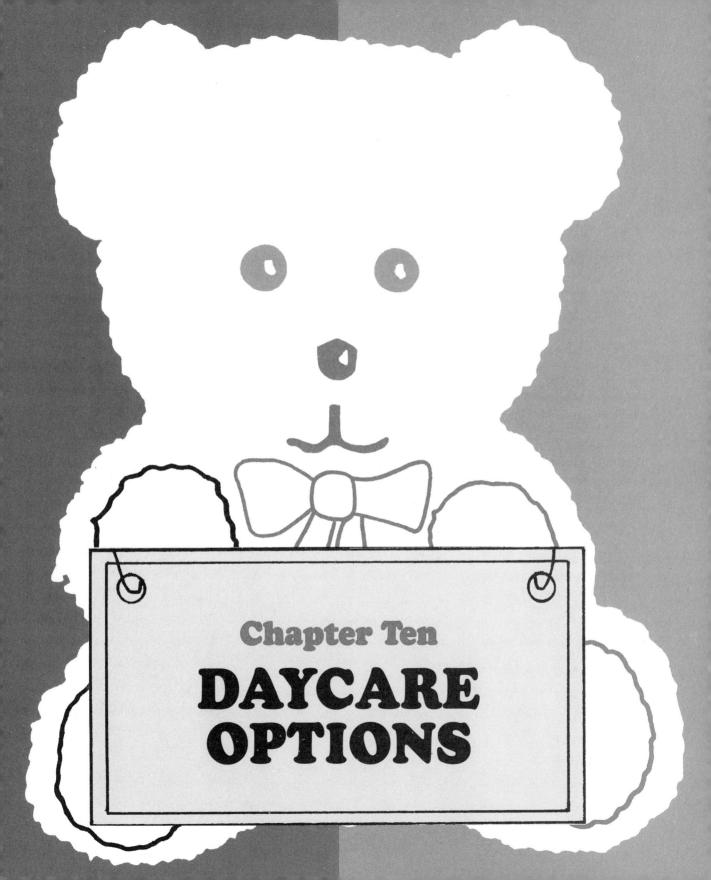

Chapter Ten

DAYCARE OPTIONS

Although you may not like the idea of having to put your baby in daycare, the reality is that many families need to rely on the incomes of both parents. Inevitably, this means you will need someone to care for baby while you're both at work.

Some parents manage to adjust the particulars of their work life so that they can both work and still spend plenty of time with their baby. Here are some ideas on how to do this:

- Ask if your company would consider a job-sharing arrangement. In this scenario, you split a full-time job with another person who can do the same kind of work into two part-time jobs. This way, you both have more time to spend with your families—and the job still gets done in the same time frame.
- Find out if your company allows for a flex-time option. A forty-hour workweek might consist of four days per week at 10 hours each—or see if you can arrange a workday that begins earlier or ends later than usual.
- Telecommute. If your job is one that can easily be accomplished at home, ask if you can work from home—and come in only for important meetings, presentations, or the like. Working from home is every bit as challenging for a telecommuter as it is for an entrepreneur, so be sure you're up to it. If you're the type who's distracted by the need to vacuum over the need to finish a report, think twice before considering the telecommuting option. And remember, just because you are at home you will probably still need child care in order to get anything done—however, your baby can be cared for in *your* own home in *your* presence.
- Hunt for a new part-time job. There may not be much part-time work available in your field, but you might consider branching out into a related field. You just might find work that you enjoy even more than your old job!
- Consider a job where you can work evenings while your partner works days (or vice versa). That way, one of you can be with the baby all the time. (The drawback to this, though, is that you will rarely see *each other.*)

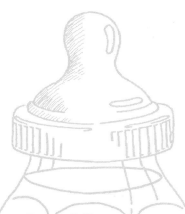

If none of these options is available to you, you may need to start your search for a quality daycare situation—one that meets all of your expectations. Planning is the key to finding good daycare; taking the time to develop your plan well in advance of your baby's birth will eliminate additional stress later on.

Start checking out daycare possibilities as soon as possible—as early as your third month of pregnancy. Quality daycare is in high demand—and some daycare centers even have waiting lists months long. If you wait until after the baby is born, you may have trouble finding a daycare situation you feel totally comfortable with: waiting too long could mean you'll have to settle for less than your ideal.

Daycare Centers

Daycare centers are one of the most popular options for working parents. In a center, your child will be cared for in a group setting by adults who are trained in childrearing and child development issues. To begin checking into daycare centers, ask your state child-care or child welfare agency for a list of licensed centers. (This is essential, because some unscrupulous daycare operators will say they are licensed when they are not. If you still have doubts or questions, you can contact the National Association for the Education of Young Children [NAEYC] for more information.)

Next call each center for basic info like fees and availability of space. Ask about the ratio of children to childcare providers. A quality daycare center should care for infants in a separate room, away from toddlers and older children (who can present safety hazards to infants). Infant childcare providers at daycare centers should care for no more than three infants apiece, and two is an even better number. Also, you should ask about how many babies are kept in each room. More than six infants in a room, whatever its size, can make for a chaotic, institutionalized setting (and you don't want your baby kept awake constantly from other babies' crying).

If the center checks out so far, you may want to schedule a visit. Ask the center director when the older children generally nap,

Initial Questions to Ask a Daycare Center Director
(continued)

Can the center accommodate special dietary requirements?
- How often are the toys cleaned? They should be cleaned and sanitized at least once a week, and preferably more often than that. How often are diapers changed? Crib sheets?
- What will baby do every day, and who will decide? Are there set routines in place, or is there room for you to provide input as to what baby likes to do during the day? Do the daycare providers seem to listen to your concerns about day-to-day operations?
- What safety precautions and policies regarding outside visitors are in existence? Are there locks on the main doors? Is there a security system in place?
- What is the center's policy for sick children?

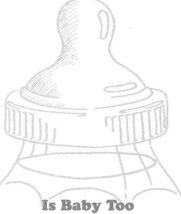

Is Baby Too Sick to Go?

One of the biggest problems associated with placing small children in a group daycare situation is that they have a higher incidence of catching everything from colds to earaches. One way to minimize such problems is for parents to keep sick children at home.

All daycare centers and family daycare providers should have policies in place to deal with sickness. For instance, they might tell you that if the baby's temperature is higher than 101 degrees, he or she should be kept at home. Other illnesses or problems that may keep baby temporarily out of daycare include the following:

- **Diarrhea.** Especially in infants, diarrhea can be highly contagious. If it's frequent or contains blood, you should call your doctor immediately—and keep your baby at home until his or her bowel movements seem normal.
- **Vomiting.** This is a sure sign that something is wrong. If your child vomits up food or formula that is already partially digested, this probably indicates illness.

and avoid visiting at that time, since you'll want to see how well the childcare providers manage when most of the children are awake.

Here are some things to look for during a visit to a daycare center:

- Do the children at the center seem happy? Do they look reasonably clean?
- Are the rooms bright and airy? Do they have natural light?
- Is there a good selection of toys? Centers should have plenty of age-appropriate, safe toys that encourage creativity and motor development.
- Is the center clean? In particular, check the bathrooms and food preparation areas. Do you detect a strong odor of urine anywhere?
- Is there a safe outdoor play area?
- Is the center thoroughly childproofed? Ask to see fire exits and first aid supplies.
- Watch the staff interact with the children. Do the childcare providers seem attentive to the children's needs?
- How noisy is the center? Happy kids do make noise—but total chaos is a problem.
- How capable do the childcare providers seem at setting limits for the children? At resolving conflicts between the children?
- Does the staff seem willing and eager to talk with you? Do they appear interested in getting to know your baby?
- Are you meeting everyone who works at the facility, from the operator to instructors to clean-up help? You should be able to meet anyone who might possibly come into contact with your baby.

Once you have narrowed your choices down to one or two centers, ask for at least three references. Call them all and ask for feedback. If they do not give you glowing reports, look elsewhere.

There are many positive aspects of using a daycare center. In a good situation, your child will have other children of a similar age to play with, facilities that are expressly designed for his or her needs, childcare providers who are knowledgeable and experienced, and a wide variety of age-appropriate activities. Daycare centers can also be moderate in price, especially when compared to the cost of hiring a trained nanny.

However, if you are choosing childcare for a young infant, you may find daycare centers a bit institutional and potentially overwhelming for your baby. Another negative consideration is the issue of staff turnover. Even good centers can experience a lot of staff turnover, and too many childcare providers in too short a time can interfere with a baby's long-term ability to form lasting attachments to other people. Finally, any time you take your child outside of your home for care, you are in for a certain amount of inconvenience. Depending on the age of your child and the center's requirements, you will need to have a diaper bag packed each day with diapers, wipes, bottles, bibs, one or more changes of clothes, etc.—and this, coupled with having to get your child fed, dressed, and ready (and getting *yourself* dressed and ready for your job), can make early mornings at your home a bit hectic.

Family Daycare

This childcare option is growing in popularity. Unlike a daycare center, a family daycare provider cares for children in her own home. Often, one or more of the children in the group are her own.

Most states have licensing requirements for family daycare, but some providers operate illegally, either because they cannot meet the health, safety, or educational requirements of their state licensing agency, or because they do not want to declare their daycare income to the IRS (these will insist that you pay them in cash). If you live in a state that licenses family daycare operations, resist the urge to check out that nice, but unlicensed, childcare provider down the street, and only consider licensed childcare providers. However, since some state requirements are fairly minimal, it is important to check out even licensed family daycare situations carefully.

Start your search by obtaining a list of licensed childcare providers in your area from your state childcare or child welfare agency. Ask friends and neighbors if they know of any good family daycare providers, and check to see if those people are on your list. Call those names first and ask if they have room for your child. It can be harder to find family daycare for an infant than for a toddler,

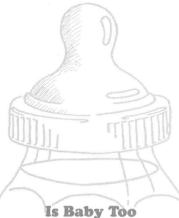

Is Baby Too Sick to Go?
(continued)

- **Pinkeye, or conjunctivitis.** If baby gets this highly contagious infection, one or both eyes will be pink and weepy. The good news is that you can call the doctor for some antibiotic drops, and once the drops have been started, baby is no longer contagious.
- **Rashes.** Ringworm is a fungus shaped like a raised ring of red skin and can be treated with antifungal cream. Impetigo (usually in the diaper area for babies) consists of itchy spots and should be treated with antibiotic ointment. Babies can usually return to daycare once they've started receiving treatment.
- **Chicken pox.** If baby has red pimples that turn into blisters, it might be chicken pox and you should call your doctor. Baby should definitely stay home until the spots crust over and scab. Count on baby being home for about a week or so.

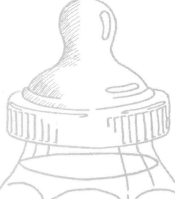

Initial Questions to Ask a Family Daycare Provider

Once you have located someone with a space for your child, try a little prescreening by phone:

- How many children do you care for? What are their ages? Consider only a provider who cares for, at the most, six children (including her own preschool-age children), of whom no more than two are infants. Of course, fewer is always better.
- What child-care related education have you had? At minimum, a provider should have formal training in infant CPR.
- How long have you been in business? Do you plan on providing family daycare on a long-term basis? It's always best to hire someone with at least a year under her belt.
- Is your home non-smoking? The dangers of secondhand smoke for infants and children have been well-documented.

since childcare providers typically can accept only one or two infants into their group. If a provider is recommended but doesn't have room for your child in the near future, ask her to recommend someone who might.

If a provider meets your requirements, make an appointment to visit her during the day. She may ask you to come during naptime, but make sure you see her in action while all the children are awake too. Spend some time there and check the following things:

- Is the house clean? The kitchen and the bathroom should be clean and sanitary. Babies and young children spend a lot of time on the floor, so carpeting should be vacuumed frequently, especially if there are pets. Also, unless you are standing right next to the diaper pail, you should not detect a strong odor of urine anywhere.
- Is the house childproofed? You should see gates on the staircases, latches on kitchen cabinets, and covers on visible electrical outlets.
- Look carefully at the area in which the children spend most of their time (most likely the living or family room). Is it light and airy? Is the furniture comfortable for small children?
- Do the children look happy? Is the atmosphere calm? Does the provider seem relaxed or tense when she is dealing with the children?
- Is there a good selection of toys? Don't expect as many toys as you might find at a daycare center, but the provider should have at least a few age-appropriate, safe toys that encourage creativity and motor development, for both the infants and the older children. The provider may also allow you to bring over some of your child's own favorite toys and leave them there.
- Is there an outdoor play space? Is it safe and fenced off? If the provider does not have an outdoor play space, ask her where she takes the children for outdoor play.

Finally, check at least three references—ideally, parents of children she cares for or has cared for in the past. If they don't seem enthusiastic about her, keep looking.

In a good family daycare situation, your child will spend his or her day in a homey atmosphere and will benefit socially by having other children to play with. If you stay with the daycare provider over the long term, your child may come to regard her as a second mom and be treated as part of the family. In many areas of the country, family daycare is also relatively inexpensive and a more economical option than are daycare centers. As with a daycare center, though, you sacrifice a certain amount of convenience when you take your children outside your home for childcare.

Childcare in Your Home

If you want your child to have one-on-one attention, childcare in your home can be a good choice. There are two basic types of home childcare providers: nannies and au pairs. While many people think the two are basically the same thing, the differences may seem startling.

Nannies

A nanny takes care of your child in your home. She may live in or live out. Many nannies have formal training in childcare and child development. Others have no formal training but rely on life experience.

There are many agencies that will, for a fee, help you find a nanny. While agencies vary in their screening and training processes, they should, at minimum, do a complete background check of potential candidates (including a police check), provide you with references, and find you at least a couple of candidates to choose from. While agency fees vary, nanny agencies in larger cities may charge you fees of $1,000 or more (although if your first choice doesn't work out, the next search may be on the house).

What if you don't want to pay a nanny agency? Ask your relatives, your friends, your neighbors, your hairdresser, or people at

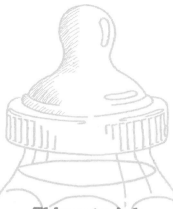

Things to Ask a Home Daycare Provider During Your Visit

- Is television allowed? Try to avoid providers who leave the TV on all day.
- What kinds of meals are served to older babies and toddlers? Are they balanced and nutritious?
- How often are the toys cleaned and sanitized? How often are diapers changed? (If a provider only replies, "Whenever they need it," press for specifics—like at least every three hours, for example.) How often are crib sheets changed?
- Where would your child sleep? Does each child have his or her own sleeping space? Infants should never share a crib, for sanitary reasons.
- Would anyone else ever take care of your child (if the provider needs to run an emergency errand, for example)? If so, what are the person's qualifications? Does the provider have a backup daycare to recommend to you if she or her children are ill and she needs to close down temporarily?

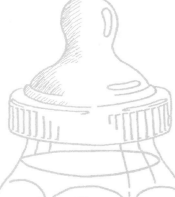

Questions You Can Ask Potential Nannies

- Why do you want to be a nanny? Try to assess whether the person has a real commitment to the care of children, or if she is just looking for something to do for a few months.
- What is your childcare experience? While a trained and experienced childcare provider is generally the best option, a less experienced childcare provider may still be a loving person and anxious to do the best job possible. At minimum you should expect substantial baby-sitting experience and a demonstrated knowledge of infant CPR.
- What kinds of activities would you like to do with my child on a typical day?

your house of worship if they have anyone to recommend. You can also place an ad in your local newspaper. Specify number of children, their ages, whether you want live in or live out care, whether the nanny will need a car, the town you live in, and the minimum amount of childcare experience you would prefer.

Nannies are in high demand in most areas and you will need to offer a competitive salary. In 1997, live-out nannies working in a major metropolitan area earned $7-$12 an hour, depending on level of experience and whether their salary was paid through an agency. You will pay less if you can find someone who is willing to live with you (you'll need an extra bedroom for this option) and take part of their compensation as room and board.

Keep your expectations realistic. Outside of hands-on childcare, a nanny should be able to prepare your children's meals and perhaps do a little light housework *that pertains to their care* (like picking up toys or doing your children's laundry). She is *not* going to clean your house from top to bottom and cook gourmet meals for you while your baby naps.

Au Pairs

Despite popular misconceptions, an au pair is not a nanny. She is typically a college-age student who comes to this country for a year to experience American culture. Au pairs agree to commit to living with a family for a year's time and provide childcare and light housework in exchange for room, board, a stipend, and sometimes tuition expenses.

If you are considering hiring an au pair, keep in mind that the program was not created to provide childcare for Americans. Instead, it was designed to provide a foreign living experience for young people. You should also keep in mind that in other countries, au pairs generally have fewer responsibilities than they are often expected to assume in this country, and rarely serve as the sole care providers for children while their parents are out of the house.

You will need to hire an au pair through an agency. The agency is supposed to do a thorough background check and provide you with references. It is also supposed to provide the au pair with a certain amount of childcare training, as well as CPR training. Make sure you know in advance exactly what experience and training you can expect an au pair to have.

While you will probably not have the opportunity to interview a potential au pair in person, you can ask some of the same questions you would ask when interviewing a nanny over the telephone. Try to get a sense of the person's experience and interests, and whether the person is interested in and likes children.

A main attraction of au pairs is cost. If you have an extra bedroom, this is almost always the cheapest childcare option short of your relatives. Even when agency fees and an au pair's transportation and tuition are factored in, costs rarely exceed $200 a week, plus room and board, for a maximum of forty-five hours of childcare and light housework. While you should be aware that while you may end up with a wonderful, nurturing, experienced live-in childcare provider, you may also spend a year trying to train a homesick teenager in the rudiments of baby care.

Making Your Final Childcare Choice

The bottom line is, if you don't feel comfortable—if something about the daycare center or individual childcare provider bothers you, no matter how small or seemingly unimportant, you owe it to yourself to either address the issue or to move on to the next center or person on the list.

You should expect the following from any childcare provider:

- **Open communication.** Providers should give you frequent and complete updates about your child's progress and problems. If they keep you informed, you can develop ways to deal with problems and build on activities and accomplishments of the day.
- **Open access to their home or center.** Parents must be welcome to visit at any time, even without calling first. Providers should also allow parents to make a reasonable number of phone calls to check on their child's well-being, especially in the case of minor illness or separation anxiety.

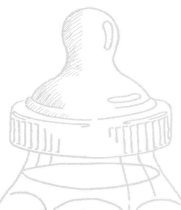

Questions You Can Ask Potential Nannies
(continued)

- Can you drive? You may not have this requirement if you live in an urban area with plenty of public transportation. However, if you don't, you will probably need a nanny who drives.
- Do you have any allergies or health problems? Any special dietary needs (if she is to live in)?
- Do you smoke?

During your interview, you can also assess the following things:

- Is she clean and dressed neatly?
- Does she have a reasonable command of English?

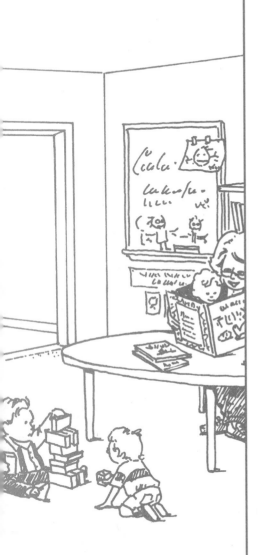

You and the provider should work out the best times for these calls and determine in advance how many are reasonable.

- **Honesty and confidence.** Childcare providers shouldn't make commitments they can't or don't intend to keep. They shouldn't cover up problems or accidents that occur.

- **Acceptance of your wishes.** Providers should abide by parents' wishes on matters such as discipline, TV viewing, food, adult smoking, and toilet training. If providers feel that they can't abide by certain wishes, they should be candid about their inability to do so.

- **Advance notice of any changes.** Since it is often very difficult to find adequate alternate care, providers should tell parents well in advance if they are going to change their hours or prices—or if they plan to close down or limit the number of children in their care. Parents need at least a month's (or, better yet, six weeks') notice if they need to find a new care provider for their child. A center or family daycare provider should also clarify holiday schedules, so parents know which days are covered and which are not. Not every calendar holiday is a paid holiday for working parents. And except in the case of emergency, parents should be given at least two weeks' notice even if the provider won't be available on a non-holiday day.

- **No advice unless asked for.** Providers shouldn't criticize or advise parents on child rearing unless parents ask for their advice. If asked, they should offer advice in a noncritical way. Of course, if providers see something that is seriously wrong (i.e., signs of child abuse, neglect, or malnutrition), they should discuss the problem with the parents and, if necessary, contact the proper authorities.

- **Assurance that everyone in contact with the child is properly trained and/or supervised.** This includes screening of custodial help, training and supervising transportation workers, and assurance that anyone who visits has been cleared for entry.

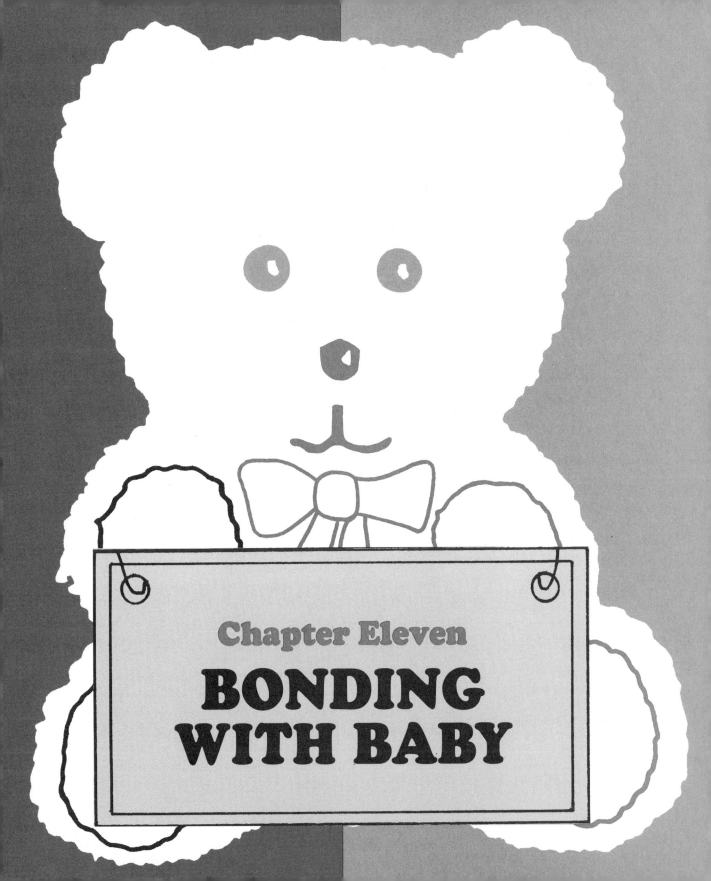

Chapter Eleven

BONDING
WITH BABY

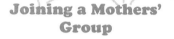

Joining a Mothers' Group

Mothers' groups are different from play groups in that they are primarily focused on the needs and concerns of the new mom. Babies are often watched by one or two parents/sitters, and mothers have discussion groups or listen to a speaker who gives them insight and ideas.

Such groups often advertise in community newspapers or at local churches; if you don't see any information about a mothers' group, ask around. Many times, the area hospital can tell you how to find such a group, and some of the more progressive hospitals even offer them.

If you don't have a mothers' group near you, you could easily start one. Send flyers out to every mother in your neighborhood or church, or even post some at grocery stores and laundromats. Select a meeting location, set a regular meeting time, and then post a sign-up sheet. If the group is large enough, arrange for one or two mothers to take turns in the day-care room.

Your baby is just waking up from a nap, and you tiptoe carefully into the room. You walk up to the crib, look over the rail, and you see a glimmer of a smile from your baby—a gift from baby to you. Is baby as attached to you as you are to him or her? Yes, but you are each attached for different reasons. Unlike adults, babies do not make attachments based solely on love; they also feel a biological imperative to bond.

Babies have a need to bond with their parents, because these are the people who help meet all of their needs. Part of comforting a hungry baby is holding the baby close to you; the other part is providing the breast or bottle.

If you're concerned about your ability to bond with your new baby, you should be relieved to know that you are not alone in your fears. Most new parents feel some uneasiness over whether they will be able to form a close family. After all, you've never had to do the work of building a family before; up until this point, you've only had to be a *member* of one.

What Baby Really Needs from You

At every stage of their tiny lives, babies will depend on you for different things. For the first two months, your baby will simply need to have basic needs met; you will bond with baby while feeding, changing, or rocking baby. Until the first spontaneous smile is given to you, you won't have tangible evidence of bonding.

After two months, baby begins to develop a personality, building on patterns established during those first few months. Baby is becoming your little buddy. At this stage, you begin to notice patterns. When baby is wet, the cry is even pitched; but when the baby is hungry, the cry becomes quite high pitched. Baby is dependent on you at this point to learn his or her signals.

Psychologists have learned that younger babies (babies less than two months old) have only a few simple emotions. Babies at this stage can show distress (e.g., when they have a wet diaper), enthusiasm or excitement (e.g., over something new), and contentment—that beautiful soft smile (e.g., after the bottle has been drained). It takes far longer for them to develop more complex emotions such as anger, fear, or happiness.

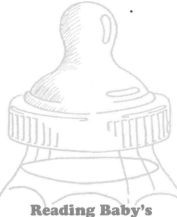

Baby's distress signals are relatively easy to deal with. All you have to do is go down the list of baby's basic needs: Does the diaper need to be changed? Is baby hungry again? Does baby need a nap?

A contented baby is a happy, quiet little one who seems perfectly at ease in whatever he or she is doing at the moment. For instance, a contented baby will swing for a half hour and not cry frantically when he or she is picked up to go to bed.

But other emotions are a little more perplexing. A baby's smile, for instance, gives rise to arguments over whether the baby is truly happy or has just passed gas.

What is baby really smiling about when he or she flashes that toothless grin? Babies begin life with little if any muscle control in their faces; thus, the first smiles are actually reflex smiles. After the baby is a few weeks old, the smile becomes more controlled but is still quite random. Baby will smile at happy voices or at tummy gas, but the smile is not directed to anything specific. The best smiles, of course, come between four and six months, when baby begins to smile at the puppy, or the toy, or directly at you (returning your smile).

And what about anger, which most parents swear their babies are feeling at an early age? Well, babies do feel anger—but not usually until they are at least six months old. This is because anger is primarily about something that has changed or been taken away, and baby doesn't usually notice such disturbances until he or she is at the six-month mark.

The emotions of an infant are, at best, crude attempts to get needs met. Keep your list of baby's needs handy, and you should have smooth sailing in those first few months.

The Ties That Bind

Creating special moments that will last a lifetime isn't a difficult thing; all you need to do is be sure to catch baby at the right time. The best time during the first few months for bonding with your baby is right after feeding and changing. At that time, most of baby's needs have been met, and baby will generally be in a happier mood.

Reading Baby's Signals

If babies could talk, what would they say? Actually, babies *do* talk—and they have a unique language of their own. The challenge is for you, the new parent, to understand what the baby needs based on nothing more than a simple cry.

As mentioned previously, a baby's cry is often different based on what it needs at the moment; a sharp, shrill cry may mean hunger; a softer cry may mean baby just wants to be rocked. There is no owner's manual to explain to you which one is which; you just have to spend enough time with your baby to get accustomed to the patterns of your baby's cries.

Another way to read your baby's signals is through body language. What is baby's body telling you? Is it stiff as a board? If so, baby needs your attention *now*—he or she could be extremely hungry or need to relieve some tummy gas.

If baby is pulling on an ear and screaming, it's a classic sign of an ear infection. Occasionally, teething will produce similar body language.

If you work outside the home, concentrate on spending quality time with your baby when you return home from work. Quality time is time you set aside for baby—and baby alone. Focus entirely on the baby, and have a great time doing so. If the phone rings while you're playing with baby, you can let the answering machine or voice mail answer it.

What can you do during quality time with baby? It needn't be anything elaborate. Many first-time parents, guilt stricken over their time away from the baby, try to fit every single activity into a half hour with baby in the early evening. This practice not only is unnecessary (since baby doesn't have a concept of time) but also can lead to overstimulation for the baby; and baby's irritability could be misread by the parents as an expression of dissatisfaction with their being away all day.

It's hard not to take baby's tears personally when you feel uneasy about your situation, but realize that the baby isn't keeping track of your hours together. All babies know (and need to know) is that there are people in the world who love them, care for them, and spend time with them.

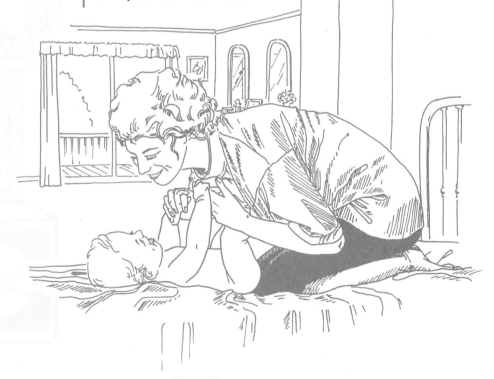

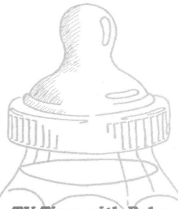

Give yourself credit for all that you do accomplish with baby, and give baby a break whenever he or she needs one. Babyhood is not about how many toys one has or how much time Mommy and Daddy have to spare. It's about the quality of the time spent and the depth of the bonds of love that are expressed between parents and their babies. Creating a lasting bond depends more on sincerity than on longevity.

What to Say When You Talk to a Baby

How many people do you know that talk baby talk to babies? More than you'd probably care to think about. Is baby talk bad for babies? Well, it doesn't really hurt, but it doesn't necessarily help baby's language development, either.

It's best to talk to a baby just as you would talk to any other person. Just work at keeping it simple. (Reading *War and Peace* to your baby isn't going to help him or her learn the language any faster.) Start with simple sounds and then build to short, concise words.

With Lilly, I started slowly saying sounds first, mouthing and saying "o-o-o" and giving her ample time to hear (and eventually repeat) it. After about a month of this, she finally did repeat the sound, and it seemed like her language development skills were off to a great start.

Here are some additional tips:

- Use short, simple words like *happy*, *ball*, *puppy*, and *kitty* when you talk to your baby. Babies can only process a few syllables at a time; so go slow and keep it simple.
- Find a toy that is a favorite of baby's to play with; tell baby the name of the toy (*bear*, *rattle*, etc.), and use its name frequently. Give the toy to baby right after saying what it is.
- Clap baby's hands along when you play word games. Physical activity can help baby associate learning new words with something that feels good to do.

TV Time with Baby

The debate over whether television is good or bad for children will likely continue as long as there is TV. Some parents would sooner die than let their children watch TV; others depend on it as a teaching tool and a way to encourage conversation with their children.

Should you decide to include television as part of your child's early learning experiences, here are some suggestions for giving baby the best in viewing pleasure:

- Keep the sound down.
- Rent movies that are geared toward small children. There are even tapes that only show faces of other babies, with music playing in the background. Babies do enjoy looking at faces.
- Put on quality public television programs that have a wide variety of activities, such as *Sesame Street* or *Mr. Rogers' Neighborhood*. Kids love these timeless shows, and they learn a lot from them, too.
- Make sure the programs you are watching with baby have lots of music in them. Babies love music, and music has been shown to enhance their brain activity.

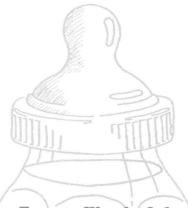

Twenty Wonderful Things to Do with Your Baby

1. Take a walk.
2. Join a play group.
3. Give baby a luxurious bath.
4. Read and sing to baby.
5. Watch kiddie TV together.
6. Enjoy doing "little" things together, such as walking around the house or going for a short drive.
7. Put on music and dance around the room with baby.
8. Play simple games, such as peek-a-boo or baby airplane.
9. Give an infant massage.
10. Use toys (such as a rattle or a music box) to entertain baby.
11. Enlist the help of a sibling to "perform" a song or miniplay for baby.
12. Play a sound game with baby, saying simple vowel sounds and encouraging baby to repeat them.
13. Take baby shopping for something special.
14. Take baby out to dinner, just the two or three of you.

⚘ Narrate the things you do during the day, for baby's sake. When baby is on the changing table, for instance, you could say "Now, I'm going to change your diaper. See, di-a-per. All clean!" When you show baby a diaper and then say the word, baby starts to associate pictures with words.

⚘ Use baby's name often; Dale Carnegie was right when he said that there is no sweeter sound to a human than the sound of his own name. This is where it all starts.

⚘ Read short, simple stories to baby. Books that have a touchy, feely approach (such as mirrors for baby to look into or fake fur to pet) are a good starting point, since much of a baby's early processing occurs through sensual, hands-on experiences. Books of rhymes are good, too, since there is repetition of sounds.

⚘ Stay encouraging and positive, even if baby doesn't show any interest in talking yet. Just because baby isn't talking at four months doesn't mean he or she isn't listening well.

⚘ Make sure baby can see your facial expression when you're communicating with him or her.

How to Have a Well-Adjusted Baby

Your baby begins life with the most important ingredient to development: love. Loving your baby is the first step in building a secure environment, one in which baby can grow and learn and feel your support every step of the way.

Here are some other ways you can encourage baby's emotional well-being:

⚘ **Take your time with day-to-day activities, such as feeding, rocking, and singing to baby.** If baby feels rushed (because you're on a cellular phone and have the baby propped up with a bottle for your own convenience), there could be emotional or eating disturbances later. Set the tone for good habits early.

⚘ **Remember that babies can do no wrong.** They aren't capable of distinguishing behaviors, so you cannot punish a

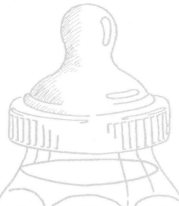

baby. Every day there are stories in the newspapers about a parent shaking a baby because it wouldn't stop crying. Don't be a statistic; be caring and supportive. You will get your chance to teach baby when he or she becomes a toddler and is more capable of processing right and wrong.

- **Encourage baby with your vocal intonation.** When baby achieves something, enthusiastically say, for example, "Good girl!" or "Good boy!" The first time baby tries to talk, encourage him or her with your voice, even though baby's sounds don't make sense yet. Have you ever known a puppy (or a person) who didn't keep trying after being positively encouraged?

- **Use your baby's name often, and associate it with different things.** Say, for example, "Kelsey is a good girl" or "Andrew can talk!" Build language skills early in your child by planting positive pictures in his or her mind.

- **Share the wealth.** Let your baby experience other gentle, loving people (and even pets). A well-balanced child can spend time with anyone and doesn't cry for Mom or Dad every time someone new comes into the room.

- **Most of all, always use a kind, soft tone of voice with your baby.** If you're having a bad day or if you need to scold another child, do so in another room of the house or as far away from baby as possible. Babies who are raised in hostile environments can grow up to be hostile adults.

How to Start (or Be in) a Play Group

All the parents sit around in a circle, babies on their laps. As they sing, "The Wheels on the Bus," they clap baby's hands together or bounce their knees in time to the music. After the song is over, the babies play "So Big," with parents stretching their arms and legs to show how big they are (and, of course, to exercise them). Someone brings out a xylophone, and babies then get to try their tiny hands at making music.

This is not a scene from a TV show, and these babies are not necessarily "gifted" children. They come from all social, economic,

Twenty Wonderful Things to Do with Your Baby
(continued)

15. Be supportive of baby's little explorations. Give lots of encouragement when you notice, for example, that baby is checking out her fingers.

16. Introduce baby to playmates, such as a puppy or another little baby.

17. Show baby your undivided attention when you can, and give lots of unconditional love.

18. Encourage baby to smile often. It exercises baby's facial muscles but can also lead to laughter—and stronger bonds with you.

19. Always provide eye contact with baby when you are talking to him or her; babies need to know who you are talking to and can't tell by any other way.

20. Make baby a part of the goings-on in your family. For example, if baby listens to the way you talk to your toddler, it can help establish positive behavior patterns.

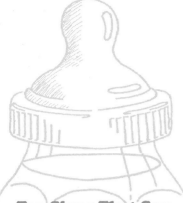

Ten Signs That Say You're Really Stuck on Your Baby

1. You have a whole gallery of baby pictures in your wallet and show them to complete strangers.
2. You can't stop reading the library of baby books you have on your bookshelf, and there are even some on your coffee table.
3. You sing the special little songs you made for baby—only baby isn't with you when you're doing it.
4. Baby has become the focus of every conversation you have (with friends, family, and strangers alike).
5. You catch yourself listening to baby's lullaby tapes, long after baby's asleep.

and ethnic groups, and from different backgrounds. The only thing they have in common is their love of play.

If you aren't a member of a play group, you might do well to consider joining one. Such groups can be a fun way to explore new activities with your baby and with other parents who may offer you interesting (and fun) suggestions. Such groups often use music, art, and educational (yet fun) toys to create new experiences—and as a bonding aid between parent and child.

Play groups are especially good for those new young families living in a place that is far away from family and friends; you can connect with others who experience the same trials and tribulations (and joys) that you do. It can be a positive experience for your baby, too, since babies love to look at and play with other little people with whom they have a lot in common.

How do you find a play group? Ask other parents you see at the park or grocery store. Find out if your church sponsors one. Often, your community newspaper is a good source for such groups. If you don't see an ad in the paper, call an editor to ask whether he or she knows of a good play group.

If all else fails, why not start one yourself? Place a classified ad in your local paper or post flyers at the grocery store or at your church. There are plenty of good resources to guide you in what games to play and what kinds of toys to have on hand. If you can get enough parents interested, you can ask for a small membership fee to cover expenses such as toys, extra diapers and wipes, snacks, and so forth.

Babies need socialization in the same way that puppies do. Finding a group you and baby feel comfortable with can be a great bonding experience for both of you.

Things That Could Upset Your Baby

Here are some things that may move baby out of his or her comfort zone during the first year:

- Approaching baby quickly and loudly can cause him or her to cry. Some people, especially those who have never had children before (but adore them nonetheless), just don't realize that excessive gushing can scare the you-know-what out of a baby.

- Separation anxiety can also cause baby to let out a wail or two. Even if the baby knows that Grandma is nice or that the baby sitter is sweet, he or she knows that you are leaving and is not happy about it. With my first baby, I was very upset by separation anxiety-related outbursts; now that I'm on my second, I leave knowing that baby will be okay again in just a few minutes. Separation anxiety can be harder on parents than on babies.

- Small children can accidentally hurt baby. They just don't understand that baby is too small yet to be a playmate.

- Pets can scare baby. Slowly integrate them, and always maintain your supervision. It is absolutely unsafe to leave pets alone with baby, even for a minute. Even the sweetest little pet can cause the baby injury—and vice versa.

- Loud music can startle or upset baby. Tell your teenagers to tone it down or go to their friend's house.

Is Baby Overstimulated?

Many first-time parents aren't sure when to stop playing with their babies; they think baby's crankiness is a signal for them to switch to yet another toy or an expression of dissatisfaction with their parenting ability. But how can you tell when enough is enough? Baby's sounds and body language will tell you all you need to know.

When a baby is overstimulated (either by too much noise or overzealous playing), you will know it by baby's crying. There may even be some rubbing of the eyes, strong kicking, and stiffness when you attempt to comfort baby through rocking or holding.

The best thing you can do is put the baby in bed, dim the lights, and put on soft, gentle music. Any other noise or fussing on the part of parents will only serve to annoy baby further. All babies need some quiet time alone (just as we adults do); so respect that need in your baby. Sometimes, fussiness is the only way baby can tell you that he or she wants to be alone for a while.

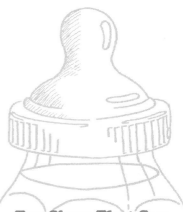

Ten Signs That Say You're Really Stuck on Your Baby
(continued)

6. You've made T-shirts with baby's picture and Web site address on them.
7. Your bedroom has become a shrine to baby's first year.
8. You've had baby's pacifiers turned into charms for your necklace.
9. You order for baby at a restaurant—even though it's only warm water to heat the bottle in. You say to the server, "And baby would like . . ."
10. Every time you gaze into baby's eyes, you can't stop saying, "Wow! Aren't we lucky?"

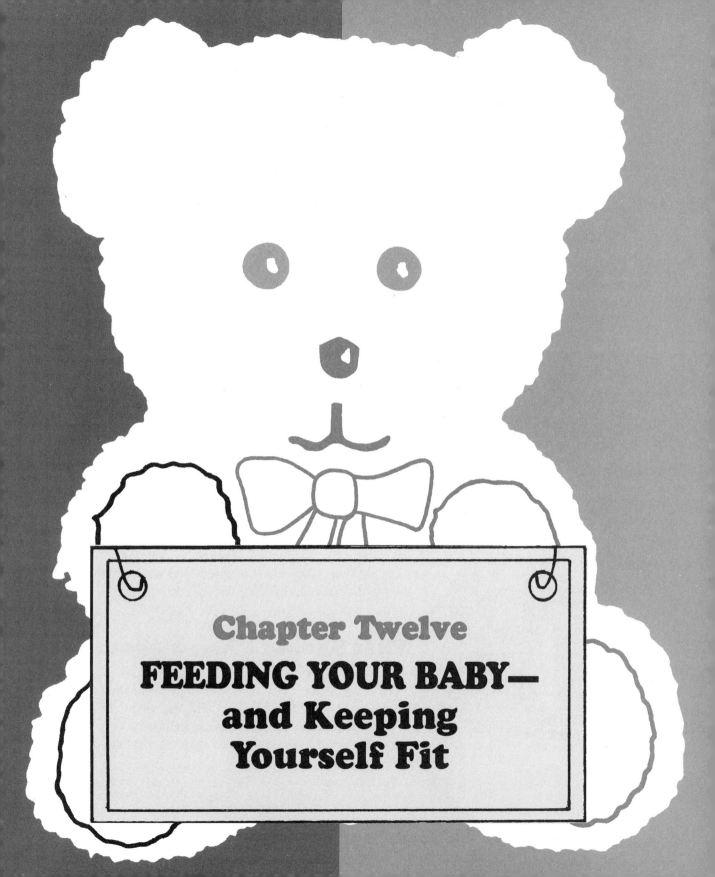

Chapter Twelve
FEEDING YOUR BABY— and Keeping Yourself Fit

Once you've had your baby, the two things you'll be most concerned with are putting weight on baby—and taking it off yourself (and not necessarily in that order!). Remember that the overall health of both you and your baby is your top priority, however you decide to get there. The postpregnancy routine for both you and baby should be focused on gradual change and development rather than on immediate results.

Baby's first-ever need from you is food. Many babies, in fact, feed in those first few moments after birth. But whether you choose to breastfeed or bottle-feed, there are plenty of important considerations to mull over prior to making a decision. You'll need as much information as possible to ensure that the final decision is one that you feel good about and that baby draws the most benefit from in the long run.

You've probably heard from both sides on the issue of breastfeeding. Some mothers (and some doctors) will tell you that breastfeeding is the only way to make sure that baby is getting proper nutrition. Others will say that formula feedings now contain better nutrients.

Both of these arguments are actually right. Formula is better than it has ever been, and breastmilk provides excellent protection against illnesses.

So, what's a new parent to do? All things being equal, it really boils down to your own personal comfort level and belief system. If you don't feel comfortable with the way you are feeding your baby, your discomfort level will become evident to the baby, and you could wind up with some feeding problems.

What Should I Know about Breastfeeding?

Breastfeeding is the most highly recommended form of providing proper nutrition for your baby. Your own milk not only has the right amount of fat and nutrients to help baby grow but also contains compounds that help build baby's immune system.

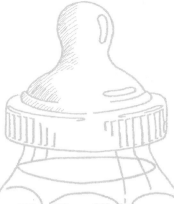

Nursing your baby should begin immediately upon birth, to give you and baby a chance to get used to this new method of meeting baby's nutritional needs. Remember that up until this point, baby has only fed on *your* food and prenatal vitamins—and had room service deliver it via the umbilical cord!

Now, baby has to work a little bit harder for his or her food. So, when you first begin to breastfeed, expect that it may take a few tries before the two of you get the hang of it. Invest in the services of a lactation consultant who can ease your mind by showing you the proper positions for breastfeeding and how to tell if baby has a good latch.

Contrary to popular belief, breastfeeding is not as easy as it looks—at first. What we are made to believe comes naturally may often be trial and error until we get used to it; so don't lose your cool until you're absolutely sure there's a problem that will permanently impede your breastfeeding efforts.

Mastitis (a painful infection of the milk ducts) is one reason mothers stop nursing their babies; the only other common reason for discontinuing nursing is the mother's belief that she'll never get it right. In the latter case, try not to give up until you've discussed the problem with your doctor or a lactation consultant, since it may be an easy problem to fix.

Here are some breastfeeding tips:

- Start in a quiet, peaceful environment. Make sure to get visitors to leave while you're nursing baby, at least until you feel more confident. There's nothing worse than being a proud new mom and then having nursing difficulty while feeling pressure to "perform." Peaceful concentration on baby will help the milk flow easily.
- Nurse as often as you can, primarily every time the baby seems hungry. At the hospital, if you are sure you want to nurse exclusively, be sure to point this out clearly to the neonatal nurses. So often, well-meaning nurses offer to feed the baby glucose water or formula so that you can rest. If you don't want this to happen, be clear and direct in your instructions that baby be brought to you every time he or

Limiting Visitors

Respiratory syncytial virus (RSV) is on the rise, especially among newborns. This disease can be dangerous because it causes inflammation of the small breathing tubes of the lungs, possibly leading to pneumonia and other respiratory problems. If your baby has a runny nose, low-grade fever, and a cough that does not appear to be getting better, call your doctor, and limit the number of visitors your baby greets until the illness goes away.

Here are some tips that can help keep baby healthy:

- Persons near the baby should wash their hands frequently.
- Keep siblings at home for a few days if a lot of children in their daycare center or school have colds.
- Keep the baby away from anyone who has flu-like symptoms.
- Disinfect your home regularly, especially when there has been an illness in your family.

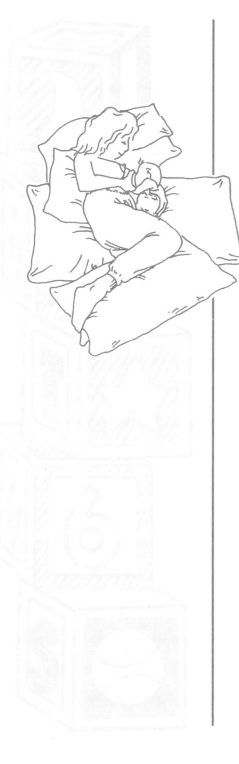

she seems hungry. The more you nurse, the more milk you will produce. Experts agree that you should try to feed at least eight times per day.

⚬ The first few days, you will not see (or feel) a whole lot of milk. However, your pre-milk has plenty of immunities in it for baby to consume, and baby actually doesn't need much more in the first days. It takes regular stimulation to make more milk. When your milk is delivered, you'll know it: Your breasts will swell, and they may even feel like cool water is running through them. Some women report a tingling feeling. Whatever symptom you experience, you'll know it's time for feeding your baby when your breasts are ready.

⚬ Pretend that your breast is a target; the nipple is the bulls-eye, but the areola surrounding it is the rest of the target. Position baby's chin and nose against your breast, and then make sure baby gets the whole target in his or her mouth. If you just let baby attach to your nipple, you will not have a good latch; and while baby can still get milk, your nipples will feel like they are nearly being pulled off of your body. If you see tiny sores on your nipples, you likely aren't positioning baby correctly, and your nipples are probably starting to abscess.

⚬ Nurse for about 10 minutes on each side to encourage milk production in both breasts. Also, drink lots of fluid before, during, and after feeding. You need to stay hydrated in order to produce more milk and to keep your own body in a healthy balance.

⚬ Hospital nurses mean well and are often quite knowledgeable about breastfeeding. Yet, there are still many who don't really know how to help you. Ask for the lactation consultant first; and if your hospital doesn't have one, ask who the best nurse is on staff to help you. Don't take the advice of just anyone passing by unless it's from someone you trust.

⚬ Once you're home, keep baby in a bassinet next to your bed. That way, you don't have far to go when baby gets hungry in the middle of the night. And breastfeeding babies nearly always will be hungry a few times at night.

- If you experience breast pain, alternate hot and cold packs on your breasts. I know some women who used frozen vegetable packages, because they are cold yet extremely flexible. Use whatever works.

- To build up nipple durability and keep from getting too tender, try expressing a little bit of breastmilk and rubbing it into your nipples. Let the milk air dry. This offers your nipples natural protection from dry or chapped skin. Another solution is to use lanolin cream on your breasts; it provides a safe, harmless barrier to skin problems.

- Cradle your baby's head, but not so closely that baby can't turn away from you when he or she is finished eating. It's baby's only way of telling you he or she is done.

- Be sure to follow your prenatal diet (and stay on the vitamins as long as you're breastfeeding). Eat a well-balanced diet, and keep the fluids coming. Don't drink too much fluid, however, since this can defeat the purpose. A dozen or more servings a day is probably too much.

- If you have problems that seem persistent or if you'd just like some friendly support, call the LaLeche League at 1-800-LALECHE (or visit their Web site at http://www.prairienet.org/llli

The benefits of breastfeeding are not limited to baby. You can also reap some rewards, including weight loss (if you breastfeed for at least three months); a uterus that contracts more quickly (since feeding stimulates contraction); and a lower chance of breast cancer (for you and, believe it or not, for female babies who were breastfed). Also, breastfed babies tend to spit up less than formula-fed babies do.

Best of all, it's free and always available, no matter where you are. You can also use a breast pump for times you can't be there, to ensure that baby is getting breastmilk at all times.

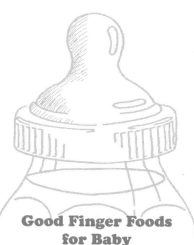

Good Finger Foods for Baby

Once your baby has a pincer grasp (ability to pick up a small object with thumb and forefinger), he's ready to try finger foods. While most babies will have a few teeth at this stage, even babies whose teeth haven't come in yet can practice chewing with their gums. Introduce new foods slowly, and serve only a few pieces of food at a time.

If you're not sure that a vegetable or fruit is tender enough for baby, try a piece yourself. If you can mash it on the roof of your mouth with your tongue, without using your teeth, baby should be able to handle it.

• Cheerios
• Soft, whole-grain bread, cut into small pieces (with butter, cream cheese, or fruit spread if desired)
• Teething biscuits
• Mild cheese, such as mozzarella or Muenster, shredded or cut into very small cubes

The Positives of Formula Feeding

What if you decide, for a health reason or just plain convenience, that baby will be formula fed? Should you feel like you have to explain it to everyone who asks? The decision to feed your baby formula is a personal one; and whether or not other folks agree, formula is better than ever at mimicking breastmilk in terms of nutrients.

The first discussion about formula feeding should be with your partner. If you both agree this is the way to go, then you need to talk with your pediatrician about the appropriate formula for your baby. Many pediatricians suggest using cow's milk formula with iron; however, if your baby has an intolerance to cow's milk, you will need to switch to a soy-based formula. Neither is a poor choice; it just depends on what baby's specific needs are.

Here are some tips for hassle-free formula feeding:

- If you can, buy the premixed cans of formula. These are the easiest to use, since they are already of perfect consistency. I've found that the powders take too long, are messy, and often don't mix well (especially after the bottles are refrigerated). The premixed formula costs a little more; but believe me, it's worth it when you have a crying baby at 2 A.M. and no bottles are ready.
- Alternate the positions you feed baby in, for variety and proper balance on your arm muscles.
- Sterilize all bottle pieces thoroughly, and always keep your hands and kitchen area clean. Use antibacterial soap to clean.
- Feed baby every three or four hours the first few months. Follow what your pediatrician tells you about increasing frequency or when to add cereal to the mix.
- Don't heat the formula in the microwave. Instead, put warm water into a dish or bowl, and then place the bottle inside. This will help the formula heat up uniformly—and prevent burns for baby.

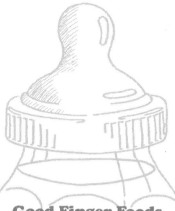

⚘ Tip the bottle over and sprinkle some formula onto your wrist to make sure it's the right temperature. Lukewarm is good.

⚘ Don't reuse formula if baby doesn't drink the whole bottle of milk. Using a bottle over again promotes bacterial growth, which is not desirable with a little one.

⚘ From birth to about four months, feed baby 4 to 6 ounces of formula at a feeding. Many doctors are starting babies on solid foods after four months.

⚘ Stop halfway throughout the feeding and burp the baby. Burp again after baby is done eating. Keep the bib on for about fifteen minutes after feeding—formula-fed babies often spit up in that time frame, and you'll want to be ready.

⚘ Enjoy your bonding time with baby every bit as much as you would if you were breastfeeding. Cuddle, kiss, and love the baby while feeding; and share the joy of bonding with baby with others in your family. Let all who ask have a try at feeding baby (with the exception of small siblings who aren't ready to hold baby yet).

Formula feeding can be a wonderful, healthy experience for you and baby, and many breastfeeding moms use formula as a supplement when they need to. I formula fed Lilly and did half-breast, half-bottle with Maddie. Neither is showing any signs of a problem.

Graduating to Solid Food

When your baby reaches the age of four months, your pediatrician may recommend that you start him or her on solid foods. That doesn't mean you're suddenly going to serve steak and potatoes, but it does mean that baby is moving on to new (and more challenging) digestibles. You'll start with something easy, such as rice or oatmeal, before moving on to jars of baby food and finger foods.

Some doctors recommend sticking with baby cereals (such as rice and oatmeal) for as long as baby will eat it. Their reasoning is that baby cereals are higher in vitamins than common adult oatmeals.

Good Finger Foods for Baby
(continued)

- Ripe banana, cut into small pieces
- Fresh blueberries
- Cooked peas
- Very ripe peaches or plums, peeled and cut into small pieces
- Other fresh fruits and vegetables, steamed until very tender and cut into small pieces (try apples, pears, carrots, or green beans)
- Cooked elbow macaroni (with butter or cheese if desired)
- Scrambled eggs, cut small

Once baby is accustomed to chewing, try adding these foods:

- Chicken or turkey, cooked until very tender and cut into small pieces
- Meat loaf or meatballs, cut into small pieces
- Graham crackers

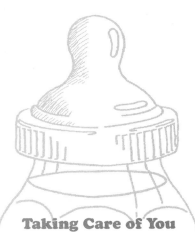

Taking Care of You

Being a new parent is a never-ending challenge; so be good to yourself and remember this advice:

- Get as much rest as you need. Yeah, right, you're probably thinking. Take your naps where you can find them—and don't be afraid to tell others you need a rest.

- Give yourself "time off." Go out for a walk, or on a shopping trip, or even to a movie if you want to. Enlist family and friends to watch the baby while you're out. Hand the baby off to Dad; he needs to bond with and care for the baby, too. Always schedule time that is yours and yours alone.

- Make regular "to do" lists. Don't list too much for one human to do on one day; going overboard will only serve to frustrate you more.

- Incorporate baby into your routine. I used a Snugli™ to carry Lilly with me while I was on assignment for a major newspaper; she had been to forty-one art galleries by the time she was a year old!

Also, many doctors recommend limiting fruit juice to only 4 ounces per day for a young baby—and diluting it to prevent diarrhea.

Finger foods can be started as early as seven months, or once baby has developed a "pincer-grasp."

Here's a quick rundown of what baby may try to eat and when he or she will probably try it:

- **Four to six months.** Breastmilk, formula, cereals (rice or oatmeal), fruits, and vegetables.

- **Six to eight months.** Breastmilk or formula (or both), cereals, fruits and vegetables, fruit and vegetable juices, and protein-rich foods such as yogurt, cheese, or egg yolks. This is the ideal time to try turkey or chicken and vegetable dinners (strained, in the jar).

- **Eight to ten months.** Breastmilk or formula, fruits and vegetables, cereals (move on to breads and muffins), and chicken or turkey meals. You could try pureed beef or lamb at this stage, too.

- **Ten months to one year.** Breastmilk, formula or whole milk; oatmeal, breads, and cereals of thicker consistency; soft-cooked fruits and vegetables cut into tiny morsels for baby to feed with his or her own hands; and tiny portions of whatever you're having for dinner, as long as baby can chew it (baby should be more interested in "Mommy" or "Daddy" food by this time, and you can let baby experiment, within reason).

Food Problems and Solutions

Some babies develop food allergies, which is why your doctor will recommend that you try a specific food for at least two days in a row before moving on to another new item. This way, if a rash develops, you'll be able to quickly identify the reason behind it. Babies can develop allergies to nuts, egg whites, strawberries, and even sweet potatoes.

If you're worried about pesticides, buy only organic baby foods (most groceries now stock some) or call the 800-number on the jar label to ask whether pesticides were used in the production of the baby food.

Of course, you could always make your own baby foods, and there are plenty of cookbooks in the baby book section of the library or bookstore. You'll need good puree equipment and perhaps a juicer. Many parents prefer this option, since it allows them to feed their babies more whole grains and less sugars.

Tackling the Diaper Dilemma

After feeding the baby, the inevitable will happen. You'll have to change a dirty diaper. One of the first choices you'll make as a new parent is which type of diaper to use on your baby. Here are your options:

- **Your own cloth diapers.** You can purchase a set of fifty or more diapers and wash them for reuse. Your baby may go through six to eight diapers per day. *Pros*: You can save a lot of money on diapers. *Cons*: It's a lot more work, and you'll go through tons of heavy-duty detergent in the process. Some reports indicate that home washing machines don't sterilize the same way commercial units do. Also, cloth diapers often leak—leading to more wet clothes.
- **A diaper service.** You can hire a service that drops off clean new diapers and removes the dirty ones once per week. *Pros*: It's convenient and environmentally responsible. *Cons*: It's costly and annoying, particularly if you miss your dirty diaper pickup.
- **Disposable diapers.** You can buy these virtually anywhere, and their manufacturers claim that they are friendlier than ever to the environment. *Pros*: They are convenient and readily available; these diapers are also great for travel. *Cons*: They can be expensive.

The "bottom" line is this: You should choose what is most comfortable for the baby and convenient for you.

Here are some tips for diapering "rookies":

Diapers can be a scary experience for first timers, since you can never really be sure what's inside a dirty diaper until you are brave enough to open it. Once you do, you will learn something you never knew before about babies: their stool can change colors dramatically.

Once you get past that initial shock, everything else becomes more practical. When changing a diaper, you should first be sure you've put all of the changing table supplies within easy reach. Never leave the baby alone on the changing table, not even if there's a safety belt on it. Babies can roll very quickly and fall off the table before you even notice a problem.

Here are some more diapering tips for "newbies" like you:

- Take off the dirty diaper, wiping away as much stool as you can with the front of the diaper and using a warm wash cloth or baby wipes for the rest.
- Be aware of the differences between boys and girls, and wipe accordingly. For girls, you should always wipe from front to back (and never in the opposite direction) to prevent any debris from getting into the vagina. Even baby girls can get bladder, urinary tract, or kidney infections, and fecal matter in the vaginal area is a primary cause. For baby boys, clean a circumcised penis with warm water and apply a thin layer of petroleum jelly to the tip. For boys who have not been circumcised, pull the foreskin back and wash with a warm cloth.
- Let the baby "air dry" without a diaper for a few minutes to minimize the chance of diaper rash. Then apply some petroleum jelly to the diaper area to keep baby's skin soft and protect it from irritation.

Making a Splash with Baby's First Bath

Bathing a newborn can be a challenge, but it can be one of the most fun times you have with your baby. Of course, when you're reading about it, it will look easy; but you may find it difficult at first if you're not used to a wet little one trying to squirm out of your arms. Try to keep calm, and have your partner with you (at least the first time) for backup assistance.

Your baby should have a complete bath about once or twice per week but should also be sponged off every day. Use a sponge or warm cloth with baby soap to wipe away any dirt, excess formula, or body oil.

Feed your baby at least an hour before the bath, so that baby can relax and go to sleep after a pleasant bathing experience—and so that you can avoid any unpleasant surprises in the diaper region.

Here are a few more tips:

- Bathe your baby in a warm bathroom. This will help drain baby's sinuses, and it will cut down on the chances of baby catching a chill.
- Keep all bath supplies within immediate reach, including that rubber ducky you've been saving for baby's special moment.
- Put baby's towel on the floor (preferably on top of the soft bathroom rug) so that you have your hands totally on baby as you take baby out of the tub. Wet babies can slip easily, and especially so if you have to let one hand go to reach for the towel.

Here are some tips on how to give baby a sponge bath:

- Fill a bowl or small bucket with lukewarm water. Put a sponge in the water, and add a little baby bath if you want to.
- Place a large bath towel on a flat surface (such as a bed, carpeted floor, or kitchen counter). Put the baby on the towel, folding a part of the towel over the baby to keep the warmth in. Be sure to keep one hand over the baby at all times.
- Wash the baby's face and the rest of his or her body. Be gentle, talk to the baby to comfort him or her, and don't move too quickly. Wipe the baby gently to dry.
- Dress the baby, and then soothe him or her by rocking and singing a lullaby. You've both earned a nice rest.

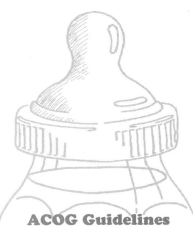

ACOG Guidelines

Here is a summary of the American College of Obstetricians and Gynecologists Guidelines (from *ACOG Technical Bulletin*, Number 189, February 1994), with exercise tips directly from doctors.

- During pregnancy, you can continue your mild-to-moderate exercise routines. It's best to exercise at least three days a week.
- Don't exercise in the supine position (flat on your back) after the first trimester. It can decrease the blood flow to the uterus. Also don't stand motionless for long periods.
- You'll have less oxygen available for aerobic exercise during pregnancy; so modify the intensity of your routine accordingly. Stop exercising when fatigued, and don't exercise to exhaustion. You might be able to continue doing weight-bearing exercise at close to your usual intensity throughout

Getting Your Body Back

We've spent a lot of time in this chapter talking about how to care for baby, but what about how to care for yourself postpregnancy? Getting your body back to its prepregnancy shape can be a challenge; after all, when do you have the time to exercise?

Hollywood and glamour magazines don't make it any easier on new moms, showing us skinny young things who claim they've just had babies and are merely returning to the gym for some "toning." These depictions only serve to antagonize us more, giving us the feeling that we are a long way off from ever wearing those size 8 jeans again.

For the best program in fitness and convenience, try a walking program. Places to walk are always available, and you can take baby along in a stroller if you need to—so there's no excuse for not doing it! Follow these tips:

Warm-up. Stretch your calves, hamstrings, quadriceps, and hip flexors, holding each stretch for about five to ten seconds.

Exercise. When you're ready to walk, put your baby in a front carrier or a stroller. Walk with even, well-paced strides and try to walk for at least fifteen minutes (for a good cardiac workout). To lose serious weight, you'll need to exercise for a longer period of time (thirty minutes to an hour per day, three or four times per week). And feel free to mix and match—walking, swimming, aerobics, or fitness equipment (such as a Nordic Track™). Join a health club that has a baby-sitting room for maximum benefit—and the option to work with a personal trainer if you decide you need one.

Cooldown. When you finish walking or exercising, you can do a few knee lifts or kicks (as high as you can) or march in place to bring your heart rate down. Then repeat the stretches you did in the warm-up, holding each for ten to fifteen seconds. Leaning against a wall in your house (or outside), push against the wall with one hand and lean your body into the wall. Feel the stretch of your back, buttock, and leg muscles; stay in this position for ten to fifteen seconds, and then breathe deeply and relax all of your muscles.

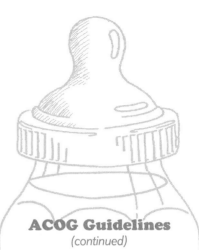

Exercise need not be a painful, miserable experience. All you need is a little encouragement, support, and direction. Of course, the motivation to return to your prepregnancy shape is what will really put you over the edge.

Here are some creative ideas for exercising with a baby:

- Do crib lifts—you lift baby up and down from the crib using the full support of your back muscles.
- Go mall walking with baby in the stroller. Do the whole mall before stopping to shop at any one store.
- Do Kegels to help your uterine muscles get back to normal.
- Lay on the floor with your knees bent and your feet flat. Lift baby up and down like a little barbell.
- Make exercise time fun time for baby, too. Prop baby up in his or her car seat while you're working out. It can be a fascinating visual experience for baby, and you won't get judged on your thigh size, either!

Most of all, don't be too hard on yourself. Just because you can't wear an evening gown the month after you've given birth doesn't mean your life is over. Losing weight and returning your body to its prepregnancy fitness takes perseverance and time. Go easy on yourself!

ACOG Guidelines
(continued)

pregnancy, but nonweight-bearing exercises such as cycling or swimming are easier to continue and carry less risk of injury.

- Don't do exercises during which you could lose your balance, especially in the third trimester. Avoid any exercise that can cause even mild abdominal trauma.
- You need an additional 300 calories a day during pregnancy, so if you're exercising, be particularly careful to ensure an adequate diet.
- During the first trimester, be sure that you stay cool when exercising; drink enough water, wear cool clothing, and don't work out in too hot an environment.

After you give birth, resume your prepregnancy exercise routine gradually, based on physical capacity. Don't push yourself.

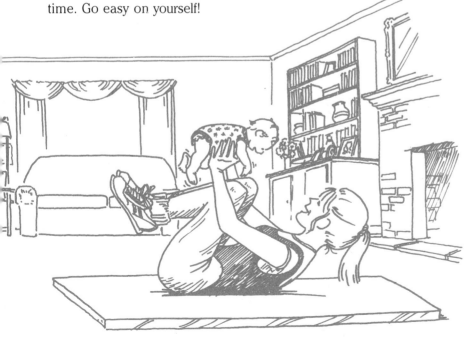

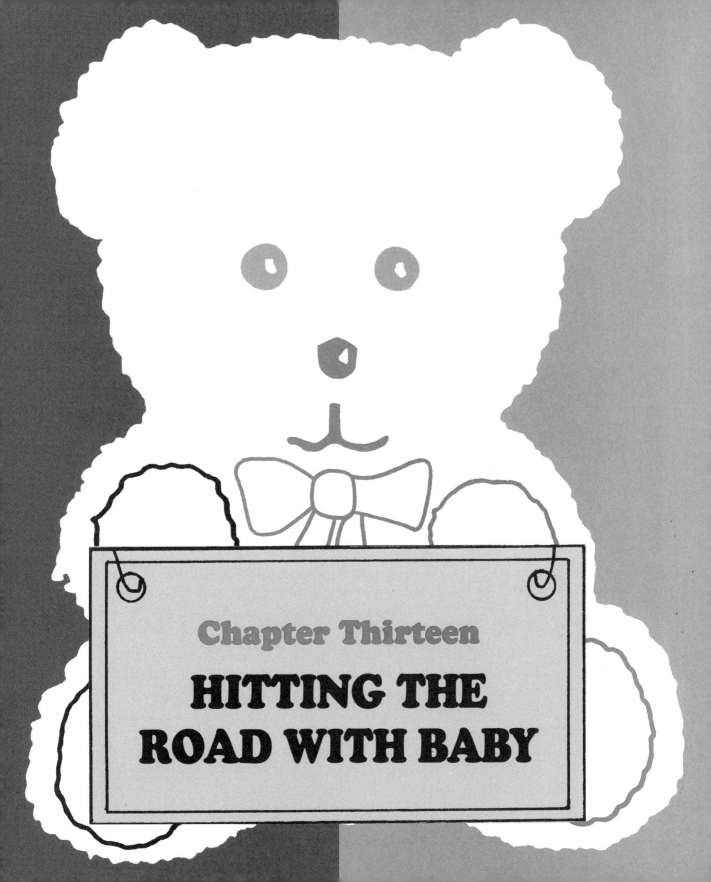

Chapter Thirteen

HITTING THE
ROAD WITH BABY

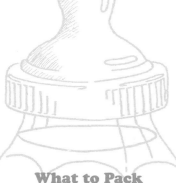

What to Pack for Baby

- Juices
- Teething toys and cookies
- Pacifiers (four—to be on the safe side)
- Bibs
- Double the amount of clothes you think you'll need (including simple outfits—the ones without a thousand buttons; lots of socks for baby, as these tend to get lost while away from home; and a complete extra set of clothes in the diaper bag!)
- A car seat (if you're flying, then renting a car)
- Music tapes for small children
- Baby books
- Diapers (and disposal bags)—you can pack some, then buy them as you need them
- A small music box (especially if baby uses one to go to sleep)

Maybe your company gives you a use-it-or-lose-it vacation option; or maybe you just plain need a break. Maybe it's a bonding thing with your new family, and you simply can't wait to get started spending some time building memories.

Whatever the reason for your vacation, you can look forward to having the time of your life traveling with your baby. And even though other folks may not understand it, it can be the most fun you've ever had on a trip. Why? Because everything, down to a blade of grass, will be a new experience for you and your baby.

Plan your trip as well as you can in advance so that you know where you want to go and when you want to go there. This doesn't mean you will actually go to all of the sites and attractions on your list, since babies don't work that way. (Remember that everything in your life will now take longer than you expect it to!)

Be as flexible as possible in your itinerary, since baby may not be on the same schedule as you. When you make your final plans, be sure to include bits and pieces of baby's regular routine. Just because you're on the road doesn't mean that baby should throw caution to the wind and give up on naptime.

Don't try to pack too much activity into your vacation, since babies can't handle too much change at one time. Do have backup ideas in mind in case you have to make a change. For instance, you might need to switch from an outdoor flea market to an indoor museum if it starts to rain.

When you travel with a baby, take the following items with you for transporting baby around: a car seat, a stroller (the umbrella type is easier for traveling), a cloth-front carrier (good for keeping baby close to you), and a backpack (if you'll be hiking or at lots of outdoor functions). You'll most likely be able to rent other equipment, such as a crib, playpen, or high chair.

Places to Go, People to See

Where are the best places to travel with a baby? Basically, anywhere you would go as an adult. But some experiences may be a little more exciting for baby:

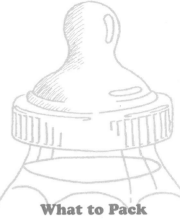

❧ A zoo or petting farm
❧ An outdoor music and arts festival
❧ A day at the beach, playing in the warm sand
❧ A park with a sandbox or swings for babies

The following experiences might not work:

❧ A European vacation
❧ A romantic bed and breakfast
❧ A bus tour with senior citizens
❧ Las Vegas
❧ Historic places (until baby is at least five years old)
❧ Places full of tourists during particular times of the year (save these places for the off-season, if you can)
❧ A Caribbean cruise

Your baby will most enjoy the experience of being with you, wherever you decide to go. It takes very little to amuse and surprise a little one, because everything is new. You can have a great time traveling with a baby for that very reason; and things you took for granted will become more appreciated as you share them with baby.

Traveling can be a wonderful bonding experience with your baby. You get to explain every new site or attraction to a captive (yet appreciative) audience. Your baby's smiles will make any minor inconveniences seem worth it. Suddenly, you won't mind the wait at airports. Room service delays won't make you pace impatiently. And baby will have the best time of all, no matter what you choose to do, because he or she will get to see plenty of new faces.

Your Baby, the Road Warrior

So, you and your partner look up from your morning paper at the same moment one day, lock eyes, and exclaim, "Road trip!" What was once easy to do is now, with a baby in tow, more difficult. How can you drive long hours to get to your destination, without enduring long hours of a crying, fussy baby?

The good news is that you can travel on the road with a baby. In fact, road travel is sometimes easier than air or sea travel, only

What to Pack for Baby
(continued)

- Baby cereals and formula
- Ice packs for baby's travel food tote
- A first-aid kit for baby (with syrup of Ipecac, bandages, antibacterial cream, a thermometer, and baby pain reliever)
- Baby bath, lotion, and oil (travel size)
- A porta-crib (if you have one; if not, call ahead to the hotel to see if it can provide one)
- An extra blanket (since you wash yours with baby-friendly detergent and most hotels use only regular detergent)
- Disinfectant spray
- A changing pad (because places on the road may not be equipped with disposable changing table covers)

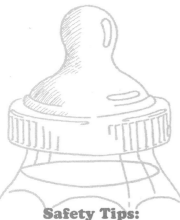

Safety Tips: Making Sure Baby Stays with You

We've all read the stories in the newspaper about babies who are kidnapped and sold on the "black market." But take some comfort in the fact that there are ways to reduce your risk of losing your baby while traveling:

1. Always be aware of your surroundings. Watch other people carefully, and don't let strangers get too close to baby.

2. Carry a recent photo of baby in both your wallet and your suitcase. If, heaven forbid, you are separated at any point, this photo will help those who are helping you.

3. Keep baby strapped into the car seat or stroller whenever you are out and around people. The best way to carry baby is in a cloth carrier; that way baby is literally strapped onto you. Backpacks are not as well recommended because you can't see behind yourself to know what others (read: weird people) are doing with baby.

because the motion of the car serves as a kind of anesthesia for babies; they almost always fall asleep in the car.

But before you hit the open road, here are some survival tips for those long trips you look forward to:

- Always use a rear-facing car seat for small infants, and position it correctly. If you're not sure of the correct position, read the manual for instructions. You'd be surprised how often well-meaning parents don't take the time to read the manual and do it right.

- Prop up the baby's head with an infant support pillow (if you think baby needs one).

- If baby starts to cry hysterically while you're on the road, pull over and tend to his or her needs. Never take baby out of the car seat—even for a few minutes—while the car is in motion.

- If you think baby just needs to see a friendly face, sit in the back with him or her for a few miles.

- Stop frequently to change baby's diaper or to feed baby. Just because baby is sleeping well doesn't mean you should try to make it to your destination nonstop. Believe me, if you let baby sleep the whole way to wherever you're going, *you* will get no sleep once you're there. Try to adhere to baby's regular schedule as much as possible.

- Attach baby's toys to the car seat or stroller so that they stay with you on most of the trip.

- Try traveling at night if your goal is to make good traveling time. Or leave just before naptime (and after a good feeding). This will cut down on motion sickness problems (yes, babies get them, too!) and will help baby to sleep better while on the road.

- Get gasoline before the trip and preferably without baby around, since babies and gasoline fumes don't mix.

- Avoid lots of starting and stopping. Take a smooth freeway ride and avoid the traffic and noise of the city whenever possible.

- Relax and enjoy your trip. The more frantic and irritable you are about getting on the road, the more upset baby will become. Babies are like mirrors of our emotions.

Feeding Your Traveling Bundle of Joy

You've got the baby all packed and ready to go on vacation . . . but what are you going to feed baby while you're out? If baby is on formula and cereal or has graduated to finger foods, you are in luck. All you have to do is pack enough bottles and snacks to feed baby during your trip. (Just be sure to keep bottles on ice until you're ready to feed; then ask an eating establishment for a cup of hot water to set the bottle in for warming.)

The best news about formula is that you can now buy it ready-made, in small, use-as-you-go sizes (8-fluid-ounce containers) or pre-bottled. It doesn't get any easier than that. If baby prefers nice, warm bottles, you can purchase a bottle warmer (they have cigarette-lighter adapters for your car).

Some parents recommend bringing along a food grinder to mash food into tiny, baby-size pieces at restaurants. I've found that this is rarely necessary, unless baby wants natural foods pureed. Otherwise, a good knife can be used to cut baby's meal into vittles.

What about breastfeeding baby while you're on the road? If you're breastfeeding, you need not feel like you are doing something indecent if you have to feed baby in a public place. Wear a loose, comfortable shirt and a nursing bra, and bring a light blanket to cover baby so you can nurse discretely.

If you feel uncomfortable feeding your baby in the middle of a busy restaurant, you can go outside with baby or even back to your car (if you're traveling with one). You don't need to go into the rest room (which can often be unclean or uncomfortable) to breastfeed your baby. Most important, if you are nursing baby while on vacation, stay well hydrated yourself. Travel can take a lot out of you—and, indirectly, the baby—if you don't get the proper food and rest.

Finally, pack the things you aren't sure you can find while out on the road; however, you can leave some things to chance. For instance, if baby likes bananas for a snack, you can locate one deli or supermarket. There's no need to pack a week's worth at one time. Snack items that do pack well (and stay fresh longer) include crackers, string cheese, cereal (such as Cheerios), apples, pretzels, and rice cakes.

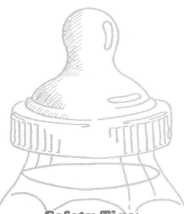

Safety Tips: Making Sure Baby Stays with You
(continued)

4. Consider keeping a chemical spray in your purse or on your key chain.
5. Travel in groups of people, preferably with other family members.
6. Try not to look like a tourist. Tuck your camera into the stroller when you're not using it, and put away maps until you really need them. Looking as though you are unfamiliar with the territory makes you appear more vulnerable to criminals.
7. Don't leave baby with strangers, even for a minute. The nicest-looking grandmotherly type could be working as part of a kidnapping ring. I know it sounds paranoid, but it could be true.
8. Always keep a close eye on baby if there is a swimming pool nearby.

Flying the (Baby) Friendly Skies

Can babies fly? Sure, if they have a seat on an airplane. It used to be that babies were allowed to sit on the laps of parents while traveling on an airplane, but the FAA has re-examined this practice and now recommends that parents purchase a seat for baby. That way, the baby can travel more safely because he or she will be fastened into a car seat. Use logic: If baby can only travel in a car seat on the ground (by law), shouldn't the same be true in the air—and for the same reasons?

If you decide to take baby on an airplane, it would probably be a good idea to postpone a feeding until you are either taking off or landing. That way, if baby's ears have difficulty popping, the swallowing will help alleviate the problem. If you can't get baby to nurse or feed in the air, try using a pacifier to solve the problem.

Bring the diaper bag and plenty of wet wipes with you on the airplane. Also, you might consider using an umbrella stroller, since these can fold easily and are lightweight enough to put in the overhead compartments on airplanes.

Most important, leave plenty of time for boarding and deplaning. Take advantage of the preboarding call for parents with small children by being at the departure gate at least thirty minutes early. And get used to being the last one off of the plane, since most folks are in a hurry and do not have the patience to wait for you to retrieve your stroller, diaper bag, and other carry-ons. There may be the occasional kind soul who will hold back the line for you, but don't count on it.

If you are traveling to a foreign country, don't forget to bring baby's immunization records and passport or birth certificate. And always ask your travel agent for information about what inoculations your baby should have before going to a specific country. However, in most cases, it is advisable that you travel within the United States until baby is two years old or older.

Baby-Friendly Hotels and Motels

Many hotel and motel chains offer to let kids under the age of twelve stay free, as long as they are in their parents' room. No matter how nice the accommodations, your first step upon check-in should always be a child-proof inspection.

Get down on all fours, just as your crawling baby would, and look at the room from a baby-eye view. Are there any electrical cords, phone cords, or other items that could lead to danger for baby? If so, move them out of the way, or decide who will take turns watching the baby while in the hotel room. You'd be surprised how easy it is for a baby to pull a heavy hotel phone onto his or her tiny head, resulting in a serious injury.

Here's a list of family-friendly accommodations:

Days Inn (1-800-325-2525). These motels offer a Kids Stay and Eat Free program for children under twelve.

Four Seasons (1-800-268-6282). These motels offer a Kids for All Seasons program (with special activities, child-proof rooms, and milk and cookies for toddlers and up). You can also get a Single Parents Weekend package.

Hilton (1-800-445-8667). Hilton offers a summer-long "vacation station" with welcome gifts and availability of toys and games.

Hyatt (1-800-233-1234). Most Hyatts offer special activities for the younger set, and some offer baby-sitting services.

Loews (1-800-23-LOEWS). Loews offers free use of cribs and child-proof kits for toddlers.

Marriott (1-800-228-9290). Call ahead for information about baby-sitting services, cribs, and toys.

Radisson (1-800-333-3333). Many Radissons offer child-proof suites and other programs.

Residence Inns (1-800-331-3131). These inns are made to look just like an apartment, and you can even leave a list of groceries for the staff to pick up and deliver directly to your room. Thus, you can have a fully stocked kitchen in which to make yourself at home.

Westin (1-800-228-3000). The new "Kids Club" program offers night-lights, juice, potty seats, and children's movies.

Home, Sweet Home

What if you decide that for financial or other reasons the best place to go on vacation this year is home? For parents who work outside of the home a lot, this is the perfect option. After all, for these parents, being home for a week can be a real novelty.

But can it be fun for baby, too? Sure it can, if you plan it right. Start off with some quality time with baby, and then do some things that are out of your ordinary routine. For instance, pretend you're a tourist in your own area—visit the area zoo, museums, restaurants, specialty shops, and so forth. Sometimes we ignore great things just because they're in our own backyards.

Get a baby sitter for part of a day so that you and your partner can get reacquainted. This will also give you a little break from baby, which is necessary every once in a while.

Another way to vacation at home is to spend a night at a friend's house—or at Grandma's— with baby. Lots of people would love to have you (and especially baby) come for an overnight visit.

Or pack a picnic and go to the park for a day of hiking and exploration. Parks are a perfect choice for a day-long excursion because babies love to see lots of people, animals, and nature. Most parks have walking trails, rest areas, and even swings and a play area for babies. Take baby to the duck pond to feed the ducks; he or she will love it, and you can take some terrific pictures of baby.

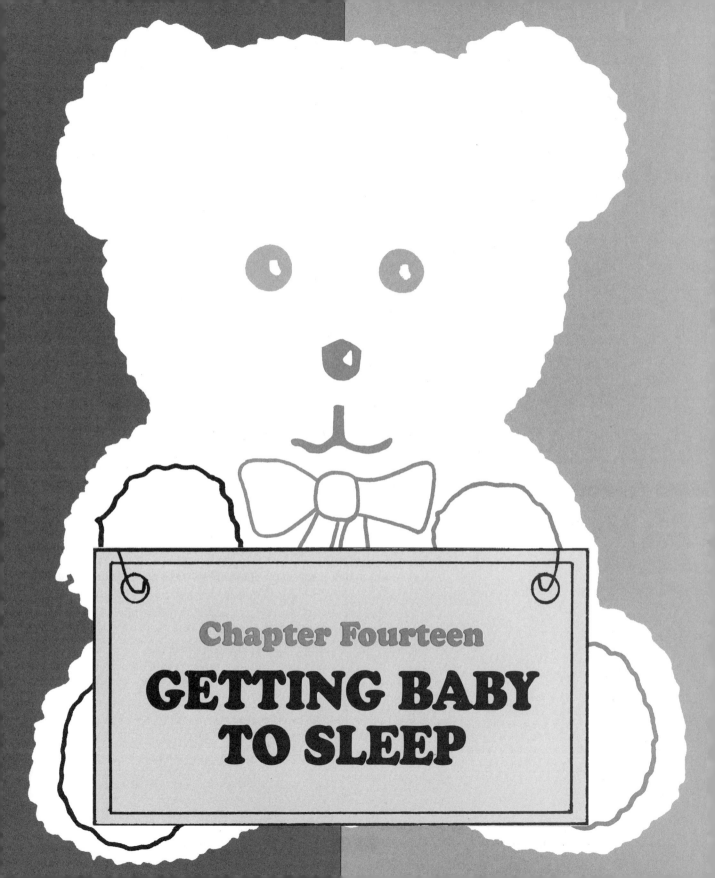

Chapter Fourteen

GETTING BABY TO SLEEP

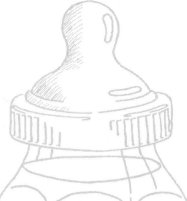

Lullabies to Sing

- "Rock-a-Bye Baby"

- "Hush, Little Baby"

- Brahms's "Lullaby"

- "Twinkle, Twinkle Little Star"

- "Golden Slumbers"

- "All Through the Night"

- "Frère Jacques"

- "Bye Baby Bunting"

- "Sleep, Baby Sleep"

- "All the Pretty Little Horses"

- "Goodnight, My Love" ("Pleasant Dreams")

You've heard the horror stories. Like the one where you put the baby to bed, and all seems well. But then you hear an unmistakable cough, then sputter—then "WAAAAAA!" You wonder what could possibly have happened in those first few minutes to make your baby change from a contented little angel to a holy terror. Or you just begin to relax and wind down for the evening, finally getting the chance to read the previous morning's paper (it's not uncommon!), when suddenly you hear the baby crying louder and louder, until you just can't stand it anymore. What can you do to get this baby back to sleep?

Getting the baby to sleep is the biggest challenge a new parent can face. It is, in fact, such a big deal that many new parents greet one another with comments like, "Oh, she's so cute . . . does she sleep through the night?" Sleeping is one of the major obsessions of new parenthood—and not without cause.

Have you noticed that there are hundreds of songs for babies containing the words *sleep* and *rest*? What about the stacks and stacks of books for babies and toddlers, all with some reference to sleep?

After visiting your local bookstore or hearing the horror stories of other parents, it wouldn't be considered crazy for you to think that your restful days are soon to be over when the blessed event occurs. My older daughter, Lilly, never slept through the night as a baby. In fact, she was two years old before she made it through an entire peaceful night's sleep. It felt like one of those psychology experiments where the researcher wakes you up every hour, and then asks whether you feel genocidal (I did).

On the other hand, my baby Maddie has slept through the night since she was in utero; I could feel her waking at the same time as me in those late-pregnancy mornings. I have no other inference to make from the difference in Lilly's and Maddie's sleep patterns except to say that perhaps there is a kind, considerate God after all— one who felt I was owed one. I am completely thankful nonetheless.

There are plenty of reasons why some babies don't sleep through the night. The baby could have gas, or have teeth coming, or just want to be rocked in your arms for comfort. Some babies don't sleep well at night because they are allowed to sleep for long stretches during the day. And some babies are just plain colicky.

Ten Ways to Calm a Crying Newborn

1. Determine whether the baby is hungry. Sixty percent of the time an empty tummy is what makes a baby cry. Offer a bottle or a breast.

2. Check baby's diaper. Change the diaper as quickly and quietly as you can; making a big fuss over the diaper can actually irritate baby more.

3. Gently rock the baby in a rocking chair. Or standing up, rock slowly back and forth, gently patting the baby's back. Maybe there's an extra burp in there that needs help getting out.

4. Swaddle or wrap the baby tightly in a blanket, just as the nurses did in the hospital nursery. Place the blanket sideways, with a point at the top. Next, place the baby at the top point, and then tuck one side under the baby's body. Pull up the bottom fold, and then wrap the remaining side over the baby's body. You're not cutting off circulation here, but you are providing that feeling of womb-like security for your baby.

5. Give the baby a pacifier. Like them or not, they are often temporary solutions to crying problems. My mother-in-law used to say that pacifiers are more for the mother than the baby, and so what if that's true? At least you've bought yourself a few moments of quiet to collect your thoughts while trying to figure out what's wrong.

6. Try to work out tummy gas. Put the baby on his or her stomach, and gently rub baby's back or pat baby's bottom. Or lay baby on his back while gently moving his legs back and forth. Use gas drops (available over the counter) as a last resort.

7. Give the baby a warm bath. There's nothing so soothing as a warm tub. Many babies calm down as soon as they hit the water. Add an infant massage (see the "spa-treatment" sidebar), and you'll have yourself one calm baby.

8. Give the baby a song and dance. Try singing to your baby, and move around the room as you do so. Babies have short attention spans, and can be easily redirected.

9. Take baby for a walk or a ride in the car. Babies love motion, and the motion of an automobile somehow serves as anesthesia for babies. You'd be surprised to know how many miles are put on a car just for a baby's sake.

10. Put baby to bed. Like all of us, baby can get irritable when tired. Since their bodies are so much smaller than ours, they process food and milk differently and thus get sleepy more quickly than you might think. Put on the baby's lullaby tape or music box, dim the lights, and then walk out. Older babies over six months can be left to cry for at least ten minutes before you return to the room (unless, of course, you're absolutely convinced there's really something wrong). Some crying before falling asleep is normal for most babies.

The Baby Sleep Cycle and How It Is Different from Ours

Many first-time parents believe (mistakenly) that babies are supposed to sleep all day and night until they are a few months old. This is not true. Babies, especially newborns, do require lots of sleep to grow, but they should only sleep at two-to-three-hour intervals during the day. The main reason for waking your baby, if it is sleeping longer than three hours at a stretch, is to make sure the baby is getting proper nourishment. If the baby is not getting enough food at regular times throughout the day, it will only serve to make your nights longer.

Do Babies Dream?

Babies do, in fact, dream, although their dreams are not as elaborate as ours. No one is really sure what they are dreaming about, since they can't tell us the details or whether or not the dream was in color. But we are sure that there is brain activity and that some babies even respond to dream-related stimuli by laughing or frowning in their sleep.

How can you know when your baby is dreaming? You can watch for signals, such as a twitching leg or mouth movements. These motor movements indicate that baby's brain is sending these signals to muscles, and brain activity is a positive sign of dream activity.

Can you give your baby good dreams? Probably not, but you can influence how secure your baby feels when asleep by providing a happy, cheerful environment during waking hours. It is a known fact that happy, secure babies calm down more quickly by themselves and that they fall asleep faster than babies who live in stressful homes.

Keys to Baby Relaxation

There are two basic words to remember when trying to calm your baby into sleeping mode: atmosphere and routine.

- **Atmosphere.** Dim the lights, put on soft lullaby-by-the-sea tapes, and rock your baby to sleep. Let your baby feel your

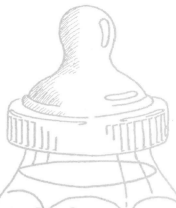

heartbeat; it's calming and comforting to the baby, reminding him or her of that special time in the womb.

꙳ **Routine.** Stick to your routine with baby as much as possible. Write it down if you find it hard to remember. Figure out ways to stick with your routine even when you're on the road—stop and feed your baby at the same time you would have at home. Routine helps a baby to feel secure, and a secure baby is a well-adjusted (and relatively quiet) one.

Understanding Colic and Related Sleeping Problems

We've all heard of colicky babies—the holy terrors of the baby world. What do you do when His Sweetness suddenly embarks on a reign of terror, complete with crying jags, pouty face, and flailing limbs? (Most new parents would say, "Run and hide?!")

Colic is a period of crying and fussiness in a baby. Pediatricians sometimes refer to colic as a baby's "daily freakout," particularly if it occurs around the same time every day. For many parents, this period of fussiness tends to occur in the 7 to 9 P.M. range.

Why do babies get fussy later in the day? Perhaps because they are at the halfway point in their eating schedule; their little bodies may have had a lot to process thus far and yet have a way to go before resting for the night. Occasionally a baby who has frequent awake times during the day will get cranky by sunset, possibly as a result of overstimulation.

An old wives' tale states that if you feed a colicky baby especially well before bedtime, you'll have a peaceful little creature who sleeps all night long. This is a fallacy. If that were true, we would have thousands of fat little babies who slept all the time.

Filling a baby chock-full of formula before going to bed, even if it is laced with infant cereal such as rice, can actually make the situation worse, since the baby's intestines get overloaded with work. Problems with tummy gas or spitting up may result from such overfeeding; so be careful how much you feed baby before bedtime.

When should you be concerned about colic or about a baby who won't calm down? When the baby cries for a prolonged period of time

The Latest on Sudden Infant Death Syndrome

It's every new parent's fear: One day, you will look into your baby's crib, only to see a lifeless little one. While the incidences of sudden infant death syndrome (SIDS) are optimistically decreasing, it is still a condition to be feared.

One way you can try to protect your child from SIDS is to buy a special pillow that positions baby to sleep on his or her side. The side position is now the recommended sleeping position for newborns. (If baby won't stay on his or her side, you don't need to worry. Just keep checking on baby, and keep trying to prop him or her up.) Rotate sides every time you put baby down, to avoid preferences later on.

Also, never leave toys in the crib while baby is sleeping or unattended.

Finally, research shows that babies who live in older homes with active (and airborne) mold spores have a greater risk of developing SIDS. Have your basement checked for mold before the baby comes home.

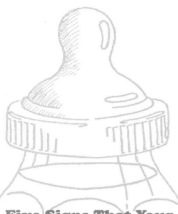

Five Signs That Your Baby Is a "Binky" Addict

1. You never leave the house without a pacifier.
2. The pacifiers you have seem to multiply by themselves. (Suddenly, there are two in the bed, two in the car seat, etc.)
3. Baby will suck on his or her fingers to the point of spitting up unless you replace fingers with a pacifier.
4. You notice that baby seems to have a "binky" museum—a growing collection of old pacifiers that have worn out before their time.
5. Baby's first word is *binky* instead of *Mama* or *Dada*.

(half an hour) or the cries seem pierced by high-pitched tones, you might decide to take a different approach. If you are worried that something is really wrong or that such crying is totally out of character for your baby, you can do the following to set your mind at ease:

- Try giving the other parent a shot at it, especially if you are tired or stressed out. You'd be surprised how much good a small break can do for you as you try to cope.
- Take baby's temperature. If your little one has a fever, crying is definitely a way of letting you know.
- Try giving the baby some infant pain reliever. There could be teeth coming soon.
- Call your pediatrician. If baby just doesn't seem right or isn't responding to any of the suggested methods of calming, your pediatrician may be able to help you with other suggestions.

Slow-to-Transition Babies

A baby who is slow to transition from one activity to the next can pose unique problems for an already harried new parent. What is a slow-to-transition baby, and how can you tell if yours is one?

A slow-to-transition baby is one who reacts negatively (crying, waving arms frantically, kicking, or even stiffening like a board) when changing from one activity to another. For instance, if you have been quietly breastfeeding and then abruptly move baby to a bouncing burp on your knee, the baby may not have had enough time to adjust to the new position. Such adjustment time, which many babies need anyway, is amazingly effective at quieting babies who only tend to cry at burping time.

Remember that they are smaller than us, and they don't know everything about the world, including what is going to happen next after they eat. Until they have a well-established routine, slow-to-transition babies need time to adjust to even the smallest change of position or scenery. Move baby slowly from position to position, or from your lap to car seat, or from crib to your loving arms, and you may notice a big difference in your little one's reaction.

Should You Stay or Should You Go?

There are two basic schools of thought on crying babies who won't sleep. The first is to simply let the baby cry itself to sleep, only returning to the crib if something seems seriously wrong. Some parents who have tried this method swear by it, saying that the crying time gets smaller and smaller each day until baby can finally go to sleep without crying. In the old days, this method was employed to keep parents from "spoiling" the baby with too much attention.

Other parents prefer a more hands-on approach and aren't afraid of spoiling a small baby with on-demand cuddling or comforting. Their point of view is that babies need to know they can depend on their parents when they need them and that babies are really too young to be manipulative about their parent's attention.

There is growing controversy over which method really works best; but the bottom line is, different approaches work for different babies. Try a few methods of calming and comforting your baby to find out which method baby seems to be most responsive to. Then be as consistent as possible in using that method.

Making Bath Time Relaxation Time

Dim the lights, put on some soft music . . . and give your *baby* a bath? We adults like quiet, soothing baths, so why wouldn't a baby like them, too? Your baby doesn't necessarily need a tubful of squeaky toys to enjoy bath time. Many babies equally enjoy a bath in peaceful surroundings, with little extra stimuli except for warm water, a few bubbles, and the soft hum of your voice.

Or you might sing to baby. I used to think that singing my own made-up bath-time songs was really kind of silly, but I've talked with many mothers who tell me they've done the same thing (and felt just as embarrassed). It doesn't matter; the baby won't mind if the song isn't record quality.

When giving baby a bath, try slowly dripping water onto baby's tummy, or rubbing baby's feet for a little longer than you normally would. Think of what is appealing to you, and then try it out on baby. If you like listening to soft, classical music while bathing, perhaps baby will, too. It might even surprise you to learn that baby recognizes some of the music you listened to while bathing during pregnancy; it happens more often than you might think.

Giving Baby the "Spa Treatment"

At our house, the "spa treatment" means that baby Maddie gets her regular, soothing bath, followed by an infant massage with baby cream. Here are some tips to help you give your baby the "spa treatment":

- Start with baby lying on his or her back. Put some baby cream in your hands and rub your hands together to create warmth. Rub some cream on baby's face, then neck, and then stomach.
- Using more cream, repeat the warming process, and then start rubbing baby's shoulders, working your way down the arms. Massage each wrist and hand, working out to the tiny fingertips.
- With additional cream, work on baby's legs. Thighs are particularly good areas to massage a little bit more deeply on a baby, since they are the largest muscles the baby has at this stage.
- If baby will let you, turn him or her over to lie on the stomach. Warm some baby cream in your hands, and then begin to massage from shoulder to buttocks. If you feel like doing it, massage the buttocks, too. Massage the legs again, and then work on the feet, beginning with the balls of the feet and gently massaging each tiny toe.

Baby should be totally and completely relaxed by the end of each treatment. If you do this at least twice per week, you will have a happy and well-adjusted baby; and, if you're lucky, you'll inspire baby's other parent to give you the "spa treatment," too.

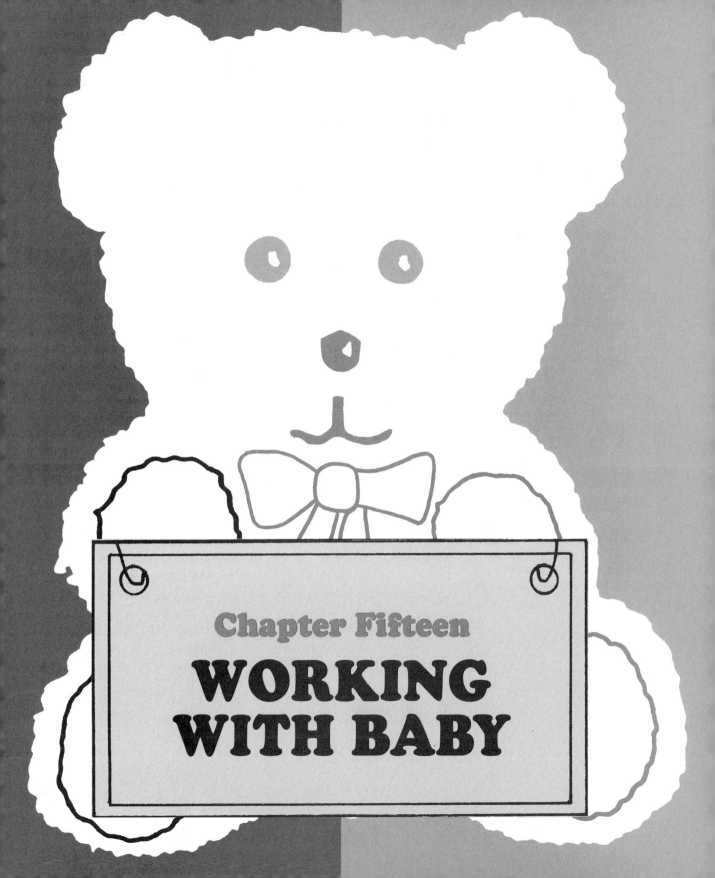

Chapter Fifteen

WORKING
WITH BABY

For most of us, the choice between staying at home as a full-time parent and returning to work after baby is born is a difficult one. It can cause lots of inner turmoil for those who grew up in a world where mommies stayed home and daddies went out to work. My own mother was a stay-at-home mom, and I feel fortunate for the great time we had together.

But we live in a world where two incomes are now the norm; and some parents have as many as two jobs each, not counting their important jobs as parents. In the '90s, we have all kinds of issues and concerns about whether we are good enough parents, or employees, or people. It's easy to get caught up in the belief that despite all the things we do we are simply not good enough. Magazines tell us that working parents don't feel they have enough time with their children and that stay-at-home parents don't feel fulfilled. Somewhere in between is the truth: There is a balance; it just takes a lot of effort to find it.

Financial Considerations: Should You Stay or Should You Go?

There are plenty of questions to ask yourself before making a decision as to whether or not to return to the work force. Weigh all factors before making a final decision. Your reasons for wanting to return to work may be for professional development purposes, but, for many people, it's a financial decision. If you don't feel comfortable analyzing your needs yourself, seek the help of a financial consultant.

Here are some starting points to consider:

- **Figure out what you need to live on.** Total up all of your monthly living expenses, and don't forget to prorate those items that you pay for once or twice per year (such as

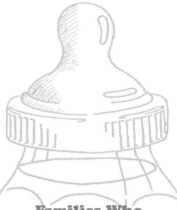

taxes and home or car insurance). Now analyze these expenses against your current and projected new incomes. Can you still meet your monthly obligations if you decide to start a business or stay at home as a full-time parent?

- **Can you live on one income?** What does a second income bring to your family each year? Is it a substantial enough amount that its absence would be harshly felt by all? What would you have to give up in your current lifestyle to stay at home, yet still be comfortable?
- **Ask yourself whether your income is compatible with your goals.** If your goal is to buy a new minivan, for instance, could you still accomplish this if your family is living on one income?
- **Look at the hidden costs of working.** Things like lunches, gas or transportation, and daycare add up. Will you still be making any money after these expenses are taken into consideration, or will you simply be paying for time away from your child? If you aren't going to benefit enough financially, ask yourself what you really want from a work situation. If it's about self-esteem and career identity, that's okay—it just needs to be profitable for your family, too.
- **Make a new budget, and stick to it.** Post it in a conspicuous place (such as on the refrigerator) for everyone in the family to see. This way, everyone knows the financial limitations of the family.

Should you decide you can afford it, staying home is a wonderful option for both parent and baby. It's a beautiful choice that can lead to many terrific memories.

As a final note, remember that in the '90s, it's not always the mommy who stays home with baby. More and more daddies are leaving the rat race to spend time as "house-dads," and they should be applauded for their willingness and effort.

Families Who Work Together

Do families who work together stay together? Research shows that they do. Entrepreneurial families typically work harder toward a common goal than other families and tend to have greater communication about financial objectives. They are also more likely to give birth to other entrepreneurs.

Ten Family-Friendly Companies

The following ten companies were profiled by *Parenting* magazine (May 1997) for their attention to the needs of growing families. Exceptional companies such as these recognize that employees can be dedicated to both job and family:

Hewlett-Packard, Palo Alto, California. This company is a pioneer of the concept of flex-time; flex-time allows parents to set their own schedules to accommodate the needs of their children and balance parenthood with work duties. In addition, this manufacturer of computer-related products allows job sharing for employees who choose it.

Patagonia, Ventura, California. This manufacturer of outdoor wear has an extensive on-site daycare facility, complete with an after-school program (with company-provided transportation from local schools) and two months' paid parental leave.

Eli Lilly and Company, Indianapolis, Indiana. This pharmaceutical maker provides financial support for parents who are adopting children.

Coach, New York City. This maker of leather goods allows its employees flexible work schedules.

Tom's of Maine, Kennebunk, Maine. This maker of natural toothpaste and personal-care products has a compressed work week, scheduling its workers ten hours per day for four days a week. This allows everyone to have Friday off.

Eddie Bauer, Redmond, Washington. The famed catalog (and now retail) shop provides on-site services for breastfeeding moms, including a refrigerator for storing breastmilk.

AT&T, Morristown, New Jersey. This company offers a summer program that gets teens involved in their communities.

Lucasfilm Ltd. and its subsidiaries, Marin County, California. Since this company has tight production schedules, it provides on-site daycare during weekend and extended hours. Daycare time is limited to a set number of hours per day; thus, children are guaranteed regular time with their parents.

First Tennessee Bank, Memphis, Tennessee. This company provides care for sick children, complete with nurses and items for the children to play with. This cuts down on sick days that parents take to care for children.

Haggar Clothing Company, Dallas, Texas. This company underwrites the cost of good prenatal care to ensure that employees have healthier pregnancies and births.

Finding a "Family-Friendly" Company to Work For

What if you discover that you *do* need two incomes in order to maintain your current lifestyle (or grow into one that better accommodates all of you)? First, you need to lay aside any guilt you might be feeling about leaving the baby to go back to work. Next, dust off your resume and brush up on your interviewing skills.

Once you're at the interview, you should be familiar with the new "ground rules." A potential employer should never ask you very much about your family life. Questions like "Are you very involved in your child's activities?" or even "How many children do you have?" can be borderline illegal for a potential employer to ask, since these types of questions can often lead to discrimination. For instance, if they ask you how many children you have, and your answer is five, they may be weighing the costs of your medical benefits in relation to those of a single nonparent job applicant. It is also an indirect way of asking about sexual orientation—another hiring taboo. A company that makes its hiring decisions based on these kinds of criteria is in violation of the Equal Opportunity clause.

Not all companies operate in a discriminatory manner against parents, but you'd be surprised how many still do it, subtly. I've even heard some women business owners declare that because they had a rough time climbing up the corporate ladder, their female employees should not expect or ask for much of a break. Some of these "super" women go back to work three days after a C-section so that others won't claim their jobs!

Because the "family friendliness" of any company is hard to judge from the outset, you might do well to ask a few questions at the interview stage:

- What kinds of policies do you have regarding family emergencies?
- Do you have on-site daycare available?
- Is flex-time an option?

Also, take a look around at the company. Ask for a tour, and make mental notes of how many folks have pictures of their children on their desks; whether there is a daycare room; and how many

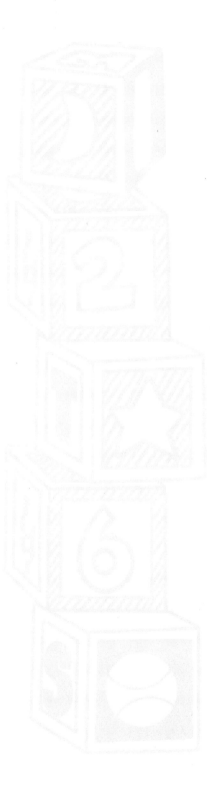

young, single people you see milling around. If you notice that most of the employees appear to be young and single—and travel frequently—you might do well to consider applying elsewhere (unless you're willing to travel frequently yourself and the childcare is already in place).

You can do some research at the library to find out which companies consider themselves to be "family-friendly" and only apply to those companies. That would limit your job search a little, but it might be worth it if you can find an excellent match. Remember that you only need one job; so limiting a search is not necessarily a bad choice to make.

Should You Start a Home-Based Business?

Maybe you've decided that the best option for you is to work your own hours, at your own pace, and still have the luxury of keeping your time with your baby. You want it all, and in the entrepreneurial '90s, you can have it all. Never has there been a friendlier environment for those who wish to escape the rat race and particularly for those who want to leave the rat race for the things that matter in their lives: their children.

Once you've decided that you'd like to start a business, you should give some thought as to whether an entrepreneurial lifestyle really suits you. Can you work on your own? Have you been self-directed and able to set and accomplish your own goals? Can you perform several tasks at one time or at least switch gears in an adaptable, highly flexible manner? If you can answer yes to any of these questions, you could enter the entrepreneurial zone with little or no problem.

If, on the other hand, you lack initiative and prefer to have others tell you what to do, you could find yourself in a stress-filled environment within your own walls. Don't take on an ambitious, time-consuming project like launching a business if you aren't 100 percent certain you can handle it. Once you've made a commitment to running a business, it isn't easy to walk away from it.

A final note to consider: Can you afford to pay self-employment taxes? You will need to do this on a quarterly basis if you choose self-employment. If this is not feasible for you, it may be worth your while to work full- or part-time for someone else and let them worry about the paperwork and taxes.

Setting up Your Home Office (and Baby-Proofing It)

If you've decided to take the plunge into entrepreneurhood, plan as much as you can about your new work situation before involving baby. Take time, for instance, to set up a baby-friendly office, one that takes baby's safety into account.

- Position as much of the baby's things in your office as you can. If you should decide to go back to work soon after the baby is born, position the bassinet next to your desk.
- If the baby is in another room, use a room monitor to keep track of what's happening with baby. When you're engulfed in your work, it's easy to forget there's a baby in your home.
- Keep electrical cords out of the way of crawling babies.
- Remember to schedule more breaks for yourself than you would normally need. You could take at least one nap that coincides with baby's and get some much-needed rest. That's why answering machines, voice mail, pagers, and fax machines were invented—so that you can run your office without always being there.

What It Means to Be a Home-Based, Working Parent

On the negative side, working at home means:

- You sneak into your office to work early in the morning—or late at night—when the little one is asleep. You often work in your pajamas, with one ear cocked for sounds from the baby's room. Eventually, you see this way of working as "normal."

Networking Tips/Resources

- Association of Part-Time Professionals, 7700 Leesburg Pike, Suite 216, Falls Church, VA 22043 (703/734-7975)
- Home-Based Working Moms, P.O. Box 500164, Austin, TX 78750 (Web site: http://www.hbwm.com)
- New Ways to Work, 785 Market Street, Suite 950, San Francisco, CA 94103
- Mothers' Home Business Network, P.O. Box 423, East Meadow, NY 11554
- Work-at-Home Moms (Web site: http://www.wahm.com)

- You can seamlessly move from breastfeeding or bottle preparation to answering the telephone in a professional manner, and no one's the wiser.
- You feel like a recording that constantly repeats the words *Even though I'm right here with you, I'm working. I can't play right now. I'm working. Pretend I'm not here. I'm working. Ask Daddy (or Mommy). I'm working. Really, I'm working.*
- You learn to work with the skill of three people and the arms of an octopus. You develop a split-brain work personality where you can negotiate a major deal on the phone while simultaneously encouraging your baby to smile again.
- You develop tremendous powers of concentration. Somehow you manage to produce good work, even when you hear a skirmish on the other side of the house between Daddy (or Mommy) and baby, or baby and baby sitter.
- You can keep your mind on your work despite loud wails and numerous interruptions ("Mama . . . hug?" "Dada, I'm hungry." "Play time?")

But on the positive side, it also means:

- Stressful moments are offset by a hug or smile that comes at a critical moment from the "junior partner."
- You have a constant reminder of what really matters most in life—your special little someone.
- You have access to an "assistant" who will basically work for hugs. From about the age of two or three, this assistant will pick up faxes (even before they're completed), use up all of your paper clips to make a chain, and drop your heaviest files while "just helping." He or she will also take all of the nicely sharpened pencils off your desk, cover your office floor with toys, and stand behind your right shoulder as you answer the phone. The crazy thing is that you'll still love this assistant anyway.

Being a home-based working parent means you must have a clear sense of priorities. Most likely your family already is a top priority, and work is a close second. However, there will be moments when this order must be reversed. A successful work-at-home parent is able to walk the daily tightrope, achieving this ever-changing balance.

Juggling Family and Work

Let's face it, both raising a family and developing a business are full-time jobs. So, how can you give 100 percent to each and still maintain your sanity?

First of all, set aside a special time each day or week that is designated as "family time." During this time, don't accept phone calls, don't set appointments, and don't even think about your business. You might not even want to stay near your office. Consider going out to dinner and sharing the three best experiences had by each family member during that week.

Or if you feel you can incorporate your family into parts of your business, you might help family members to better understand your needs and constraints. It's one thing for your spouse or children to see you completely stressed out; it's quite another for them to be in your office when that high-volume order comes in on short notice. It would be a positive experience for your children to observe your commitment to your work.

Smaller children, particularly females, need positive workplace role models—and who better to pave the way than Mom or Dad? Historically, children who are raised by entrepreneurs tend to become entrepreneurs themselves.

What should you do in the event that a client or customer wants to meet during one of your special family times? You can handle it one of two ways: You could rearrange your family time; or, better yet, you could simply say, "I already have a meeting at that time . . . is there another time that works for you?" Others will respect your attention to commitments, and you never have to offer any further

Famous (and Infamous) Working Families

With careers in common or common goals in minds, here are some famous siblings and family members who have worked together on some famous (and infamous) projects. Some are fictional; some we only wish were fictional:

- The Partridge Family (based on the real-life Cowsills)
- The Brady Bunch
- The Von Trapp Family Singers
- The Jacksons
- The Osmonds
- The Dalton Gang
- Frank and Jesse James
- Martin Sheen, Emilio Estevez, and Charlie Sheen
- Eric and Julia Roberts
- Kirk and Michael Douglas
- The Fondas (Peter, Jane, Bridget, and the late Henry)
- The Rockefeller family

explanation as to whom you're meeting with. However you decide to work your children into your business life, one thing is for sure: There will never be a time without challenges or interruptions.

You will need to develop the skill to work around any obstacle or challenge, and the best way to accomplish a good balance between work and home life is to learn to follow a time-management program. Scheduling your time is the best way to make sure that everything gets done. The rest is just recognizing that it is possible to have two loves: your business and your family.

If you do run into problems with time management, consider hiring a baby sitter to work with you at home, caring for the baby while you tend to business. This way, you're still able to do your work, and you're only an arm's length away from baby.

Five Steps to Better Time Management

1. Know your goals and set your priorities accordingly. Give your tasks priority according to what must be done today and what can be done tomorrow.
2. Delegate responsibility wherever possible. Invest the time at the outset to explain the task, the results you expect, and the deadline. You'll soon notice the benefit.
3. Clear your desk each day, at a time when you can prevent interruptions or before they begin. You can manage interruptions by using voice mail to prioritize your calls and by focusing on completing tasks by the end of each day. 4. Make "wasted" time as productive as possible. This may call for an investment in a cellular phone or a laptop computer; however, much of the time you spend, for example, sitting in lobbies will become more productive as a result. Even driving time can be more productive if you make calls along the way.
5. Give yourself creative time. Spend this time alone or having coffee with an employee; just be sure to fit this time into your schedule.

How to Feel "Connected" When You're Home-Based

You work anywhere from thirty to sixty hours per week in your cozy little home office. You can curl up with a cup of coffee and enjoy the solitude of working for yourself. You don't have to deal with office politics, petty disagreements, corporate pressure, and, in particular, someone telling you that you can't stay home when your child needs you.

But too much of this paradise can get tedious. When the sounds of silence start to get to you, what can you do to become revitalized? Here are some tips for beating the boredom:

- Take a play break with your baby.
- Chat on-line with other work-at-home parents (use keywords such as *home business* and *entrepreneur* to locate chat rooms).

One Hundred Home-Based Businesses You Can Start

If you've decided to work at home, there's never been a better time to become an entrepreneur. Granted, it's a little more challenging with small children at home, but that's what makes it interesting, right? Following is a list of potential businesses you can start on your own with little or no seed money. For more detailed information on each, consult the *Adams Businesses You Can Start Almanac*. The book is also available in CD-ROM format.

Bookkeeping service
Secretarial service
Writer/editor
Laundry service
Graphic artist/illustrator
Arts festival promoter
Apartment preparation service
Book indexer
Cake decorator/baker
Calligrapher
Child care referral service
Child care provider
Errand service
College application consultant
Commercial plant watering service
Coupon/newspaper distributor
Doll repair service
Etiquette advisor/finishing school for adults and/or children
Genealogical service/family history writer
Graphologist (handwriting analyst)*
In-home mail service
Incorporation service for businesses

Jewelry design/sales
Lactation (breastfeeding) consultant*
Makeup artist/cosmetics representative
Literary agent
Multilevel marketing
Mystery shopper
Nutrition consultant*
Party planner
Packing service (for movers)
Gourmet foods-to-go/ meal-planning service
Professional organizer
Reminder service
Storyteller
Stress management counselor*
Toy cleaning service
Vacation rentals broker
Adoption search service
Art broker/dealer
Alterations/seamstress/tailoring business
Bridal consultant
Web site developer/layout specialist
Computer consultant/trainer
Clip art service

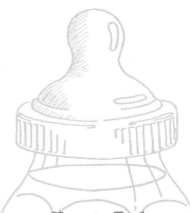

How to Feel "Connected" When You're Home-Based
(continued)

- Join a professional organization made up of professionals like you; check with the Chamber of Commerce for such groups.
- Join Toastmasters International for a chance to get out and improve your speaking skills.
- Volunteer at your child's daycare to come in and read stories to all of the youngsters.
- Take yourself out for a "working" lunch.
- Form a "buddy system" with other work-at-home parents; you can go on family outings together or help each other with childcare.

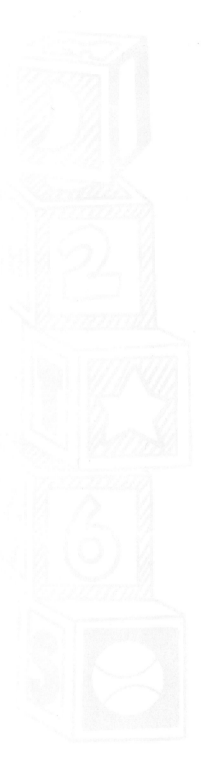

Daycare service*
Desktop publisher
Dog trainer/breeder
Grants/proposal writer
Fund-raising specialist
Interior designer/decorator
Image consultant
Internet marketing/promotions
    specialist
On-line services consultant
Personality testing service
Personalized check printing
    service
Resume service
Reunion organizer
Manicurist
Translation services
Sales trainer
Business plan writer/packager
Upholsterer
Window treatment designer
Public relations company
Balloon delivery service
Gift basket service
Technical writer
    (software documentation,
    procedures, etc.)
Database consultant
Dog walker/pet sitter
Doula/midwife*

Executive search firm
Fax-on-demand service
Gardening consultant
Greeting card mailing service
Herbal products distributor
Home office consultant
Commercial space design/office
    ergonomics specialist
Marketing consultant
Insurance broker
Locksmith service
Maid/cleaning service
Mailing list service
Medical claims processing
Medical transcriptionist
Monogramming service
New product researcher
On-line researcher
Personalized children's books
Pet groomer
Rare book dealer/search
    service
Speakers bureau
Talent agent
Tax preparation service
Benefits administrator/consultant
Assembly work at home
Nanny service
Child ID products
Caterer

(Note: An asterisk (*) denotes a business that will likely require a license or professional certification.)

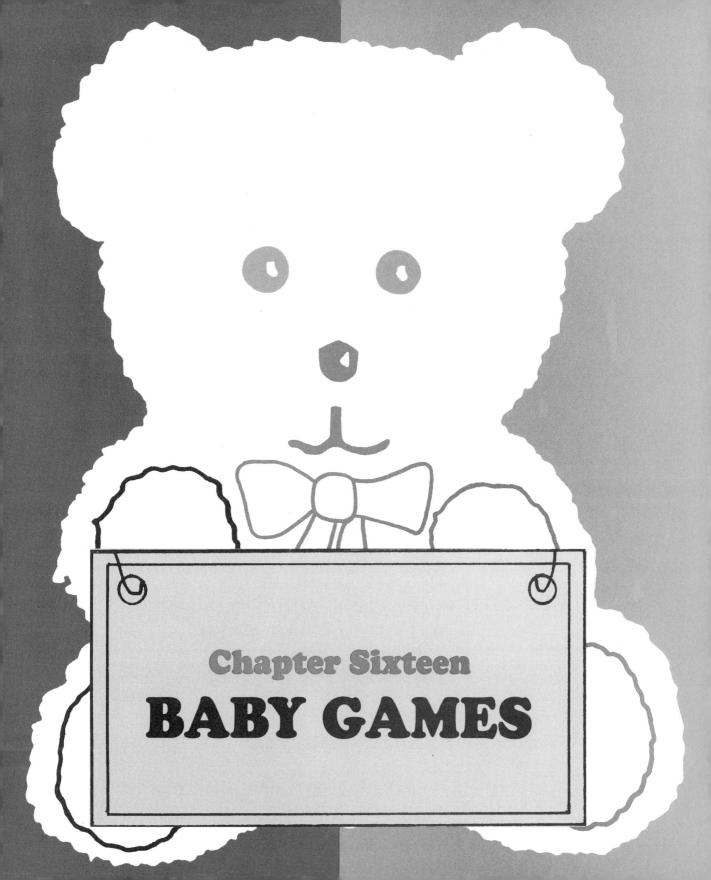

Chapter Sixteen
BABY GAMES

You'll probably want to learn a few nursery rhymes and games to play with baby. Both have a long-standing history of helping babies to develop. And some stay forever etched in our memories, sending us on a sentimental journey every time we hear them.

Even though at first you may feel self-conscious about tugging at baby's toes and playing peek-a-boo over and over again, nursery rhymes and games can be a good way to bond with your child. Just because you're a little self-conscious doesn't mean baby is; and baby will learn the value and joy of laughing out loud.

You can learn traditional rhymes and games, or you can purchase state-of-the-art stimulators, such as flash cards that come in black, red, and white and feature very simple shapes for baby to stare at. Also available are videos featuring the faces of other babies or animated characters, cassette tapes with funny songs for babies, and even computer games for babies (believe it or not, these do exist).

In addition, there are tapes that simulate the sounds of the womb—to help baby adjust to life outside it—and tapes that give you step-by-step game instructions.

Nursery Rhyme Games

For the more traditional minded, here are some tried-and-true nursery rhyme games you can play with your baby. If you start to get bored with these, try some personal adaptations (like the ones I've thrown in, for example).

This Little Pig Went to Market
(Traditional, North American)

This little pig went to market.
This little pig stayed home.
This little pig ate roast beef.
This little pig had none.
This little pig cried, "Wee, wee, wee"—all the way home!

I did a '90s version of this for my daughter, Lilly, who liked me to do it on her fingers and her toes (start with the thumb or big toe, of course).

This little piggy went to the mall.
This little piggy stayed home.
This little piggy had roast beef at Arby's.
This little piggy had none.
And this little piggy went, "Wee, wee, wee"—all the way home.

Hush, Little Baby
(Traditional, United States)

Hush, little baby, don't say a word,
Papa's gonna buy you a mockingbird.
If that mockingbird don't sing,
Papa's gonna buy you a diamond ring.
If that diamond ring turns brass,
Papa's gonna buy you a looking glass.
If that looking glass gets broke,
Papa's gonna buy you a billy goat.
If that billy goat don't pull,
Papa's gonna buy you a cart and bull.
If that cart and bull turn over,
Papa's gonna buy you a dog named Rover.
If that dog named Rover don't bark,
Papa's gonna buy you a horse and cart.
If that horse and cart fall down,
You'll still be the sweetest baby in town.

Hey Diddle Diddle, the Cat and the Fiddle
(Traditional, English)

Hey diddle diddle, the cat and the fiddle,
The cow jumped over the moon.
The little dog laughed to see such sport
And the dish ran away with the spoon.

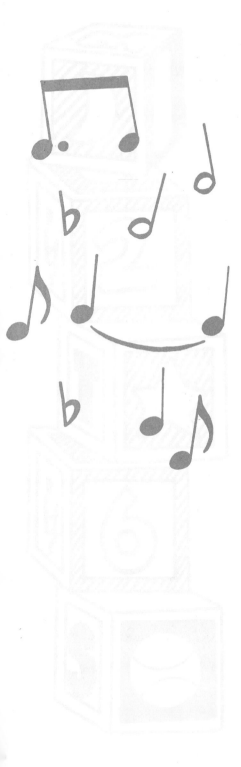

Sleep, Baby Sleep

(Traditional, English)

Sleep, baby sleep,
Your father tends the sheep.
Your mother shakes the dreamland tree,
Down falls a dream for thee.
Sleep, baby sleep.

To Market, to Market

(Traditional, English)

To market, to market, to buy a fat pig,
Home again, home again, jiggety-jig.
To market, to market, to buy a fat hog,
Home again, home again, jiggety-jog.
To market, to market, to buy a plum bun,
Home again, home again, marketing's done.

Rub-a-Dub-Dub

(Traditional, English)

Rub-a-dub-dub,
Three men in a tub.
And who do you think they be?
The butcher, the baker, and
The candlestick maker.
Turn 'em out,
Knaves all three!

Ring around a Rosy

(Traditional, English/American)

Ring around a rosy,
A pocket full of posies,
Ashes, ashes
We all fall down!

The Itsy, Bitsy Spider

(Traditional, English/American)

The itsy, bitsy spider
Climbed up the waterspout.
Down came the rain and
Washed the spider out.
Out came the sun and
Dried up all the rain.
And the itsy, bitsy spider
Climbed up the spout again.

There Was a Crooked Man

(Traditional, English)

There was a crooked man, and he walked a crooked mile,
He found a crooked sixpence against a crooked stile;
He bought a crooked cat, which caught a crooked mouse,
And they all lived together in a little crooked house.

Old King Cole

(Traditional, English)

Old King Cole was a merry old soul,
And a merry old soul was he.
He called for his pipe and
He called for his bowl and
He called for his fiddlers three.

Pat-a-Cake

(Traditional, English/American)

Pat-a-cake, pat-a-cake, baker's man.
Bake me a cake as fast as you can.
Pat it and roll it, and mark it with a "B,"
And put it in the oven for baby and me.

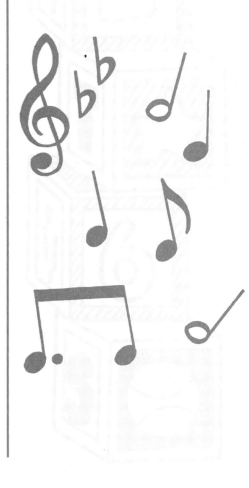

Row, Row, Row Your Boat

(Traditional, English/American)

Row, row, row your boat
Gently down the stream,
Merrily, merrily, merrily, merrily,
Life is but a dream.

Old MacDonald

(Traditional, American)

Old MacDonald had a farm,
E-i-e-i-o!
And on that farm he had a (pig, cat, cow, chick, etc.)
E-i-e-i-o!
With an oink, oink here, an oink, oink there
Here an oink, there an oink
Everywhere an oink, oink
Old MacDonald had a farm,
E-i-e-i-o!

The Wheels on the Bus

(Traditional, English/American)

The wheels on the bus go round and round
Round and round, round and round
Wheels on the bus go round and round
All through the town.

The people on the bus go up and down . . .
The wipers on the bus go swish, swish, swish . . .
The babies on the bus go "Wah, wah, wah!" . . .
The mommies on the bus go "Sh-sh-shh!" . . .

My own variation is much more simple:

We're going for a ride in the Mommy car,
The Mommy car, the Mommy car
Goin' for a ride in the Mommy car
Yes we, yes we are!

Silly as that may seem, my daughter still sings that tune when we're alone in the car.

London Bridge
(Traditional, English)

London Bridge is falling down,
Falling down, falling down.
London Bridge is falling down,
My fair lady.

Build it up with iron bars,
Iron bars, iron bars.
Build it up with iron bars,
My fair lady.

The more physically expressive you are for these nursery rhymes, the more your baby (and you) will enjoy them. And the more expressive he or she will grow to be.

Other Games to Play with Baby

Here is a list of tried-and-true games that baby will enjoy:

- **Peek-a-boo.** Put your hands over your face for a few seconds, and then remove them quickly and say, "Peek-a-boo."
- **I'm Gonna Get You.** I always thought the "got-your-nose" game was a little on the gory side, but small babies don't seem to think so. They laugh at this game until they are at least two or three years old—so it must be worth something. So, put your thumb between your first two fingers and say, "Got-your-nose!" Make your own variations. My mother used to creep up my stomach with her fingers, like a spider, while saying, "I'm gonna get you!"—scary, yet a fun kind of scary.
- **Hiding things.** The object is for you to show baby a brightly colored object or toy, and then hide it under a blanket or pillow. Ask baby, "Where did it go?" and baby will probably respond with smiles or giggles. Because they don't understand the concept of object permanence yet, babies find this one hilarious.

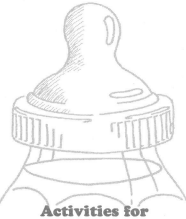

Activities for Baby and You

There are plenty of things that you and baby can do besides playing games and going shopping. Here are just a few "bonding" activities:

- **Bubble fest.** Take baby outside, and blow soap bubbles toward baby or up in the air.
- **Zoo visit.** Babies love to ride around in their strollers, looking at all of the animals. You could tell baby the names of all of the animals and perhaps the sound each makes (if the animals don't oblige).
- **Music or art festival.** Babies love to be out around people. It's where they take their best notes about the human experience.
- **Go for a stroll.** Take baby for a daily stroller ride around the neighborhood or at your local shopping mall. It can be great exercise for you and a nice change of pace for the baby.

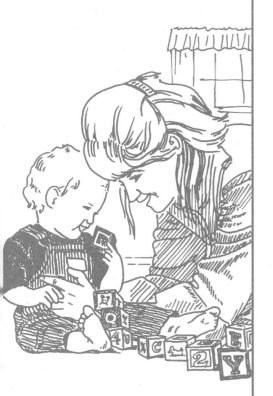

- **Sit-ups, knee bends, tug-of-war, and so forth.**
These games are a little more physical, with baby relying on you to move his or her legs. Or you can give baby a blanket or toy to hold onto while you pull him or her up. If you have a padded surface below, you can pull baby up a bit and let him or her fall gently back down on it, saying the word *boom* each time. Babies also think this one is really funny.

- **Animal noises, vehicle sounds, and so forth.** Babies love to learn the sounds that other creatures make, and it helps them learn how to make sounds, too. Don't be surprised if one of baby's first words is *kitty* or *moo*.

- **Where's Mommy?** Hide around the corner, and ask, "Where's Mommy?" or "Where's Daddy?" (Depending on who or what you have in the room, you could use variations from kitty to grandma.) If the baby starts to cry when you disappear, he or she might still be too young for this one. Generally, the three-to-eight-month crowd finds this one entertaining.

- **Playing music.** If you have an instrument such as a piano or drums, let baby tap out a few notes occasionally. You don't have to start with formal classes, unless your child appears to be a prodigy. For most of us, it's just a lot of meaningless (yet fun) noise that baby gets to make. It does, however, teach baby a little about cause and effect. If you don't have musical instruments, give baby a pot or pan and a wooden spoon—many babies enjoy these even more than the real thing.

- **Art time.** Give baby a big, fat crayon and paper or a bowl of colored Jello® for finger painting. This activity should be closely supervised and is expressly for those babies who are six to eight months or older. Any sooner and they're just not interested; the advantage to the Jello® is that it's completely edible, should your child decide that he or she is not Picasso.

Chapter Seventeen

KEEPING THE RECORDS STRAIGHT

Putting It All Together: A Diary of Baby's First Year

Making a permanent record of your baby's important milestones can be an incredibly daunting task. You may be unsure about what to put in and what to leave out. And you may be afraid to miss something that will later be of significance to your baby.

However, there are many resources available to help you in this endeavor. You can ask other parents how they preserved their babies' collections of "favorite things," or you can surf the Internet for a wider range of ideas. Some of you artsy, nontraditional types may choose to capture your baby's precious memories in your own personal style.

One popular method is to dry mount all of the items in a large binder with plastic page protectors. This method will keep all of your papers neatly preserved for many years. You can add pages when necessary or remove some for show. Or you could preserve each item in a clear plastic bag (the ones that are self-sealing work best), placing the bags on top of one another in a large decorated box. Be careful to store your book or box of memories in a dry place. Excessive heat or cold could damage your materials, making them musty or unsalvageable. Taking the time to store your memories properly now can save you both time and tears later.

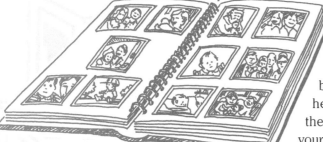

No matter how you decide to do it, putting all of your baby's special moments into one space will undoubtedly help you when baby grows up and asks you that age-old question, "What was I like when I was a baby?"

The next step is to decide what to include in baby's keepsake. Here are some suggestions:

- Early photos
- Baby's birth statistics
- Details about the birth experience
- Lists of well-wishers (and perhaps a collection of greeting card wishes sent to baby upon arrival)

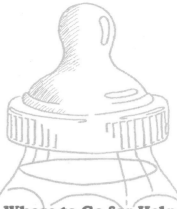

- Information about baby's looks: What color hair and eyes did baby have? Whom did you think baby looked most like? Whom did other people think baby looked most like?
- A list of baby's first gifts
- Details about baby's ride home: What kind of car did you bring baby home in? Did you stop anywhere first? Did baby seem to enjoy his or her first ride?
- A photo and the address of baby's first home
- A list of first visitors (it would be nice to ask each to write a welcome note for baby)
- A copy of baby's first footprints and birth certificate
- Newspaper clippings announcing baby's arrival
- A printout of baby's Web page (if applicable)
- One birth announcement (if you had some made)
- Answers to questions about "firsts": When did baby first sleep through the night? When did the first smile happen, and the first sounds? When did baby discover his or her hands? When did he or she first recognize a sibling? When was the first tooth evident?
- Brief stories about baby's favorite things: songs, toys, people, stories, and activities
- Favorite (and not-so-favorite) foods
- The time, date, and place of baby's first steps
- Baby's first words and nicknames for siblings (especially if the sibling has a hard-to-pronounce first name)
- Items related to baby's first holidays (Halloween costume, Christmas photos, Hanukkah celebration, or other event)
- Special trips baby took (to Grandma's, to Disney World, etc.)
- Handmade items from siblings or relatives that carry a special significance
- Room for stray notes and small (yet important) memories

Letting the World Know about Baby's Firsts

Some cyber-savvy parents post all of the important updates about their baby's "firsts" on a Web site designed especially for baby. All

Where to Go for Help in Preserving Memories

- America Online Scrapbooking Forum (keyword: *creative scrapbooking*), offers a chat room where you can share ideas about putting together memory books.
- Family Treasures is a business dedicated to helping families preserve memories; this company sells everything from scissors to acid-free paper. Call 1-800-413-2645 for information.
- Creative Memories has consultants who offer classes and a complete related product line. Call 1-800-468-9335 for information.
- Creating Keepsakes is a bimonthly magazine offering advice on layout and content for scrapbooks. Call 1-888-247-5282 or http://www.creatingkeepsakes.com for information.
- Memory Makers is a quarterly publication that showcases submissions from readers. Call 1-800-366-6465 or http://www.memorymakers.com for information.

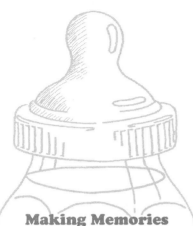

Making Memories

If you're looking for other things to put in your baby's first year diary, check out this list for some ideas:

Write down your thoughts about the world when your baby was young; cut out newspaper clippings about world events and tape them to a piece of paper. Put your comments about the event on the piece of paper (yes, it is a lot like your high-school civics class!).

One of the nicest baby gifts I ever received was a "time capsule" from the day my daughter Lilly was born; it contained everything from a "welcome" letter to newspaper clips, lists of bestsellers and TV shows, and a few product samples. It has made for a lot of memories for us to share now that she's older.

Take along a tape recorder when you go to the park or for a walk. If ideas occur to you while you're out, you'll have a handy, convenient way of recording them. I keep mine in the car for many of the moments I hope not to miss.

you have to do is find a host (usually, this can be provided by an on-line service, such as America Online) and use a template to design the Web site.

You can accomplish a beautiful, near-professional quality Web page in a matter of minutes from good templates. If you don't feel comfortable doing it yourself, there are plenty of on-line businesses that specialize in designing Web pages for babies. (See Chapter 18 for more information about these services.)

How should you set up your baby's Web page? Try to include as many "click-ons" as you can, with buttons for things like baby's first sounds, handprints, pictures, and, of course, statistics (height, weight, etc.). Create links to other Web sites that you find enjoyable or interesting, or even to Web pages of other family members.

Recording Your Family History

What will baby want to know about his or her first days on the planet? You may want to find a special place or book to keep your family memories in for later reference.

What do you put into a family history?

- Letters from grandparents telling about their own childhood, how they met, and what baby's parents were like as babies
- Pictures from everyone in the family, including group shots from family reunions
- Any mementos from great moments in the family history, including, for example, a baseball Grandpa caught at a major league baseball game or a celebrity photo autographed expressly for Grandma—or anything that other members in the family might like to preserve for future generations
- A family tree that shows where the family came from and how they got to where they are now (include tombstone rubbings, if you can get them)
- Newspaper clippings relating to family "passages"—births, deaths, graduations, and so on

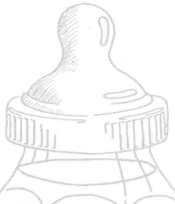

How to Make a Scrapbook of Baby's First Year

Here's what you will need to make a homemade scrapbook full of baby's "firsts":

- Scissors, tape, and glue
- A computer and printer (there are software programs available for keeping family records and milestones)
- Wrapping paper, tissue, and stickers
- Mounting spray
- Photo holders
- Labels (for photo captions)
- Plastic page covers
- A notebook (for scribbling ideas)
- A storage box (a shoe box will do to start)
- An X-acto knife (for trimming edges of photos neatly)
- A binder with extra filler pages (large photo albums work best)
- Colored pens (to add narrative throughout the scrapbook)

Creative Ways to Immortalize Baby

Whether you choose to bronze baby's first shoes (as was so popular in the '50s and '60s) or to mount a small collection of baby things to hang in your living room, you will want to find some unusual ways to remember those beautiful and loving early days.

- Have a local artist paint your baby's portrait. It doesn't have to be the standard, run-of-the-mill pastel (unless that's what you want); it can even be an abstract or computer graphic.
- Have a professional photographer shoot black-and-white photos of baby dressed as an angel, or wearing an unusual hat, or with a puppy. I had a picture done of Lilly wearing a hat with a huge flower on it and sitting on the bench where her dad and I had our first kiss. It is something that she will always treasure because it has such meaning.

Making Memories
(continued)

Videotape baby's firsts, and try to keep as many as possible on one tape. If you can afford it, locate an editing service that can dub your commentary (written or audio).

Take baby to the park or for a ride on a carousel at the local mall or at a fair. Have your partner or family friend take photos.

Babies love baby animals. A trip to the zoo might be worth a lot to your developing baby; it is a place full of sounds, sights, and smells—a great place to create memories.

The most important way to make memories with your baby is to spend quality time together—time when you're not focused on anything but your little precious one. These are the times that build a lifetime.

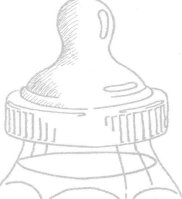

Celebrating Baby's "Monthly" Birthdays

Some parents like to celebrate each monthly "birthday" as a special event. If, for instance, your baby was born on the first of July, you would celebrate the first day of every month thereafter (until, of course, the more traditional annual birthday).

Should you have a party each month? Such celebrations are often marked quietly by both parents, either by a simple birthday kiss or by a mini-party (if you have other children who would like to take part). Some parents choose to wait until the baby reaches three, six, and nine months to celebrate mini-birthdays, and this is acceptable if you both agree.

Whatever you choose to do, be sure to take a picture of baby on each monthly birthday; it is an excellent way to stay on track in terms of the photo library of your baby's development.

❦ Collect a few items that are of sentimental value to you from baby's first days. Have them mounted and framed in a Plexiglas frame, with a printed note card explaining the significance of each item and giving the date. Suggestions include a favorite photo, baby's birth certificate, baby's hospital cap, dad's hospital shirt from the delivery room (some even have the baby's footprints on them), baby's first rattle, and a christening gown with the invitation next to it.

How to Write Your Baby's Story

❦ Choose a tense, and stay in it. If you choose to write everything in active, present tense, you should be consistent throughout the diary. If you choose past tense, keep it in the past.

❦ Include the daily, mundane activities along with the interesting or funny episodes you have with baby. You'd be surprised how important those seemingly insignificant little details will become after your baby has grown.

❦ Just because baby is small doesn't mean you have to write in baby-talk. Remember, baby will likely read this with you when he or she is much older.

❦ Illustrate your diary with plenty of pictures, and write lively, interesting captions for them. Some parents do thought-clouds (as in cartoons), in which they provide baby's imagined dialogue. Captions and/or thought-clouds can be extremely entertaining for others who read the diary.

❦ Set aside a regular time at least once per month to update your baby's diary. If you let a few months' worth of writing pile up, you may forget some precious little memories; and it's hard to remember tiny details for long periods of time. Make diary time a habit, and you'll be happier with the results.

Baby's Growth Stages: What Happens When

Part of being successful at capturing your baby's milestones is knowing when they are likely to occur. Following is a list of typical turning points in a baby's first year.

One month. Babies still sleep more than they are awake at this stage. They should be able to lie on their stomachs and lift their heads for brief moments. A one-month-old can usually recognize the voices of his or her parents and perhaps a sibling or two. Babies at this early stage are good listeners, since they are just beginning to learn the language.

Two months. Two-month-olds can often roll from a side position to their backs. They are beginning to make simple vowel sounds, most often after watching their parents' lips and mimicking them. Smiles begin this month.

Three months. Babies get more of a personality and seem to smile at more specific things (such as a parent's smile, a toy, or a sibling). Now is a good time to start playing more music or to sing around your baby, if you haven't already. Babies react more to music at three months.

Four months. A four-month-old is much more lively and will likely have longer awake periods than younger babies. At four months, a baby can usually roll from stomach to back on his or her own. Laughter begins, and sounds begin to be more refined than in the previous month.

Five months. Many babies begin to sleep through the night at five months; and their sleep patterns become more regular. With some support from you, baby should stand on his or her feet and bounce for a few minutes at a time. Five-month-olds should also be able to lie on their back and raise their heads and shoulders a little. Teeth begin to sprout this month.

Six months. Six months is a real turning point for babies, since they begin to sit briefly by themselves. Babies' noises begin to sound a little more like complete sentences, even though the sounds still don't amount to much more than cooing or simple words (*dada* or *mama*). Six-month-olds can reach for toys or other objects that they find interesting (such as earrings). Watch out!

Seven months. Your seven-month-old is becoming more mobile, with rocking motions, more grasping with hands, and the ability to sit up all by himself or herself. If you have gone back to work or even leave the room for a spell, you may notice that baby isn't very thrilled at your leaving. This is when separation anxiety starts.

Eight months. Eight-month-olds sit up for longer periods of time by themselves and can even pull themselves up to a standing position, although they don't typically hold this position too long. They show more interest in learning to walk and may even start crawling. Also, a new study suggests that babies can remember things you say from this point on—so watch your language!

Nine months. Your nine-month-old can crawl into the most unusual places, such as up a small staircase or under furniture. Some babies at this stage can even walk while holding onto a parent or some furniture. There is even growing evidence that baby actually understands many of the words you use.

Ten months. At ten months, your baby can wave (and possibly even say) bye-bye; crawl nearly everywhere in the house; and form crude, two-word sentences (e.g., *pretty dog*). The baby can pull himself or herself into sitting position, sometimes by rolling up. Baby has probably been eating solids for four months now, graduating to chewier vegetables for a toothier mouthful.

Eleven months. Baby can walk with you, as long as you hold his or her hand. He or she can also call for "Mama" and "Dada," play simple hand clapping games, and sometimes stand

by himself or herself for longer than one minute. Walking, of course, is still another matter. Expect baby to collapse back to the ground easily or to wind up in a squatting position.

One year. Baby is one year old! Now, you need to get those video cameras rolling, since baby is likely walking for three to ten minutes at a time.

The Journey That Lies Ahead

It may be hard to believe right now that your baby is actually going to grow up. In all honesty, your days with baby will pass too quickly. Someday, in the not-too-distant future, those tiny hands will be grasping for your car keys instead of the ones attached to the baby rattle. Those tiny feet will walk down the aisle on the arm of another whom you do not know yet. That tiny mouth will tell you incredible stories, and pass yours on to another tiny little soul.

Listen to the parents who tell you that this time is precious and short lived. It absolutely is. Enjoy the moments you share with your new baby, and remember to reflect back on those moments at times when you are feeling overwhelmed or in despair.

Good luck as you embark on a journey that is beyond words and beyond any experience you've ever known before. May you live to see your grandchildren's children, and may you share your own stories with them as life goes on and as they grow!

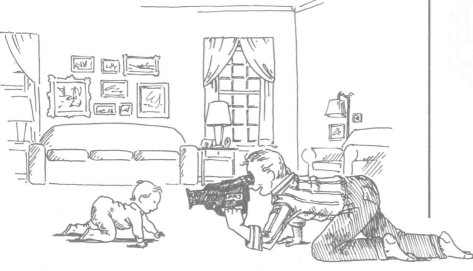

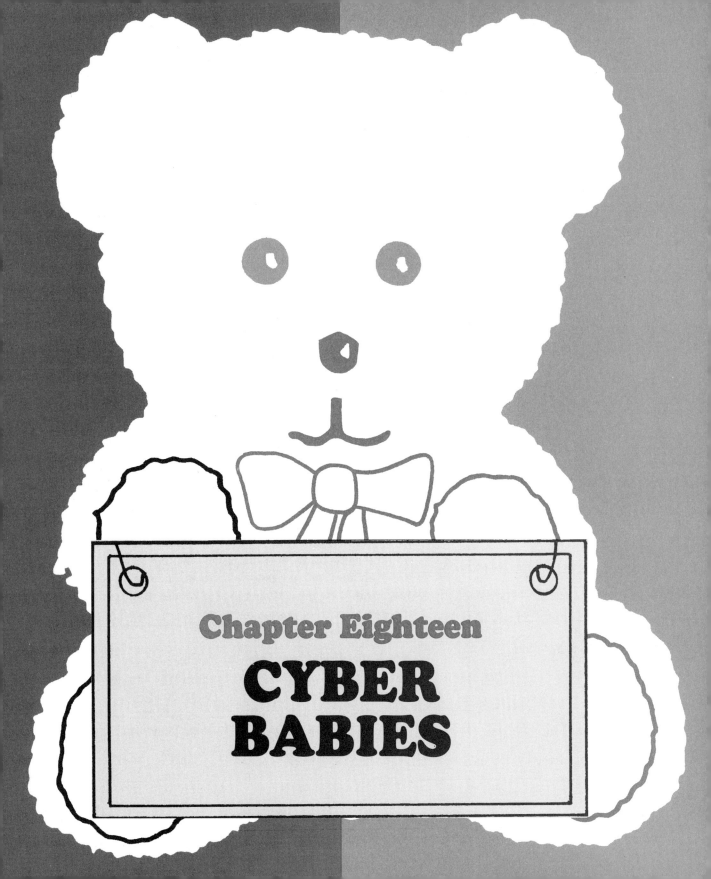

Chapter Eighteen

CYBER
BABIES

The times, they are a-changin'. In the past, parents scanned bookshelves at the library looking for the latest information about babies. Most of it was written by doctors, and much of it was written by Dr. Benjamin Spock. Today, in this age of the World Wide Web, you don't even have to leave home to access thousands of words of advice. You can surf the 'Net in your pajamas and ask for on-line help with your baby in your arms.

You can surf the hundreds of Web sites and hyperlinks related to pregnancy, newborns, and infants and find information on everything from what to eat during pregnancy to how to ease your baby into toddlerhood to how to baby proof your house. So, get out baby's "surfboard" and cruise the following interesting and useful Web sites.

Pregnancy-Related Sites

The following sites are dedicated mostly, if not entirely, to the pregnancy and birthing processes:

Childbirth.org @ http://www.childbirth.org
This fabulous resource offers a home page with a library link and plenty of opportunity for discussion. It covers virtually every aspect of giving birth.

Babyonline @ http://www.babyonline.com
This site is packed with articles (and an extensive archive) related to everything from getting pregnant to baby safety and the latest on postpartum issues for new mothers. There are even items geared especially for the new dad. This site hails from the United Kingdom, the country that is always on the cutting edge of pregnancy and women-related issues. It's a great site to bookmark.

Interactive Pregnancy Calendar @ http://www.olen.com/baby
This innovative site allows you to enter your due date for a more personalized pregnancy calendar. You get a detailed, day-to-day account of your baby's development that you can print out each month as a keepsake or launch pad for your pregnancy journal. What a neat idea!

Pillow Talk's Stork Site @ http://www.storksite.com
Here you'll find lots of useful (and supportive) information regarding most common concerns of pregnancy. Much of this site has the feel of a childbirth education class; and that's no accident, since the site is maintained by a registered nurse. One of the best features of this site is its chat room, where pregnant women can voice their concerns, hopes, or fears with others who understand and can sympathize.

Midwifery.com @ http://www.midwifery.com
Although this site is mostly geared toward educating midwives in their profession, there are plenty of articles that pregnant couples might find informative.

Birth Stories @ http://www.geocities.com/Heartland/7269
Read the birth stories of other parents, or post your own birth story (once you've had the baby, of course!).

Baby Announcement @ http://www.ARGO.NET.AU/ALEX
Parents offer a free spot for other parents to post "the news."

The Baby Bag @ http://www.babybag.com
This site includes product reviews, shopping links, a section for birth announcements, tips on safety, surveys and articles, and, of course, a place to share your birth story.

Parent Soup @ http://www.parentsoup.com
Here you'll find discussion groups, chat rooms, an articles library with extensive archives, book and product reviews by parents for parents, and much more. This site covers everything from pregnancy to baby naming to discipline tactics. It's a popular site; definitely bookmark this one.

The Babies Planet @ http://www.TheLastPlanet.com/babyhp.html
This site is cool, interesting, and informative, with plenty of links to related sites. In addition to health and general parenting tips, on this "planet" you'll learn how your pets will be affected by the "newbie." There are very nice graphics, and the information is current, too.

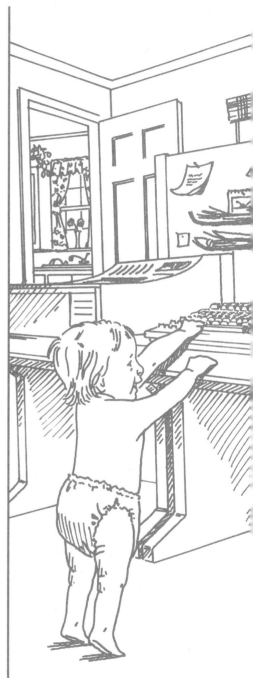

The Visible Embryo @ http://www.visembryo.ucsf.edu
Covering only about the first four weeks of pregnancy, this tutorial for medical students can also be accessed by curious parents. It's amazing stuff, if you can understand it all.

ASPO/Lamaze Web Site
@ http://www.lamaze-childbirth.com
This site has everything you need to know about the Lamaze method of childbirth. It's educational and useful to those still trying to decide on a method, too.

The Whole Nine Months
@ http://www.homearts.com/depts/health/00ninec1.htm
This fun, interactive site features everything from baby's horoscope to information on postpartum depression; and it links to an interactive, personalized pregnancy calendar. It's a fun way to learn about your body's nine-month adventure.

Obstetric Ultrasound
@ http://www.hkstar.com/~joewoo/joewoo2.html
Ever wonder how the doctors can make heads or tails of those ultrasound pictures? Here, a doctor explains it to you; and he uses some fascinating pictures.

The Planned Parenthood National Site
@ http://www.igc.apc.org/ppfa
This site offers a special section on pregnancy and related issues.

Online Birth Center
@ http://www.efn.org/~djz/birth/birthindex.html
This site is dedicated largely to the cause of international midwifery; yet it provides plenty of good information and is highly searchable.

Names! @ http://members.aol.com/fishware/name.html
This is an extensive dictionary for those still trying to pick out the right name. It has original meanings of names, too.

Jellinek's Baby Name Chooser
@ http://www.jellinek.com/baby
This innovative site lets the computer choose names for your baby; some are quite unusual. It's a place for the unique-minded.

Moms Online @ http://www.momsonline.com
A virtual community and supportive site for moms, this site includes helpful tips from other moms, a cyber shop, and a daily chronicle of the editor's son Alex. One of the nicest features is a Mom of the Week.

Newborn and Beyond

These sites cover general parenting issues, from baby care to teen years:

Baby Web: The Internet Parenting Resource
@ http://www.netaxs.com/~iris/infoweb/baby.html
This site has news groups, literature, tips on baby care, and more. Babies can even get their own home page with 'Net Babies. There's also a Baby Web Store and a cool Baby Art Gallery with simple, high-contrast designs for baby to view on the computer. There's nothing like starting them early.

New Parent Talk @ http://www.newparentalk.com
This site focuses on the myriad of new and changing relationships as a result of a new baby; its primary goal is to coach the new parent through a "new inner life." It's a little New Age-y but extremely sensitive to emotional issues in ways that other sites are not. I recommend this site, particularly for first-time parents.

Family.com @ http://www.family.com
Useful bulletin boards and chat rooms abound in this Disney-run site.

Zero to Three @
http://www.zerotothree.org
Run by a child advocacy group, this site has much in the way of research and information related to child development.

The Mommy Page @
http://www.rahul.net/jacbop/lisa
A London-based mom is still adding to this site, but you can contribute or peruse the useful list of related sites.

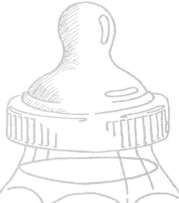

Avoiding 'Net Scams

As sad as it might seem, there are lots of cyber punks out there who prey on new parents. These scam artists offer all kinds of products and services, and many an unsuspecting parent has given out a credit card number only to find that he or she has been ripped off. How can you avoid such treachery? Follow these guidelines:

• **Purchase only from established, reputable sources.** The bigger the name, the lower the odds that you'll be ripped off.

• **Ignore attached files on unsolicited e-mail.** If you don't recognize the source, it's safe to look at the message but *not* at any attached files. There could possibly be a virus encoded in the attachment, and, if this is the case, opening it could completely erase your hard drive. Unfortunately, there's no way to know until you open the file. Pitch it first.

• **Never give out any critical information unless you know where it's going.** Your name, address,

Parenting Twins or Other Multiples
@ http://www.parentsplace.com/readroom/multiples.html
This is one of the most comprehensive sites so far on the challenging role of parenting more than one baby at a time.

Parenthood Web @ http://www.parenthoodweb.com
Here you can find good advice for new parents, offered by a panel of experts. A special feature is an "I Wish I Knew" section, which tells you the things other new parents wish they had known before their babies were born.

Parents Place @ http://www.parentsplace.com
This site was begun by parents who wanted to offer others the advice they wish they had gotten. The site has now become a great resource for beleaguered parents who are hungry for information and tips on everything from what to feed their kids to teething and health issues.

Parents at Home Page @ http://www.quest.com/~jsn/moms/
The emphasis here is on at-home parenting as a positive choice (although employed parents are also welcome). This site offers useful information, especially about finances.

Work-at-Home Moms @ http://www.wahm.com
This site is geared toward the growing number of mothers for whom every day is "Take Your Child to Work Day." You'll find lots of good advice from other moms in similar situations; it also has a classified section and profiles area to promote your business. The encouraging, networking environment is a plus.

The Baby Care Corner @ http://www.familynet.com/babycare
This site offers health tips and more for the new parent.

The Baby Page @ http://www.ultranet.ca/baby
You'll find parent-to-parent discussions at this resource site.

The Bored Mom @ http://www.cyberus.ca/~cmclaren/karen.html
Developed by a stay-at-home mom, this site shares tips and is particularly noted as a favorite among parents because of its list of product recalls. It hails from Canada.

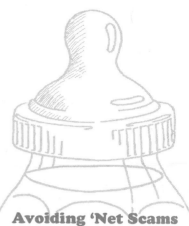

FatherNet @ http://www.cyfc.umn.edu/fathernet.html
Here you'll find supportive data and literature for involved fathers; the site also offers a discussion group, valuable links to related sites, and more.

At-Home Dads
@ http://www.parentsplace.com/readroom/father.html
Articles, tips, and general information for stay-at-home dads can be found here. It's also a terrific place for dads to "bond" with each other.

National Center for Fathering @ http://www.fathers.com
This site offers advice and detailed information for fathers who consider their roles in their babies' lives to be critical. You'll also find feature articles from *Today's Father* magazine.

La Leche League International
@ http://www.prairienet.org/llli/
Anything you ever wanted to know about breastfeeding is on this site. It also contains valuable links to other baby-related sites.

Resources and Publications

Knowing where to look for information and ideas is key to good parenting. Here are some starting points on the Internet:

U.S. Consumer Product Safety Commission
@ http://www.cpsc.gov
Before purchasing toys and furniture for baby, check out this site for the latest in safety information and product recalls. It's a definitive source.

American Baby **magazine**
@ http://www.enews.com:80/magazines/baby/
Subscribe to this highly regarded magazine for parents and parents-to-be, or access articles through the archives.

Depression after Delivery
@ http://www.behavenet.com/dadinc/
This site is dedicated to the 20 percent of new moms who

Avoiding 'Net Scams
(continued)

social security number, phone number, and on-line password should *always* remain private. Credit card numbers should not be given out unless you feel 100 percent sure about the merchant.

- **Never do a direct debit unless you're absolutely sure about the merchant's reputation.** Allowing someone free access to your checking account is never a good idea, unless you know who it is and have assurance that it's a one-time deal. Always ask for a way to contact them back, and do so before committing to the sale. That way, you can be sure the access works both ways.

- **When in doubt, clear out.** If there's something that makes you feel uncomfortable about the site, vacate it. The beauty of the Internet is you can leave without saying good-bye.

- **Shop around.** There are plenty of items on the Internet that you can get for free if you surf around enough. Do a search for related items or sites before committing to a purchase.

experience postpartum depression—the condition beyond the "baby blues." It's a valuable resource for you or any other new mother you know who's feeling like her depression is insurmountable. Here you find local chapters of support groups that can be extremely helpful.

The Mommy Times @ http://www.mommytimes.com
For stressed-out moms, here's a publication that aims to preserve your sanity while informing you at the same time. It's a welcome relief.

ParenTalk newsletter
@ http://www.tnpc.com/parentalk/index.html
This site features articles by psychologists and other professionals; but don't worry, you'll be able to understand the language, since it's well written and expressly for the lay person.

Parent News
@ http://www.moss.fgreen.com/parent/parent/index.html
The best feature of this psychologist-run site is a section for stepparents and families in transition.

Usenet @ http://alt.parenting *and* http://misc.kids
This site offers a good starting point on the Internet's newsgroup collection; you can search for lots of discussion areas related to parenting and babies. You can also get tips from other parents on everything from breastfeeding to getting baby to sleep through the night.

The National Parenting Center @ http://www.tnpc.com
Here is a terrific resource for parenting questions of all kinds, from newborn concerns to teen issues. It offers an extensive library, too.

***Fathering* magazine** @ http://www.fathermag.com
This publication is expressly for actively involved dads. After you've visited it, you'll see why these '90s men don't want to be known as "Mr. Moms." They are parents in their own right and every bit as competent as moms.

All about Kids @ http://www.aak.com
The Cincinnati-based *All about Kids* newspaper has a Web

site with an interactive forum and a library with an archive for back issues.

Positive Parenting Online
@ http://www.positiveparenting.com
This site contains resources and plenty of information in the form of a newsletter; you'll also find a bulletin board, a chat room, articles, and a list of experts on a variety of subjects.

The Nanny Network @ http://www.nannynetwork.com
This site helps you locate child-care professionals in your area.

I Love My Nanny @ http://www.ilovemynanny.com
Here you'll find a nanny placement agency. This site is a member of Parents Place.com.

The Daycare Page @ http://www.thegrapevine.com
If you're looking for the right daycare provider, this resource (with more than 10,000 entries) is an excellent place to start.

American Childcare Solutions
@ http://www.parentsplace.com/readroom/ACS
Visit this site if you're concerned about the legalities of hiring child-care assistance.

Toys/Products/Catalogs
Shopping on-line has the advantage of saving time and sometimes money. The only disadvantage is that you're buying an item you can see but can't touch; so be careful about your purchases and make sure there's a clear return policy, just in case the product doesn't meet your expectations.

E-toys @ http://www.etoys.com
Choose from hundreds of quality toys. Selections are organized by age group.

Cybercalifragilistic @ http://www.webcom/getagift
Order unique shower gifts here, or purchase those things you didn't get at your own shower and have them shipped to you. You'll appreciate the ease and convenience of shopping on-line.

My-Kids.Com @ http://www.my-kids.com
Create baby's own Web site through this company; you send them the pictures and they put up a professionally designed site for a fee. You can update as often as you like, and you receive fifteen announcement cards to let friends and family know where to find baby's Web site.

The Breastfeeding Mother @ http://members.aol.com/bestfed
Here's an on-line shopping center for breastfeeding mothers.

Stork Net @ http://www.pages.prodigy.com/gifts/stork
Subscribe to the Stork Net newsletter; or go directly to the shopping area to buy gifts for baby.

Little Tikes Web Site @ http://www.littletikes.com
Order a catalog on-line, or make a purchase directly from the site. You can also access a list of stores nearest you that carry Little Tikes products.

Combi Home Page @ http://www.combi-intl.com
Check out the various styles and designs in Combi strollers.

Baby Depot @ http://www.coat.com/babydepot
Order products on-line; or locate the store nearest you. This site features clothes, furniture, and accessories for baby.

Pampers Web Site @ http://www.totalbabycare.com
In addition to advertisements for diapers, you'll find some good general baby care advice from experts.

Stork Avenue @ http://www.storkavenue.com
Order birth announcements from this site.

H&F Announcements @ http://www.hfproducts.com
Here's another source for birth announcements.

The Baby Jogger @ http://www.babyjogger.com
Select a jogger from the company catalog, and have it delivered to your door.

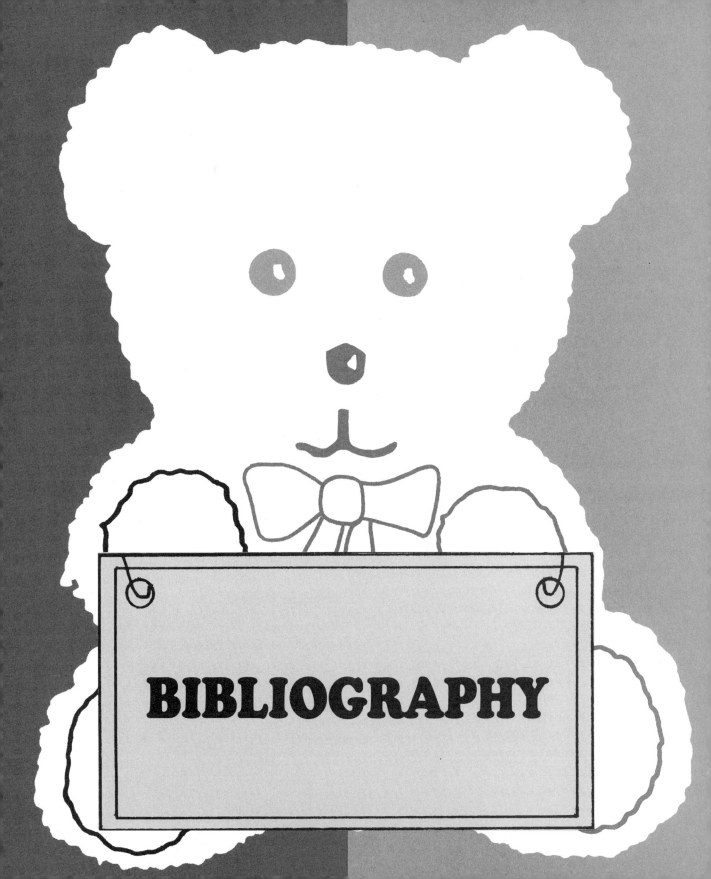

Acredolo, Linda, and Susan Goodwyn. *Baby Signs: How to Talk with Your Baby Before Your Baby Can Talk.* Contemporary Books, New York: 1996.

Bernstein, Sara. *Hand Clap!: "Miss Mary Mack" and 42 Other Hand Clapping Games for Kids.* Adams Media Corporation, Holbrook, MA: 1994.

Bigner, Jerry J. *Parent-Child Relations: An Introduction to Parenting.* Macmillan Publishing Company, New York: 1989.

Boates, Karen Scott. *Letters to a Child Being Born.* Running Press, Philadelphia: 1991.

Brazelton, T. Berry, M.D. *Toupoints: Your Child's Emotional and Behavioral Development.* Addison-Wesley Publishing Company, Boston: 1994.

Carpenter, Humphrey, and Mari Prichard. *The Oxford Companion to Children's Literature.* Oxford University Press, London: 1984.

The Complete Book of Fortune. Crescent Books, New York: 1990.

Davis, Laura, and Janis Keyser. *Becoming the Parent You Want to Be: A Sourcebook of Strategies for the First Five Years.* Broadway Books, New York: 1997.

DeFrancis, Beth. *The Parents' Resource Almanac.* Adams Media Corporation, Holbrook, MA: 1994.

Dunham, Caroll, Frances Myers, Neil Barnden, and Alan McDougall. *Mamatot: A Celebration of Birth.* Viking Press, New York, NY 1992.

Eisenberg, Arlene, Heidi Eisenberg Murkoff, and Sandee Eisenberg Hathaway, R.N., B.S.N. *What to Expect During the First Year.* Workman Publishing, New York: 1988.

Eisenberg, Arlene, Heidi Eisenberg Murkoff, and Sandee Eisenberg Hathaway, R.N., B.S.N. *What to Expect When You're Expecting.* Workman Publishing, New York: 1988.

Engber, Andrea, and Leah Klungness, Ph.D. *The Complete Single Mother.* Adams Media Corporation, Holbrook, MA: 1995.

Ferber, Richard. *Solve Your Child's Sleep Problems.* Simon & Schuster, New York: 1986.

Green, Diana Huss (ed.), and the editors of *Consumer Reports. Parents' Choice Guide to Video-Cassettes for Children.* Consumers Union, Mount Vernon, NY: 1989.

Harris, A. Christine, Ph.D. *The Pregnancy Journal: A Day-to-Day Guide to a Healthy and Happy Pregnancy.* Chronicle Books, San Francisco: 1996.

Huggins, Kathleen. *The Nursing Mother's Companion.* Harvard Common Press, Cambridge, MA: 1995.

Jacob, Dr. S. H. *Your Baby's Mind.* Adams Media Corporation, Holbrook, MA: 1992.

Kiester, Edwin, Jr., Sally Valente Kiester, et al. *New Baby Book.* Meredith Corporation, Des Moines, IA: 1979.

Kiley, Susan. *Baby Love: A Treasury for New Mothers.* Andrews & McMeel, New York: 1994.

Kopp, Claire B., Ph.D., and Donna L. Bean. *Baby Steps: The "Whys" of Your Child's Behavior in the First Two Years.* W. H. Freeman, New York: 1993.

La Leche League International. *The Womanly Art of Breastfeeding.* Plume, New York: 1997.

Lansky, Bruce. *Mother Murphy's Law and Other Perils of Parenthood.* Meadowbrook, Inc., Deephaven, MN: 1986.

Lansky, Vicki. *A Parent's Guide to Child Safety.* Safety First, Chestnut Hill, MA: 1991.

Lau, Theodora. *The Handbook of Chinese Horoscopes.* Harper Colophon Books, New York: 1979.

Leach, Penelope. *Your Baby and Child: From Birth to Age Five.* Alfred A. Knopf, New York: 1989.

Lipper, Ari, and Joanna Lipper. *Baby Stuff: A No-Nonsense Shopping Guide for Every Parent's Lifestyle.* A Balliett & Fitzgerald Book/Dell Trade Paperback, New York: 1997.

MacGregor, Cynthia. *Free Family Fun.* Berkley Books, New York: 1994.

Martin, Elaine. *Baby Games: The Joyful Guide to Child's Play from Birth to Three Years.* Running Press, Philadelphia: 1988.

Morris, Desmond. *Illustrated Babywatching.* Crescent Books, New York: 1995.

Neifert, Marianne. *Dr. Mom's Parenting Guide: Commonsense Guidance for the Life of Your Child.* Plume, New York: 1996.

Podell, Susan Kagen, M.S., R.D. *Checklist for Your First Baby.* Main Street Books/Doubleday, New York: 1997.

Reid, Lori. *The Complete Book of Chinese Horoscopes.* Barnes & Noble, New York: 1997.

Riverside Mothers Group, The. *Entertain Me!* Pocket Books, New York: 1993.

Saltman, Judith. *The Riverside Anthology of Children's Literature.* Houghton Mifflin Company, Boston: 1985.

Sears, William, M.D. and Martha Sears, R.N. *The Baby Book.* Little, Brown and Company, New York: 1993.

Shaw, Lisa. *The Everything Baby Names Book.* Adams Media Corporation, Holbrook, MA: 1997.

Spock, Benjamin, M.D., and Michael B. Rothenberg, M.D. *Dr. Spock's Baby and Child Care.* Pocket Books, New York: 1992.

Tamaro, Janet. *So That's What They're For: Breastfeeding Basics.* Adams Media Corporation, Holbrook, MA: 1996.

Verny, Thomas, M.D., with John Kelly. *The Secret Life of the Unborn Child.* A Delta Book/Dell Publishing, New York: 1981.

Verrilli, George E., M.D., F.A.C.O.G., and Anne Marie Mueser, Ed.D. *While Waiting: A Prenatal Guidebook.* St. Martin's Press, New York: 1987.

INDEX